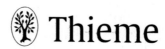

Color Atlas of Pharmacology

3rd edition, revised and expanded

Heinz Lüllmann, M.D.

Former Professor and Chairman
Department of Pharmacology
University of Kiel
Germany

Klaus Mohr, M.D.

Professor
Department of Pharmacology
and Toxicology
University of Bonn
Germany

Lutz Hein, M.D.

Professor
Department of Pharmacology
University of Freiburg
Germany

Detlef Bieger, M.D.

Professor Emeritus
Division of Medical Sciences
Faculty of Medicine
Memorial University of
Newfoundland
St. John's, Newfoundland
Canada

With 170 color plates by Jürgen Wirth

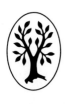

Thieme
Stuttgart · New York

IV

Library of Congress Cataloging-in-Publication Data

Taschenatlas der Pharmakologie. Englisch.
Color atlas of pharmacology/Heinz Luellmann ...
[et al.]; 172 color plates by Juergen Wirth.—
3rd ed., rev. and expanded
    p. ; cm.
Rev. and expanded translation of: Taschenatlas
der Pharmakologie. 5th ed. c2004.
Includes bibliographical references and index.
ISBN 3-13-781703-X (GTV: alk. paper)—
ISBN 1-58890-332-X (alk. paper)
1. Pharmacology—Atlases. 2. Pharmacology—
Handbooks, manuals, etc. [DNLM: 1. Pharma-
cology—Atlases. 2. Pharmacology—Handbooks.
3. Drug Therapy—Atlases. 4. Drug Therapy—
Handbooks. 5. Pharmaceutical Preparations—
Atlases. 6. Pharmaceutical Preparations—Hand-
books. QV 17 T197c 2005a] I. Lüllmann, Heinz.
II. Title.

RM301.12.T3813 2005
615'.1—dc22
                                2005012554

Translator: Detlef Bieger, M.D.

Illustrator: Jürgen Wirth, Professor of Visual
Communication, University of Applied Sciences,
Darmstadt, Germany

© 2005 Georg Thieme Verlag,
Rüdigerstrasse 14, 70469 Stuttgart, Germany
http://www.thieme.de
Thieme New York, 333 Seventh Avenue,
New York, NY 10001 USA
http://www.thieme.com

Cover design: Cyclus, Stuttgart
Typesetting by primustype Hurler GmbH,
Notzingen
Printed in Germany by Appl, Wemding

ISBN 3-13-781703-X (GTV)
ISBN 1-58890-332-X (TNY)

Important note: Medicine is an ever-changing science undergoing continual development. Research and clinical experience are continually expanding our knowledge, in particular our knowledge of proper treatment and drug therapy. Insofar as this book mentions any dosage or application, readers may rest assured that the authors, editors, and publishers have made every effort to ensure that such references are in accordance with **the state of knowledge at the time of production of the book.**

Nevertheless, this does not involve, imply, or express any guarantee or responsibility on the part of the publishers in respect to any dosage instructions and forms of applications stated in the book. **Every user is requested to examine carefully** the manufacturers' leaflets accompanying each drug and to check, if necessary in consultation with a physician or specialist, whether the dosage schedules mentioned therein or the contraindications stated by the manufacturers differ from the statements made in the present book. Such examination is particularly important with drugs that are either rarely used or have been newly released on the market. Every dosage schedule or every form of application used is entirely at the user's own risk and responsibility. The authors and publishers request every user to report to the publishers any discrepancies or inaccuracies noticed.

Preface to the 3rd edition

In many countries, medicine is at present facing urgent political and economic calls for reform. These socioeconomic pressures notwithstanding, pharmacotherapy has always been an integral part of the health care system and will remain so in the future. Well-founded knowledge of the preventive and therapeutic value of drugs is a sine qua non for the successful treatment of patients entrusting themselves to a physician or pharmacist.

Because of the plethora of proprietary medicines and the continuous influx of new pharmaceuticals, the drug market is difficult to survey and hard to understand. This is true not only for the student in search of a logical system for dealing with the wealth of available drugs, but also for the practicing clinician in immediate need of independent information.

Clearly, a pocket atlas can provide only a basic framework. Comprehensive knowledge has to be gained from major textbooks. As is evident from the drug lists included in the Appendix, some 600 drugs are covered in the present Atlas. This number should be sufficient for everyday medical practice and could be interpreted as a Model List. The advances in pharmacotherapy made in recent years have required us to incorporate new plates and text passages, and to expunge obsolete approaches. Several plates needed to be brought in line with new knowledge.

As the new edition was nearing completion, several high-profile drugs experienced withdrawal from the market, substantive change in labeling, or class action litigation against their manufacturers. Amid growing concern over effectiveness of drug safety regulations, "pharmacovigilance" has become a new priority. It is hoped that this compendium may aid in promoting the critical awareness and rational attitude required to meet that demand.

We are grateful for comments and suggestions from colleagues, and from students, both doctoral and undergraduate. Thanks are due to Professor R. Lüllmann-Rauch for histological and cell-biological advice. We are indebted to Ms. M. Mauch and Ms. K. Jürgens, Thieme Verlag, for their care and assistance and to Ms. Gabriele Kuhn for harmonious editorial guidance.

Heinz Lüllmann, Kiel
Klaus Mohr, Bonn
Lutz Hein, Freiburg
Detlef Bieger, St. John's, Canada
Jürgen Wirth, Darmstadt

Disclosure: The authors of the *Color Atlas of Pharmacology* have no financial interests or other relationships that would influence the content of this book.

Contents

Systems Pharmacology   83

Therapy of Selected Diseases 313

Further Reading   349

Drug Indexes   351

Subject Index   381

Abbreviations

6-APA	6-aminopenicillanic acid		ER	endoplasmic reticulum
AA	amino acid		FSH	follicle stimulating hormone
ABP	arterial blood pressure		GABA	γ-aminobutyric acid
AC	adrenal cortex		GDP	guanosine diphosphate
ACE	angiotensin-converting enzyme		GnRH	gonadotropin-releasing hormone = gonadorelin:
ACh	acetylcholine		GRH	growth hormone-releasing
AChE	acetylcholinesterase			hormone = somatorelin
ADH	antidiuretic hormone (= vasopressin, AVP)		GRIH	growth hormone release-inhibiting hormone
AH	adenohypophyseal			= somatostatin
AP	action potential		GTP	guanosine triphosphate
ATP	adensosine triphosphate		HCG	human chorionic gonadotropin
AVP	vasopressin (= antidiuretic hormone, ADH)		HIT II	heparin-induced thrombocytopenia type II
BMI	Body-Mass-Index		HMG	human menopausal
BP	blood pressure			gonadotropin
BP	boiling point		i.m.	intramuscular(ly)
CAH	carbonic anhydrase		i.v.	intravenous(ly)
cAMP	cyclic adenosine monophosphate		IFN	interferon
CG	cardiac glycoside		IFN-α	interferon alpha
cGMP	cyclic guaniidine monophosphate		IFN-β	interferon beta
			IFN-γ	interferon gamma
CHH	corticotropin-releasing hormone		IGF-1	insulin-like growth factor 1
			IL	interleukins
CHO	Chinese hamster ovary		IOP	intraocular pressure
CHT	specific choline-transporter		IP$_3$	inositol trisphosphate
CML	chronic myeloic leukemia		ISA	intrinsic sympathomimetic activity
CNS	central nervous system			
COMT	catecholamine O-methyl transferase		ISDN	isosorbide dinitrate
			ISMN	5-isosorbide mononitrate
CRH	corticotropin-releasing hormone		LH	luteinizing hormone
			M	moles/liter, mol/l
DAG	diacylglycerol		MAC	minimal alveolar concentration
DHF	dihydrofolic acid, dihydrofolate			
			MAO	monoamine oxidase
DHT	dihydrotestosterone		mesna	sodium 2-mercaptoethane-sulfonate
DNA	deoxyribonucleic acid			
DPTA	diethylenetriaminopentaacetic acid		MHC	major histocompatibility complex
DRC	dose–response curves		MI	myocardial infarction
ECL	enterochromaffin-like		mM	millimoles/liter, mmol/l
EDRF	endothelium-derived relaxant factor		mmHg	millimeters of mercury
			mRNA	messenger RNA
EEG	electroencephalogram		mTOR	mammalian target of rapamycin
EFV	extracellular fluid volume			
EMT	extraneuronal monoamine transporter		MW	molecular weight
			NAChR	nicotinic receptor

NAT	norepinephrine transporter
NE	norepinephrine
NFAT	nuclear factor of activated T cells
NH	neurohypophyseal
NMDS	N-methyl-d-asparate
NSTEMI	non-STEMI (non-ST elevation MI)
NTG	nitroglycerin
NYHA	New York Heart Association
PABA	p-aminobenzoic acid
PAMBA	p-aminomethylbenzoic acid
PDE	phosphodiesterase
PF3	platelet factor 3
PL	phospholipid
PLC	phospholipase C
PPARα	peroxisome proliferator-activated receptor alpha
PPARγ	peroxisome proliferator-activated receptor gamma
PRIH	prolactin release inhibiting hormone = dopamine
REM	rapid eye movement
rER	rough endoplasmic reticulum
RNA	ribonucleic acid
rt-PA	recombinant tissue plasminogen activator
RyR	ryanodine receptors
s.c.	subcutaneous(ly)
sER	smooth endoplasmic reticulum
SERM	selective estrogen receptor modulators

SJS	Steven–Johnson syndrome
TEN	toxic epidermal necrolysis
SR	sarcoplasmic reticulum
SSRI	selective serotonin reuptake inhibitors
STEMI	ST elevation MI
THF	tetrahydrofolic acid, tetrahydrofolate
TIVA	total intravenous anaesthesia
TMPT	thiopurine methyltransferase
TNFα	necrosis factor α
t-PA	tissue plasminogen activator
TRH	thyrotropin-releasing hormone = protirelin
VAChT	vesicular ACh transporter
VMAT	vesicular monoamine transporter

Pharmacokinetic parameters

B

B_{max}

c_0

Cl_{tot}

c_{max}

c_t

F

k

K_D

$t_{1/2}$

V_{app}

General Pharmacology

□ History of Pharmacology

Since time immemorial, medicaments have been used for treating disease in humans and animals. The herbal preparations of antiquity describe the therapeutic powers of certain plants and minerals. Belief in the curative powers of plants and certain substances rested exclusively upon traditional knowledge, that is, empirical information not subjected to critical examination.

The Idea

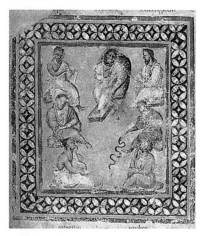

Claudius Galen (AD 129–200) first attempted to consider the theoretical background of pharmacology. Both theory and practical experience were to contribute equally to the rational use of medicines through interpretation of the observed and the experienced results:

The empiricists say that all is found by experience. We, however, maintain that it is found in part by experience, in part by theory. Neither experience nor theory alone is apt to discover all.

The Impetus

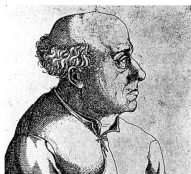

Theophrastus   von   Hohenheim (1493–1541), called Paracelsus, began to question doctrines handed down from antiquity, demanding knowledge of the active ingredient(s) in prescribed remedies, while rejecting the irrational concoctions and mixtures of medieval medicine. He prescribed chemically defined substances with such success that professional enemies had him prosecuted as a poisoner. Against such accusations, he defended himself with the thesis that has become an axiom of pharmacology:

If you want to explain any poison properly, what then is not a poison? All things are poison, nothing is without poison; the dose alone causes a thing not to be poison.

Early Beginnings

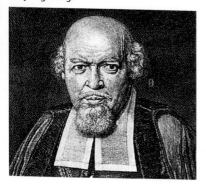

Johann Jakob Wepfer (1620–1695) was the first to verify by animal experimentation assertions about pharmacological or toxicological actions.

I pondered at length. Finally I resolved to clarify the matter by experiments.

Foundation

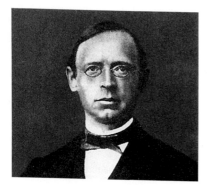

Rudolf Buchheim (1820–1879) founded the first institute of pharmacology at the University of Dorpat (Tartu, Estonia) in 1847, ushering in pharmacology as an independent scientific discipline. In addition to a description of effects, he strove to explain the chemical properties of drugs.

The science of medicines is a theoretical, i. e., explanatory, one. It is to provide us with knowledge by which our judgment about the utility of medicines can be validated at the bedside.

Consolidation—General Recognition

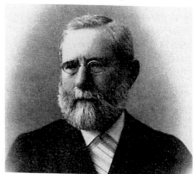

Oswald Schmiedeberg (1838–1921), together with his many disciples (12 of whom were appointed to chairs of pharmacology), helped establish the high reputation of pharmacology. Fundamental concepts such as structure–activity relationships, drug receptors, and selective toxicity emerged from the work of, respectively, T. Frazer (1840–1920) in Scotland, J. Langley (1852–1925) in England, and P. Ehrlich (1854–1915) in Germany. Alexander J. Clarke (1885–1941) in England first formalized receptor theory in the early 1920s by applying the Law of Mass Action to drug–receptor interactions. Together with the internist Bernhard Naunyn (1839–1925), Schmiedeberg founded the first journal of pharmacology, which has been published since without interruption. The "Father of American Pharmacology," John J. Abel (1857–1938) was among the first Americans to train in Schmiedeberg's laboratory and was founder of the *Journal of Pharmacology and Experimental Therapeutics* (published from 1909 until the present).

Status Quo

After 1920, pharmacological laboratories sprang up in the pharmaceutical industry outside established university institutes. After 1960, departments of clinical pharmacology were set up at many universities and in industry.

□ Drug and Active Principle

Until the end of the 19th century, medicines were natural organic or inorganic products, mostly dried, but also fresh, plants or plant parts. These might contain substances possessing healing (therapeutic) properties, or substances exerting a toxic effect.

In order to secure a supply of medically useful products not merely at the time of harvest but year round, plants were preserved by drying or soaking them in vegetable oils or alcohol. Drying the plant, vegetable, or animal product yielded a drug (from French "drogue" = dried herb). Colloquially, this term nowadays often refers to chemical substances with high potential for physical dependence and abuse. Used scientifically, this term implies nothing about the quality of action, if any. In its original, wider sense, *drug* could refer equally well to the dried leaves of peppermint, dried lime blossoms, dried flowers and leaves of the female cannabis plant (hashish, marijuana), or the dried milky exudate obtained by slashing the unripe seed capsules of *Papaver somniferum* (raw opium).

Soaking plants or plant parts in alcohol (ethanol) creates a *tincture*. In this process, pharmacologically active constituents of the plant are extracted by the alcohol. Tinctures do not contain the complete spectrum of substances that exist in the plant or crude drug, but only those that are soluble in alcohol. In the case of opium tincture, these ingredients are alkaloids (i. e., basic substances of plant origin) including morphine, codeine, narcotine = noscapine, papaverine, narceine, and others.

Using a natural product or extract to treat a disease thus usually entails the administration of a number of substances possibly possessing very different activities. Moreover, the dose of an individual constituent contained within a given amount of the natural product is subject to large variations, depending upon the product's geographical origin (biotope), time of harvesting, or conditions and length of storage. For the same reasons, the relative proportions of individual constituents may vary considerably. Starting with the extraction of morphine from opium in 1804 by F.W. Sertürner (1783–1841), the active principles of many other natural products were subsequently isolated in chemically pure form by pharmaceutical laboratories.

□ The Aims of Isolating Active Principles

1. Identification of the active ingredient(s).
2. Analysis of the biological effects (pharmacodynamics) of individual ingredients and of their fate in the body (pharmacokinetics).
3. Ensuring a precise and constant dosage in the therapeutic use of chemically pure constituents.
4. The possibility of chemical synthesis, which would afford independence from limited natural supplies and create conditions for the analysis of structure–activity relationships.

Finally, derivatives of the original constituent may be synthesized in an effort to optimize pharmacological properties. Thus, derivatives of the original constituent with improved therapeutic usefulness may be developed.

Modification of the chemical structure of natural substances has frequently led to pharmaceuticals with enhanced potency. An illustrative example is fentanyl, which acts like morphine but requires a dose only 0.1–0.05 times that of the parent substance. Derivatives of fentanyl such as carfentanyl (employed in veterinary anesthesia of large animals) are actually 5000 times more potent than morphine.

A. From poppy to morphine

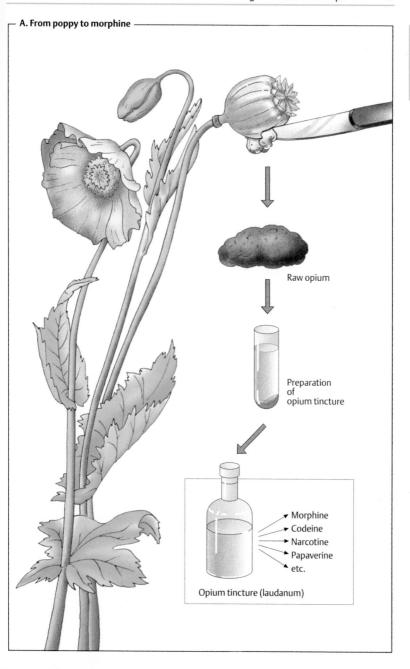

Raw opium

Preparation
of
opium tincture

Morphine
Codeine
Narcotine
Papaverine
etc.

Opium tincture (laudanum)

□ European Plants as Sources of Effective Medicines

Since prehistoric times, humans have attempted to alleviate ailments or injuries with the aid of plant parts or herbal preparations. Ancient civilizations have recorded various prescriptions of this kind. In the herbal formularies of medieval times numerous plants were promoted as remedies. In modern medicine, where each drug is required to satisfy objective criteria of efficacy, few of the hundreds of reputedly curative plant species have survived as drugs with documented effectiveness. Presented below are some examples from local old-world floras that were already used in prescientific times and that contain substances that to this day are employed as important drugs.

A. A group of local plants used since the middle ages to treat "dropsy" comprises foxglove (digitalis sp.), lily of the valley (*Convallaria majalis*), christmas rose (*Helleborus niger*), and spindletree (*Evonymus europaeus*). At the end of the 18th century the Scottish physician William Withering introduced **digitalis leaves** as a tea into the treatment of "cardiac dropsy" (edema of congestive heart failure) and described the result. The active principles in these plants are steroids with one or more sugar molecules attached at C3 (see p. 135). Proven clinically most useful among all available cardiac glycosides, **digoxin** continues to be obtained from the plants *Digitalis purpurea* or *D. lanata* because its chemical synthesis is too difficult and expensive.

B. The **deadly nightshade** of middle Europe (*Atropa belladonna*, a solanaceous herb)[1] contains the alkaloids **atropine**, in all its parts, and **scopolamine**, in smaller amounts. The effects of this drug were already known in antiquity; e. g., pupillary dilation resulting from the cosmetic use of extracts as eye drops to enhance female attractiveness. In the 19th century, the alkaloids were isolated, their structures elucidated, and their specific mechanism of action recognized. Atropine is the prototype of a competitive antagonist at the acetylcholine receptor of the muscarinic type (cf. p. 108).

C. The **common white** and **basket willow** (*Salix alba*, *S. viminalis*) contain salicylic acid derivatives in their bark. Preparations of willow bark were used from antiquity; in the 19th century, **salicylic acid** was isolated as the active principle of this folk remedy. This simple acid still enjoys use as an external agent (keratolytic action) but is no longer taken orally for the treatment of pain, fever, and inflammatory reactions. Acetylation of salicylic acid (introduced around 1900) to yield **acetylsalicylic acid** (ASA, Aspirin®) improved oral tolerability.

D. The **autumn crocus** (*Colchicum autumnale*) belongs to the lily family and flowers on meadows in late summer to fall; leaves and fruit capsules appear in the following spring. All parts of the plant contain the alkaloid **colchicine**. This substance inhibits the polymerization of tubulin to microtubules, which are responsible for intracellular movement processes. Thus, under the influence of colchicine, macrophages and neutrophils lose their capacity for intracellular transport of cell organelles. This action underlies the beneficial effect during an acute attack of gout (cf. p. 326) Furthermore, colchicine prevents mitosis, causing an arrest in metaphase (spindle poison).

---

[1] This name reflects the poisonous property of the plant: Atropos was the one of the three Fates (moirai) who cut the thread of life.

A. European plants as sources of drugs

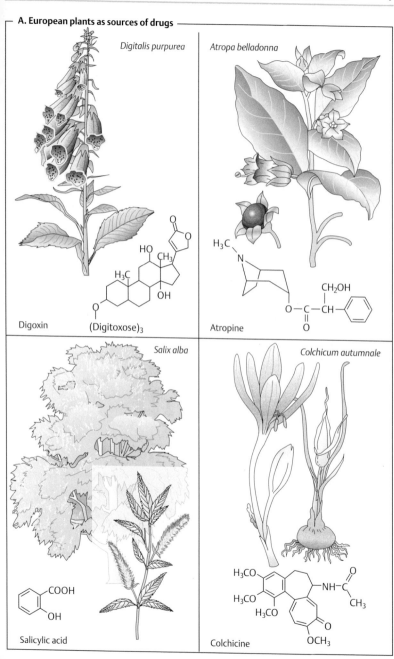

Digitalis purpurea

Digoxin (Digitoxose)₃

Atropa belladonna

Atropine

Salix alba

Salicylic acid

Colchicum autumnale

Colchicine

□ Drug Development

The drug development process starts with the **synthesis** of novel chemical compounds. Substances with complex structures may be obtained from various sources, e. g., plants (cardiac glycosides), animal tissues (heparin), microbial cultures (penicillin G) or cultures of human cells (urokinase), or by means of gene technology (human insulin). As more insight is gained into structure–activity relationships, the search for new agents becomes more clearly focused.

Preclinical testing yields information on the biological effects of new substances. Initial screening may employ *biochemical-pharmacological investigations* (e. g., receptor binding assays, p. 56) or experiments on cell cultures, isolated cells, and isolated organs. Since these models invariably fall short of replicating complex biological processes in the intact organism, any potential drug must be tested in the whole animal. Only animal experiments can reveal whether the desired effects will actually occur at dosages that produce little or no toxicity. *Toxicological investigations* serve to evaluate the potential for: (1) toxicity associated with acute or chronic administration; (2) genetic damage (genotoxicity, mutagenicity); (3) production of tumors (oncogenicity or carcinogenicity); and (4) causation of birth defects (teratogenicity). In animals, compounds under investigation also have to be studied with respect to their absorption, distribution, metabolism, and elimination (*pharmacokinetics*). Even at the level of preclinical testing, only a very small fraction of new compounds will prove potentially fit for use in humans.

Pharmaceutical technology provides the methods for drug formulation.

Clinical testing starts with **Phase I** studies on healthy subjects and seeks to determine whether effects observed in animal experiments also occur in humans. Dose–response relationships are determined. In **Phase II**, potential drugs are first tested on selected patients for therapeutic efficacy in those disease states for which they are intended. If a beneficial action is evident, and the incidence of adverse effects is acceptably small, **Phase III** is entered, involving a larger group of patients in whom the new drug will be compared with conventional treatments in terms of therapeutic outcome. As a form of human experimentation, these clinical trials are subject to review and approval by institutional ethics committees according to international codes of conduct (Declarations of Helsinki, Tokyo, and Venice). During clinical testing, many drugs are revealed to be unusable. Ultimately, only one new drug typically remains from some 10 000 newly synthesized substances.

The decision to **approve a new drug** is made by a national regulatory body (Food and Drug Administration in the United States.; the Health Protection Branch Drugs Directorate in Canada; the EU Commission in conjunction with the European Agency for the Evaluation of Medicinal Products, London, United Kingdom) to which manufacturers are required to submit their applications. Applicants must document by means of appropriate test data (from preclinical and clinical trials) that the criteria of efficacy and safety have been met and that product forms (tablet, capsule, etc.) satisfy general standards of quality control.

Following approval, the new drug may be marketed under a trade name (pp. 10, 352) and thus become available for prescription by physicians and dispensing by pharmacists. As the drug gains more widespread use, regulatory surveillance continues in the form of postlicensing studies (**Phase IV** of clinical trials). Only on the basis of long-term experience will the risk–benefit ratio be properly assessed and, thus, the therapeutic value of the new drug be determined. If the new drug offers hardly any advantage over existing ones, the cost–benefit relationship needs to be kept in mind.

A. From drug synthesis to approval

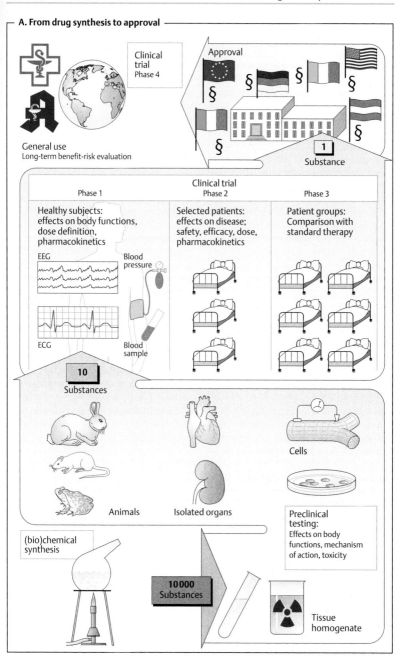

Clinical trial
Phase 4

Approval

General use
Long-term benefit-risk evaluation

1
Substance

Clinical trial

Phase 1

Phase 2

Phase 3

Healthy subjects:
effects on body functions,
dose definition,
pharmacokinetics

EEG

Blood pressure

ECG

Blood sample

Selected patients:
effects on disease;
safety, efficacy, dose,
pharmacokinetics

Patient groups:
Comparison with
standard therapy

10
Substances

Cells

Animals

Isolated organs

Preclinical
testing:
Effects on body
functions, mechanism
of action, toxicity

(bio)chemical
synthesis

10000
Substances

Tissue
homogenate

☐ Congeneric Drugs and Name Diversity

The preceding pages outline the route leading to approval of a new drug. The pharmaceutical receives an **International Nonproprietary Name** (INN) and a brand or trade name chosen by the innovative pharmaceutical company. Patent protection enables the patent holder to market the new substance for a specified period of time. As soon as the patent protection expires, the drug concerned can be put on the market as a generic under a nonproprietary name or as a successor preparation under other brand names. Since patent protection is generally already sought during the development phase, protected sale of the drug may occur only for a few years.

The value of a **new drug** depends on whether one deals with a novel active principle or merely an analogue (or congeneric) preparation with a slightly changed chemical structure. It is of course much more arduous to develop a substance that possesses a novel mechanism of action and thereby expands therapeutic possibilities. Examples of such fundamental innovations from recent years include the ACE inhibitors (p. 128), the lipid-lowering agents of the statin type (p. 158), the proton pump inhibitors (p. 170), the gonadorelin superagonists (p. 238), and the gyrase inhibitors (p. 276).

Much more frequently, "new drugs" are analogue substances that imitate the chemical structure of a successful pharmaceutical. These compounds contain the requisite features in their molecule but differ from the parent molecule by structural alterations that are biologically irrelevant. Such **analogue substances**, or "me-too" preparations, do not add anything new regarding the mechanism of action. A model example for the overabundance of analogue substances are the β-blockers: about 20 individual substances with the same pharmacophoric groups differ only in the substituents at the phenoxy residue. This entails small differences in pharmacokinetic behavior and relative affinity for β-receptor subtypes (examples shown in **A**). A small fraction of these substances would suffice for therapeutic use. The WHO Model formulary names only one β-blocker from the existing profusion, marked in **A** by an asterisk. The corresponding phenomenon is evident among various other drug groups (e. g., benzodiazepines, nonsteroidal anti-inflammatory agents, and cephalosporins). Most analogue substances can be neglected.

After patent protection expires, competing drug companies will at once market successful (i. e., profitable) pharmaceuticals as second-submission **successor** (or "follow-on") **preparations**. Since no research expenses are involved at this point, successor drugs can be offered at a cheaper price, either as **generics** (INN + company name) or under new fancy names. Thus some common drugs circulate under 10 to 20 different trade names. An extreme example is presented in **B** for the analgesic ibuprofen.

The excess of analogue preparations and the unnecessary diversity of trade names for one and the same drug make the pharmaceutical markets of some countries (e. g., Germany) rather perplexing. A critical listing of **essential drugs** is a prerequisite for optimal pharmacotherapy and would be of great value for medical practice.

A. β-Blockers of similar basic structure

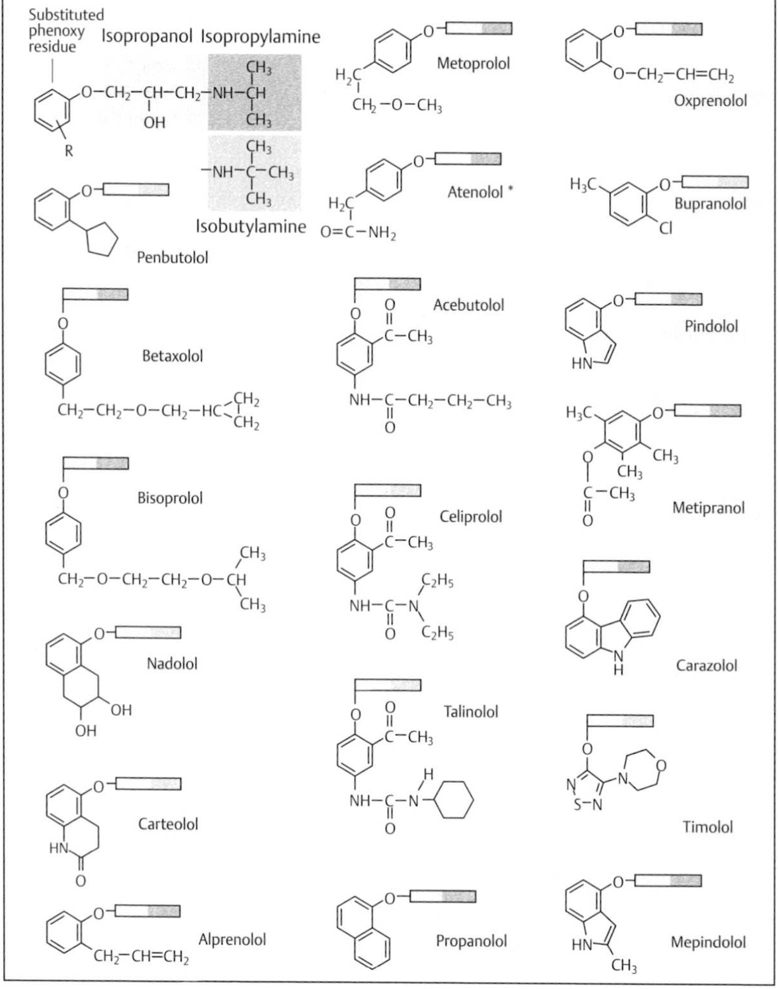

Substituted phenoxy residue   Isopropanol Isopropylamine

Metoprolol

Oxprenolol

Atenolol *

Bupranolol

Isobutylamine

Penbutolol

Betaxolol

Acebutolol

Pindolol

Bisoprolol

Celiprolol

Metipranol

Nadolol

Talinolol

Carazolol

Carteolol

Timolol

Alprenolol

Propanolol

Mepindolol

B. Successor preparations for a pharmaceutical

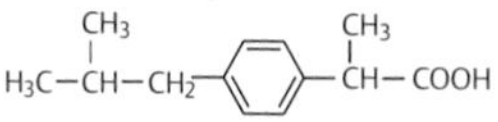

Ibuprofen = 2-(4-isobutylphenyl)propionic acid
1. Generic ibuprofen from eight manufacturers
2. Ibuprofen under different brand names; introduced as Brufen® (no longer available)

$H_3C-CH-CH_2$ —⟨phenyl⟩— $CH-COOH$ (with CH_3 substituents)

Aktren®, Contraneural®, Dismenol®, Dolgit®, Dolodoc®, Dolopuren®, Dolormin®, Dolosanol®, Esprenit®, Eudorlin®, Gynofug®, Gynoneuralgin®, Ibu®, Ibu-acis®, Ibu-Attritin®, Ibubeta®, Ibudolor®, Ibu-Eu-Rho®, Ibuflam®, Ibuhemo-pharm®, Ibuhexal®, Ibu-KD®, Ibumerck®, Ibuphlogont®, Ibupro®, Iburatiopharm®, Ibu-TAD®, Ibutop®, Ilvico®, Imbun®, Jenaprofen®, Kontragripp®, Mensoton®, Migränin®, Novogent®, Nurofen®, Optalidon®, Opturem®, Parsal®, Pharmaprofen®, Ratiodolor®, Schmerz-Dolgit®, Spalt-Liqua®, Tabalon®, Tempil®, Tispol®, Togal®, Trauma-Dolgit®, Urem®

□ Oral Dosage Forms

The **coated tablet** contains a drug within a core that is covered by a shell, e.g., wax coating, that serves (1) to protect perishable drugs from decomposing, (2) to mask a disagreeable taste or odor, (3) to facilitate passage on swallowing, or (4) to permit color coding.

Capsules usually consist of an oblong casing—generally made of gelatin—that contains the drug in powder or granulated form.

In the **matrix-type tablet**, the drug is embedded in an inert meshwork, from which it is released by diffusion upon being moistened. In contrast to *solutions*, which permit direct absorption of drug (**A**, track 3), the use of solid dosage forms initially requires *tablets* to break up and *capsules* to open (**disintegration**), before the drug can be dissolved (**dissolution**) and pass through the gastrointestinal mucosal lining (**absorption**). Because disintegration of the tablet and dissolution of the drug take time, absorption will occur mainly in the intestine (**A**, track 2). In the case of a solution, absorption already starts in the stomach (**A**, track 3).

For acid-labile drugs, a coating of wax or of a cellulose acetate polymer is used to prevent disintegration of solid dosage forms in the stomach. Accordingly, disintegration and dissolution will take place in the duodenum at normal rate (**A**, track 1) and drug liberation per se is not retarded.

The **liberation** of drug, and hence the site and time-course of absorption, are subject to modification by appropriate production methods for matrix-type tablets, coated tablets, and capsules. In the case of the matrix tablet, this is done by incorporating the drug into a lattice from which it can be slowly leached out by gastrointestinal fluids. As the matrix tablet undergoes enteral transit, drug liberation and absorption proceed en route (**A**, track 4). In the case of coated tablets, coat thickness can be designed such that release and absorption of drug occur either in the proximal (**A**, track 1) or distal (**A**, track 5) bowel. Thus, by matching dissolution time with small-bowel transit time, drug release can be timed to occur in the colon.

Drug liberation and, hence, absorption can also be spread out when the drug is presented in the form of a granulate consisting of pellets coated with a waxy film of graded thickness. Depending on film thickness, gradual dissolution occurs during enteral transit, releasing drug at variable rates for absorption. The principle illustrated for a *capsule* can also be applied to tablets. In this case, either drug pellets coated with films of various thicknesses are compressed into a tablet or the drug is incorporated into a *matrix-type* tablet. In contrast to timed-release capsules *slow-release tablets* have the advantage of being divisible ad libitum; thus fractions of the dose contained within the entire tablet may be administered.

This kind of **retarded drug release** is employed when a rapid rise in blood levels of drug is undesirable, or when absorption is being slowed in order to prolong the action of drugs that have a short sojourn in the body.

A. Oral administration: drug release and absorption

Administration

| Enteric coated tablet | Tablet, capsule | Drops, mixture, effervescent solution | Matrix tablet | Coated tablet with delayed release |

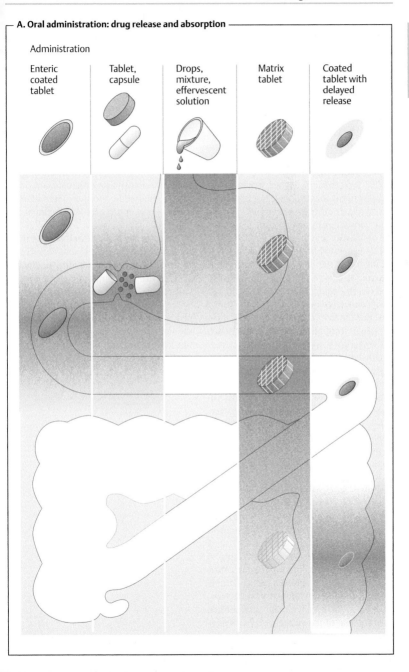

□ Drug Administration by Inhalation

Inhalation in the form of an aerosol, a gas, or a mist permits drugs to be applied to the bronchial mucosa and, to a lesser extent, to the alveolar membranes. This route is chosen for drugs intended to affect bronchial smooth muscle or the consistency of bronchial mucus. Furthermore, gaseous or volatile agents can be administered by inhalation with the goal of alveolar absorption and systemic effects (e. g., inhalational anesthetics, p. 216). **Aerosols** are formed when a drug solution or micronized powder is converted into a mist or dust, respectively.

In conventional sprays (e. g., nebulizer), the air blast required for the aerosol formation is generated by the stroke of a pump. Alternatively, the drug is delivered from a solution or powder packaged in a pressurized canister equipped with a valve through which a metered dose is discharged. During use, the inhaler (spray dispenser) is held directly in front of the mouth and actuated at the start of inspiration. The effectiveness of delivery depends on the position of the device in front of the mouth, the size of the aerosol particles, and the coordination between opening the spray valve and inspiration. The size of the aerosol particles determines the speed at which they are swept along by inhaled air, and hence the **depth of penetration into the respiratory tract**. Particles > 100 μm in diameter are trapped in the oropharyngeal cavity; those having diameters between 10 and 60 μm will be deposited on the epithelium of the bronchial tract. Particles < 2 μm in diameter can reach the alveoli, but they will be exhaled again unless they settle out.

Drug deposited on the mucous lining of the bronchial epithelium is partly absorbed and partly transported with bronchial mucus toward the larynx. Bronchial mucus travels upward owing to the orally directed undulatory beat of the epithelial cilia. Physiologically, this mucociliary transport functions to remove inspired dust particles.

Thus, only a portion of the drug aerosol (~ 10%) gains access to the respiratory tract and just a fraction of this amount penetrates the mucosa, whereas the remainder of the aerosol undergoes mucociliary transport to the laryngopharynx and is swallowed. The advantage of inhalation (i. e., localized application without systemic load) is fully exploited by using drugs that are poorly absorbed from the intestine (tiotropium, cromolyn) or are subject to first-pass elimination (p. 42); for example, glucocorticoids such as beclomethasone dipropionate, budesonide, flunisolide, and fluticasone dipropionate or β-agonists such as salbutamol and fenoterol.

Even when the swallowed portion of an inhaled drug is absorbed in unchanged form, administration by this route has the advantage that drug concentrations at the bronchi will be higher than in other organs.

The efficiency of mucociliary transport depends on the force of kinociliary motion and the viscosity of bronchial mucus. Both factors can be altered pathologically (e. g., by smoker's cough or chronic bronchitis).

A. Application by inhalation

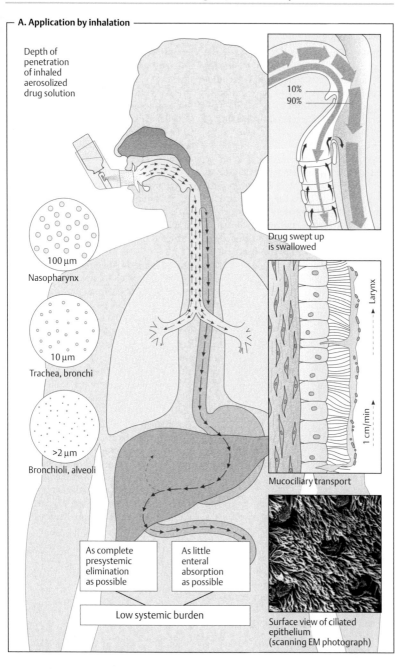

Depth of penetration of inhaled aerosolized drug solution

100 μm
Nasopharynx

10 μm
Trachea, bronchi

>2 μm
Bronchioli, alveoli

10%
90%

Drug swept up is swallowed

Larynx

1 cm/min

Mucociliary transport

As complete presystemic elimination as possible

As little enteral absorption as possible

Low systemic burden

Surface view of ciliated epithelium (scanning EM photograph)

□ Dermatological Agents

Pharmaceutical preparations applied to the outer skin are intended either to provide skin care and protection from noxious influences (**A**) or to serve as a vehicle for drugs that are to be absorbed into the skin or, if appropriate, into the general circulation (**B**).

Skin Protection (A)

Protective agents are of several kinds to meet different requirements according to skin condition (dry, low in oil, chapped vs. moist, oily, elastic), and the type of noxious stimuli (prolonged exposure to water, regular use of alcohol-containing disinfectants, intense solar irradiation). Distinctions among protective agents are based upon consistency, physicochemical properties (lipophilic, hydrophilic), and the presence of additives.

Dusting powders are sprinkled onto the intact skin and consist of talc, magnesium stearate, silicon dioxide (silica), or starch. They adhere to the skin, forming a low-friction film that attenuates mechanical irritation. Powders exert a drying (evaporative) effect.

Lipophilic ointment (oil ointment) consists of a lipophilic base (paraffin oil, petroleum jelly, wool fat) and may contain up to 10% powder materials, such as zinc oxide, titanium oxide, starch, or a mixture of these. Emulsifying ointments are made of paraffins and an emulsifying wax, and are miscible with water.

Paste (oil paste) is an ointment containing more than 10% pulverized constituents.

Lipophilic (oily) cream is an emulsion of water in oil, easier to spread than oil paste or oil ointment.

Hydrogel and **water-soluble ointment** achieve their consistency by means of different gel-forming agents (gelatin, methylcellulose, polyethylene glycol). **Lotions** are aqueous suspensions of water-insoluble and solid constituents.

Hydrophilic (aqueous) cream is an oil-in-water emulsion formed with the aid of an emulsifier; it may also be considered an oil-in-water emulsion of an emulsifying ointment.

All dermatological agents having a lipophilic base adhere to the skin as a water-repellent coating. They do not wash off and they also prevent (**occlude**) outward passage of water from the skin. The skin is protected from drying, and its hydration and elasticity increase. Diminished evaporation of water results in warming of the occluded skin. Hydrophilic agents wash off easily and do not impede transcutaneous output of water. Evaporation of water is felt as a cooling effect.

Dermatological Agents as Vehicles (B)

In order to reach its site of action, a drug must leave its pharmaceutical preparation and enter the skin if a local effect is desired (e.g., glucocorticoid ointment), or be able to penetrate it if a systemic action is intended (transdermal delivery system, e.g., nitroglycerin patch, p.124). The tendency for the drug to leave the drug vehicle is higher the more the drug and vehicle differ in lipophilicity (high tendency: hydrophilic drug and lipophilic vehicle; and vice versa). Because the skin represents a closed lipophilic barrier (p.22), only lipophilic drugs are absorbed. Hydrophilic drugs fail even to penetrate the outer skin when applied in a lipophilic vehicle. This formulation can be useful when high drug concentrations are required at the skin surface (e.g., neomycin ointment for bacterial skin infections).

A. Dermatologicals as skin protectants

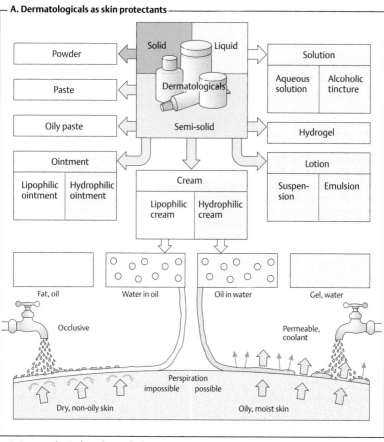

Solid   Liquid

Dermatologicals

Semi-solid

Powder

Paste

Oily paste

Ointment

| Lipophilic ointment | Hydrophilic ointment |

Cream

| Lipophilic cream | Hydrophilic cream |

Solution

| Aqueous solution | Alcoholic tincture |

Hydrogel

Lotion

| Suspension | Emulsion |

Fat, oil   Water in oil   Oil in water   Gel, water

Occlusive   Permeable, coolant

Perspiration
impossible   possible

Dry, non-oily skin   Oily, moist skin

B. Dermatologicals as drug vehicles

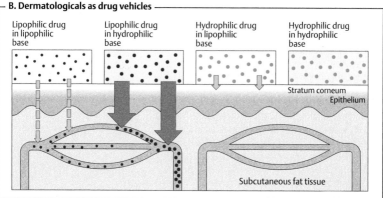

Lipophilic drug in lipophilic base

Lipophilic drug in hydrophilic base

Hydrophilic drug in lipophilic base

Hydrophilic drug in hydrophilic base

Stratum corneum
Epithelium

Subcutaneous fat tissue

☐ From Application to Distribution in the Body

As a rule, drugs reach their target organs via the blood. Therefore, they must first enter the blood, usually in the venous limb of the circulation. There are several possible sites of entry.

The drug may be injected or infused **intravenously**, in which case it is introduced directly into the bloodstream. In **subcutaneous** or **intramuscular** injection, the drug has to diffuse from its site of application into the blood. Because these procedures entail injury to the outer skin, strict requirements must be met concerning technique. For this reason, the **oral** route (i.e., simple application by mouth) involving subsequent uptake of drug across the gastrointestinal mucosa into the blood is chosen much more frequently. The disadvantage of this route is that the drug must pass through the liver on its way into the general circulation. In all of the above modes of application, this fact assumes practical significance for any drug that may be rapidly transformed or possibly inactivated in the liver (first-pass effect, presystemic elimination, bioavailability; p. 42). Furthermore, a drug has to traverse the lungs before entering the general circulation. Pulmonary tissues may trap hydrophobic substances. The lungs may then act as a buffer and thus prevent a rapid rise in drug levels in peripheral blood after i.v. injection (important, for example, with i.v. anesthetics). Even with rectal administration, at least a fraction of the drug enters the general circulation via the portal vein, because only blood from the short terminal segment of the rectum drains directly into the inferior vena cava. Hepatic passage is circumvented when absorption occurs buccally or sublingually, because venous blood from the oral cavity drains into the superior vena cava. The same would apply to administration by **inhalation** (p. 14). However, with this route, a local effect is usually intended, and a systemic action is intended only in exceptional cases. Under certain conditions, drug can also be applied percutaneously in the form of a **transdermal** delivery system (p. 16). In this case, drug is released from the reservoir at constant rate over many hours, and then penetrates the epidermis and subepidermal connective tissue where it enters blood capillaries. Only a very few drugs can be applied transdermally. The feasibility of this route is determined by both the physicochemical properties of the drug and the therapeutic requirements (acute vs. long-term effect).

Speed of absorption is determined by the route and method of application. It is *fastest* with *intravenous injection, less fast* with *intramuscular injection*, and *slowest* with *subcutaneous injection*. When the drug is applied to the oral mucosa (**buccal**, **sublingual** routes), plasma levels rise faster than with conventional oral administration because the drug preparation is deposited at its actual site of absorption and very high concentrations in saliva occur upon the dissolution of a single dose. Thus, uptake across the oral epithelium is accelerated. Furthermore, drug absorption from the oral mucosa avoids passage through the liver and, hence, presystemic elimination. The buccal or sublingual route is not suitable for poorly water-soluble or poorly absorbable drugs. Such agents should be given orally because both the volume of fluid for dissolution and the absorbing surface are much larger in the small intestine than in the oral cavity.

A. From application to distribution

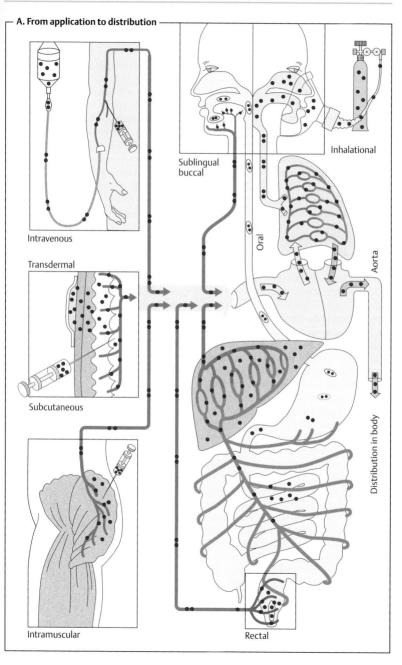

Intravenous

Transdermal

Subcutaneous

Intramuscular

Sublingual buccal

Inhalational

Oral

Aorta

Rectal

Distribution in body

☐ Potential Targets of Drug Action

Drugs are designed to exert a selective influence on vital processes in order to alleviate or eliminate symptoms of disease. The smallest basic unit of an organism is the **cell**. The outer cell membrane, or plasmalemma, effectively demarcates the cell from its surroundings, thus permitting a large degree of internal autonomy. Embedded in the plasmalemma are **transport proteins** that serve to mediate *controlled metabolic exchange with the cellular environment*. These include energy-consuming pumps (e.g., Na$^+$,K$^+$-ATPase, p.134), carriers (e.g., for Na$^+$/glucose co-transport, p.180), and ion channels (e.g., for sodium (p.138) or calcium (p.126) (**1**).

Functional coordination between single cells is a prerequisite for the viability of the organism, hence also the survival of individual cells. Cell functions are coordinated by means of cytosolic contacts between neighboring cells (gap junctions, e.g., in the myocardium) and messenger substances for the transfer of information. Included among these are "transmitters" released from nerves, which the cell is able to recognize with the help of specialized membrane binding sites or **receptors**. Hormones secreted by endocrine glands into the blood, then into the extracellular fluid, represent another class of chemical signals. Finally, signaling substances can originate from neighboring cells: paracrine regulation, for instance by the prostaglandins (p.196) and cytokines.

The **effect of a drug** frequently results from interference with cellular function. Receptors for the recognition of endogenous transmitters are obvious sites of drug action (receptor agonists and antagonists, p.60). Altered activity of membrane transport systems affects cell function (e.g., cardiac glycosides, p.134; loop diuretics, p.166; calcium-antagonists, p.126). Drugs may also directly interfere with intracellular metabolic processes, for instance by inhibiting (phosphodiesterase inhibitors, pp.66, 122) or activating (organic nitrates, p.124) an enzyme (**2**);

even processes in the cell nucleus can be affected (e.g., DNA damage by certain cytostatics).

In contrast to drugs acting from the outside on cell membrane constituents, agents acting in the cell's interior need to penetrate the cell membrane.

The **cell membrane** basically consists of a **phospholipid bilayer** (50 Å = 5 nm in thickness), embedded in which are proteins (integral membrane proteins, such as receptors and transport molecules). Phospholipid molecules contain two long-chain *fatty acids* in ester linkage with two of the three hydroxyl groups of *glycerol*. Bound to the third hydroxyl group is *phosphoric acid*, which, in turn, carries a further *residue*, e.g., choline (phosphatidylcholine = lecithin), the amino acid serine (phosphatidylserine), or the cyclic polyhydric alcohol inositol (phosphatidylinositol). In terms of solubility, phospholipids are amphiphilic: the tail region containing the apolar fatty acid chains is lipophilic; the remainder—the polar head—is hydrophilic. By virtue of these properties, phospholipids aggregate spontaneously into a bilayer in an aqueous medium, their polar heads being directed outward into the aqueous medium, the fatty acid chains facing each other and projecting into the inside of the membrane (**3**).

The **hydrophobic interior** of the phospholipid membrane constitutes a diffusion barrier virtually impermeable to charged particles. Apolar particles, however, are better able to penetrate the membrane. This is of major importance with respect to the absorption, distribution, and elimination of drugs.

A. Site at which drugs act to modify cell function

1

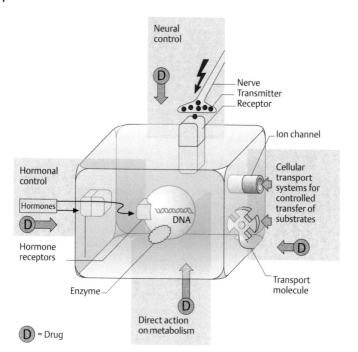

Neural control

Nerve

Transmitter

Receptor

Ion channel

Hormonal control

Hormones

DNA

Cellular transport systems for controlled transfer of substrates

Hormone receptors

Enzyme

Transport molecule

Direct action on metabolism

D = Drug

2

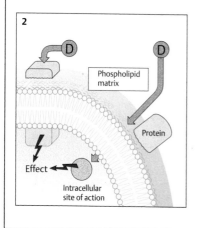

Phospholipid matrix

Protein

Effect

Intracellular site of action

3

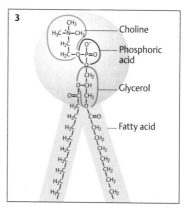

Choline

Phosphoric acid

Glycerol

Fatty acid

☐ External Barriers of the Body

Prior to its uptake into the blood (i. e., during absorption), the drug has to overcome barriers that demarcate the body from its surroundings, that is, that separate the internal from the external milieu. These boundaries are formed by the skin and mucous membranes.

When absorption takes place in the **gut** (enteral absorption), the intestinal epithelium is the barrier. This single-layered epithelium is made up of enterocytes and mucus-producing goblet cells. On their luminal side, these cells are joined together by *zonulae occludentes* (indicated by black dots in the inset, bottom left). A *zonula occludens*, or tight junction, is a region in which the phospholipid membranes of two cells establish close contact and become joined via integral membrane proteins (semicircular inset, left center). The region of fusion surrounds each cell like a ring such that neighboring cells are welded together in a continuous belt. In this manner, an unbroken phospholipid layer is formed (yellow area in the schematic drawing, bottom left) and acts as a continuous barrier between the two spaces separated by the cell layer—in the case of the gut, the intestinal lumen (dark blue) and interstitial space (light blue). The efficiency with which such a barrier restricts exchange of substances can be increased by arranging these occluding junctions in multiple arrays, as for instance in the endothelium of cerebral blood vessels. The connecting proteins (connexins) furthermore serve to restrict mixing of other functional membrane proteins (carrier molecules, ion pumps, ion channels) that occupy specific apical or basolateral areas of the cell membrane.

This phospholipid bilayer represents the intestinal mucosa–blood barrier that a drug must cross during its enteral absorption. Eligible drugs are those whose physicochemical properties allow permeation through the lipophilic membrane interior (yellow) or that are subject to a special inwardly directed carrier transport mechanism. Conversely, drugs can undergo backtransport into the gut by means of efflux pumps (P-glycoprotein) located in the luminal membrane of the intestinal epithelium. Absorption of such drugs proceeds rapidly because the absorbing surface is greatly enlarged owing to the formation of the epithelial brush border (submicroscopic foldings of the plasmalemma). The absorbability of a drug is characterized by the *absorption quotient*, that is, the amount absorbed divided by the amount in the gut available for absorption.

In the **respiratory tract**, cilia-bearing epithelial cells are also joined on the luminal side by zonulae occludentes, so that the bronchial space and the interstitium are separated by a continuous phospholipid barrier.

With sublingual or buccal application, the drug encounters the nonkeratinized, multilayered squamous epithelium of the **oral mucosa**. Here, the cells establish punctate contacts with each other in the form of desmosomes (not shown); however, these do not seal the intercellular clefts. Instead, the cells have the property of sequestering polar lipids that assemble into layers within the extracellular space (semicircular inset, center right). In this manner, a continuous phospholipid barrier arises also inside squamous epithelia, although at an extracellular location, unlike that of intestinal epithelia. A similar barrier principle operates in the multilayered keratinized squamous epithelium of the **skin**.

The presence of a continuous phospholipid layer again means that only lipophilic drugs can enter the body via squamous epithelia. Epithelial thickness, which in turn depends on the depth of the stratum corneum, determines the extent and speed of absorption. Examples of drugs that can be conveyed via the skin into the blood include scopolamine (p. 110), nitroglycerin (p. 124), fentanyl (p. 212) and the gonadal hormones (p. 250).

A. External barriers of the body

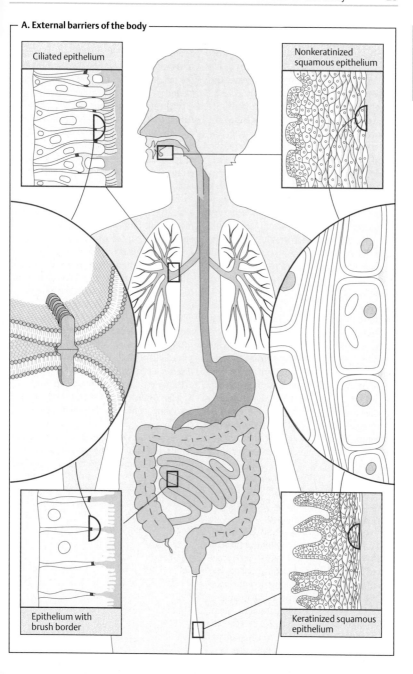

Ciliated epithelium

Nonkeratinized squamous epithelium

Epithelium with brush border

Keratinized squamous epithelium

☐ Blood–Tissue Barriers

Drugs are transported in the blood to different tissues of the body. In order to reach their sites of action, they must leave the bloodstream. Drug permeation occurs largely in the capillary bed, where both surface area and time available for exchange are maximal (extensive vascular branching, low velocity of flow). The capillary wall forms the blood–tissue barrier. Basically, this consists of an endothelial cell layer and a basement membrane enveloping the latter (solid black line in the schematic drawings). The endothelial cells are "riveted" to each other by tight junctions or occluding zonulae (labeled Z in the electron micrograph, upper left) such that no clefts, gaps, or pores remain that would permit drugs to pass unimpeded from the blood into the interstitial fluid.

The blood–tissue barrier is developed differently in the various capillary beds. Permeability of the capillary wall to drugs is determined by the structural and functional characteristics of the endothelial cells. In many capillary beds, e. g., those of **cardiac muscle**, endothelial cells are characterized by pronounced **endocytotic** and **transcytotic** activity, as evidenced by numerous invaginations and vesicles (arrows in the electron micrograph, upper right). Transcytotic activity entails transport of fluid or macromolecules from the blood into the interstitium and vice versa. Any solutes trapped in the fluid, including drugs, may traverse the blood–tissue barrier. In this form of transport, the physicochemical properties of drugs are of little importance.

In some capillary beds (e. g., in the **pancreas**), endothelial cells exhibit **fenestrations**. Although the cells are tightly connected by continuous junctions, they possess pores (arrows in electron micrograph, lower left) that are closed only by diaphragms. Both the diaphragm and basement membrane can be readily penetrated by substances of low molecular weight—the majority of drugs—but less so by macromolecules, e.g.,

proteins such as insulin (G: insulin storage granule). Penetrability of macromolecules is determined by molecular size and electric charge. Fenestrated endothelia are found in the capillaries of the *gut* and *endocrine glands.*

In the central nervous system (**brain** and **spinal cord**), capillary endothelia lack pores and there is little transcytotic activity. In order to cross the **blood–brain barrier**, drugs must diffuse transcellularly, i. e., penetrate the luminal and basal membrane of endothelial cells. Drug movement along this path requires specific physicochemical properties (p. 26) or the presence of a transport mechanism (e. g., L-dopa, p. 188). Thus, the blood–brain barrier is permeable only to certain types of drugs.

Drugs exchange freely between blood and interstitium in the liver, where endothelial cells exhibit large fenestrations (100 nm in diameter) facing Disse's spaces (D) and where neither diaphragms nor basement membranes impede drug movement.

Diffusion barriers are also present beyond the capillary wall; e. g., *placental barrier* of fused syncytiotrophoblast cells; *blood–testicle barrier*, junctions interconnecting Sertoli cells; brain *choroid plexus–blood barrier*, occluding junctions between ependymal cells.

(Vertical bars in the electron micrographs represent 1 μm; E, cross-sectioned erythrocyte; AM, actomyosin; G, insulin-containing granules.)

A. Blood-tissue barriers

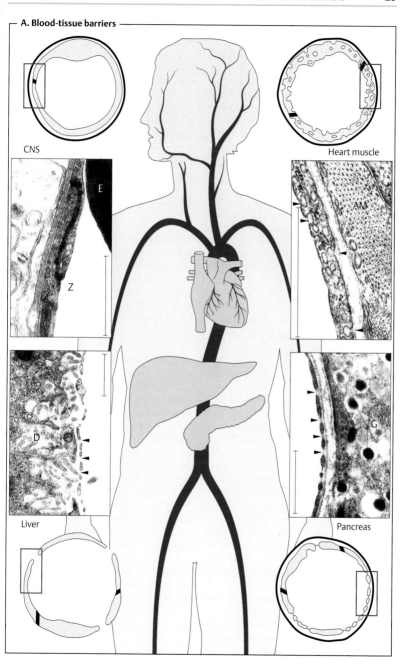

CNS

Heart muscle

Liver

Pancreas

☐ Membrane Permeation

An ability to penetrate lipid bilayers is a prerequisite for the absorption of drugs, their entry into cell or cellular organelles, and passage across the blood–brain barrier. Owing to their amphiphilic nature, phospholipids form bilayers possessing a hydrophilic surface and a hydrophobic interior (p. 20). Substances may traverse this membrane in three different ways.

Diffusion (A). Lipophilic substances (red dots) may enter the membrane from the extracellular space (area shown in ochre), accumulate in the membrane, and exit into the cytosol (blue area). Direction and speed of permeation depend on the relative concentrations in the fluid phases and the membrane. The steeper the gradient (concentration difference), the more drug will be diffusing per unit of time (Fick's law). The lipid membrane represents an almost insurmountable obstacle for hydrophilic substances (blue triangles).

Transport (B). Some drugs may penetrate membrane barriers with the help of transport systems (carriers), irrespective of their physicochemical properties, especially lipophilicity. As a prerequisite, the drug must have affinity for the carrier (blue triangle matching recess on "transport system") and, when bound to the carrier, be capable of being ferried across the membrane. Membrane passage via transport mechanisms is subject to competitive inhibition by another substance possessing similar affinity for the carrier. Substances lacking in affinity (blue circles) are not transported. Drugs utilize carriers for physiological substances: e.g., L-dopa uptake by L-amino acid carrier across the blood–intestine and blood–brain barriers (p. 188); uptake of aminoglycosides by the carrier transporting basic polypeptides through the luminal membrane of kidney tubular cells (p. 280). Only drugs bearing sufficient resemblance to the physiological substrate of a carrier will exhibit affinity to it.

The distribution of drugs in the body can be greatly changed by transport glycoproteins that are capable of moving substances out of cells against concentration gradients. The energy needed is produced by hydrolysis of ATP. These P-glycoproteins occur in the blood–brain-barrier, intestinal epithelia, and tumor cells, and in pathogens (e.g., malarial plasmodia). On the one hand, they function to protect cells from xenobiotics; on the other, they can cause drug resistance by preventing drugs from reaching effective concentrations at intracellular sites of action.

Transcytosis (vesicular transport, C). When new vesicles are pinched off, substances dissolved in the extracellular fluid are engulfed and then ferried through the cytoplasm, unless the vesicles (phagosomes) undergo fusion with lysosomes to form phagolysosomes and the transported substance is metabolized.

Receptor-mediated endocytosis (C). The drug first binds to membrane surface receptors (1, 2) whose cytosolic domains contact special proteins (adaptins, 3). Drug–receptor complexes migrate laterally in the membrane and aggregate with other complexes by a clathrin-dependent process (4). The affected membrane region invaginates and eventually pinches off to form a detached vesicle (5). The clathrin and adaptin coats are shed (6), resulting in formation of the "early" endosome (7). Inside this, proton concentration rises and causes the drug–receptor complex to dissociate. Next, the receptor-bearing membrane portions separate from the endosome (8). These membrane sections recirculate to the plasmalemma (9), while the endosome is delivered to the target organelles (10).

A. Membrane permeation: diffusion

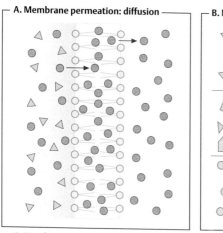

B. Membrane permeation: transport

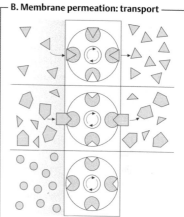

C. Membrane permeation: vesicular uptake, and transport

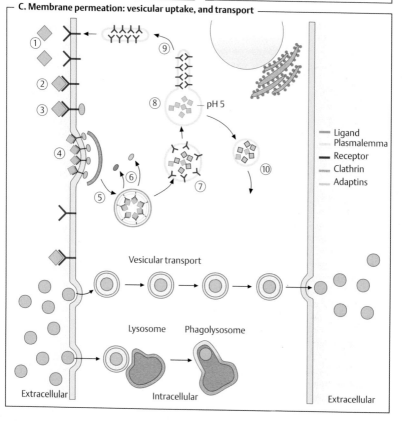

pH 5

Ligand
Plasmalemma
Receptor
Clathrin
Adaptins

Vesicular transport

Lysosome   Phagolysosome

Extracellular   Intracellular   Extracellular

□ Possible Modes of Drug Distribution

Following its uptake into the body, the drug is distributed in the blood (**1**) and through it to the various tissues of the body. Distribution may be restricted to the extracellular space (plasma volume plus interstitial space) (**2**) or may also extend into the intracellular space (**3**). Certain drugs may bind strongly to tissue structures so that plasma concentrations fall significantly even before elimination has begun (**4**).

After being distributed in blood, macromolecular substances remain largely confined to the vascular space, because their permeation through the blood–tissue barrier, or endothelium, is impeded, even where capillaries are fenestrated. This property is exploited therapeutically when loss of blood necessitates refilling of the vascular bed, for instance by infusion of dextran solutions (p. 156). The vascular space is, moreover, predominantly occupied by substances bound with high affinity to plasma proteins (p. 30; determination of the plasma volume with protein-bound dyes). Unbound, free drug may leave the bloodstream, albeit with varying ease, because the blood–tissue barrier (p. 24) is differently developed in different segments of the vascular tree. These regional differences are not illustrated in the accompanying figures.

Distribution in the body is determined by the ability to penetrate membranous barriers (p. 20). Hydrophilic substances (e. g., inulin) are neither taken up into cells nor bound to cell surface structures and can thus be used to determine the extracellular fluid volume (**2**). Lipophilic substances diffuse through the cell membrane and, as a result, achieve a uniform distribution in body fluids (**3**).

Body weight may be broken down as illustrated in the pie-chart. Further subdivisions are shown in the panel opposite.

The volume ratio of interstitial: intracellular water varies with age and body weight. On a percentage basis, interstitial fluid vol-

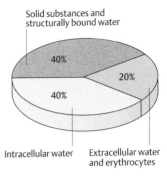

Solid substances and structurally bound water

40%

20%

40%

Intracellular water

Extracellular water and erythrocytes

ume is large in premature or normal neonates (up to 50% of body water), and smaller in the obese and the aged.

The concentration (c) of a solution corresponds to the amount (D) of substance dissolved in a volume (V); thus, $c = D/V$. If the dose of drug (D) and its plasma concentration (c) are known, a volume of distribution (V) can be calculated from $V = D/c$. However, this represents an *apparent* (notional) volume of distribution (V_{app}), because an even distribution in the body is assumed in its calculation. Homogeneous distribution will not occur if drugs are bound to cell membranes (**5**) or to membranes of intracellular organelles (**6**) or are stored within organelles (**7**). In these cases, plasma concentration c becomes small and V_{app} can exceed the actual size of the available fluid volume. Conversely, if a major fraction of drug molecules is bound to plasma proteins, c becomes large and the calculated value for V_{app} may then be smaller than that attained biologically.

A. Compartments for drug distribution

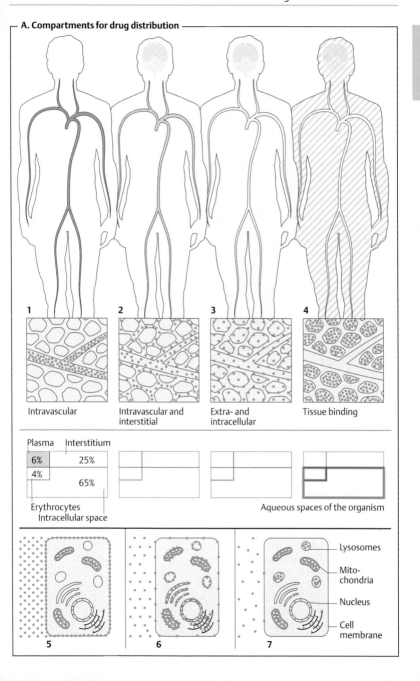

1 Intravascular

2 Intravascular and interstitial

3 Extra- and intracellular

4 Tissue binding

Plasma   Interstitium
6%   25%
4%
65%
Erythrocytes
Intracellular space

Aqueous spaces of the organism

Lysosomes

Mito-chondria

Nucleus

Cell membrane

5   **6**   **7**

□ Binding to Plasma Proteins

Having entered the blood, drugs may bind to the protein molecules that are present in abundance, resulting in the formation of drug–protein complexes.

Protein binding involves primarily albumin and, to a lesser extent, β-globulins and acidic glycoproteins. Other plasma proteins (e.g., transcortin, transferrin, thyroxin-binding globulin) serve specialized functions in connection with specific substances. The degree of binding is governed by the concentration of the reactants and the affinity of a drug for a given protein. Albumin concentration in plasma amounts to 4.6 g/100 ml, or 0.6 mM, and thus provides a very high binding capacity (two sites per molecule). As a rule, drugs exhibit much lower affinity (K_D ~10^{-5}–10^{-3} M) for plasma proteins than for their specific binding sites (receptors). In the range of therapeutically relevant concentrations, protein binding of most drugs increases linearly with concentration (exceptions: salicylate and certain sulfonamides).

The albumin molecule has different binding sites for anionic and cationic ligands, but *van der Waals* forces also contribute (p. 58). The extent of binding correlates with drug hydrophobicity (repulsion of drug by water).

Binding to plasma proteins is instantaneous and reversible, i.e., any change in the concentration of unbound drug is immediately followed by a corresponding change in the concentration of bound drug. Protein binding is of great importance because it is the concentration of free drug that determines the intensity of the effect. At a given total plasma concentration (say, 100 ng/ml) the *effective* concentration will be 90 ng/ml for a drug 10% bound to protein, but 1 ng/ml for a drug 99% bound to protein. The reduction in concentration of free drug resulting from protein binding affects not only the intensity of the effect but also biotransformation (e.g., in the liver) and elimination from the kidney, because only free drug will enter hepatic sites of metabolism or undergo glomerular filtration. When concentrations of free drug fall, drug is resupplied from binding sites on plasma proteins. Binding to plasma protein is equivalent to a depot in prolonging the duration of the effect by retarding elimination, whereas the intensity of the effect is reduced. If two substances have affinity for the same binding site on the albumin molecule, they may compete for that site. One drug may displace another from its binding site and thereby elevate the free (effective) concentration of the displaced drug (a form of **drug interaction**). Elevation of the free concentration of the displaced drug means increased effectiveness and accelerated elimination.

A decrease in the concentration of albumin (in liver disease, nephrotic syndrome, poor general condition) leads to altered pharmacokinetics of drugs that are highly bound to albumin.

Plasma protein-bound drugs that are substrates for transport carriers can be cleared from blood at high velocity; e.g., *p*-aminohippurate by the renal tubule and sulfobromophthalein by the liver. Clearance rates of these substances can be used to determine renal or hepatic blood flow.

A. Importance of protein binding for intensity and duration of drug effect

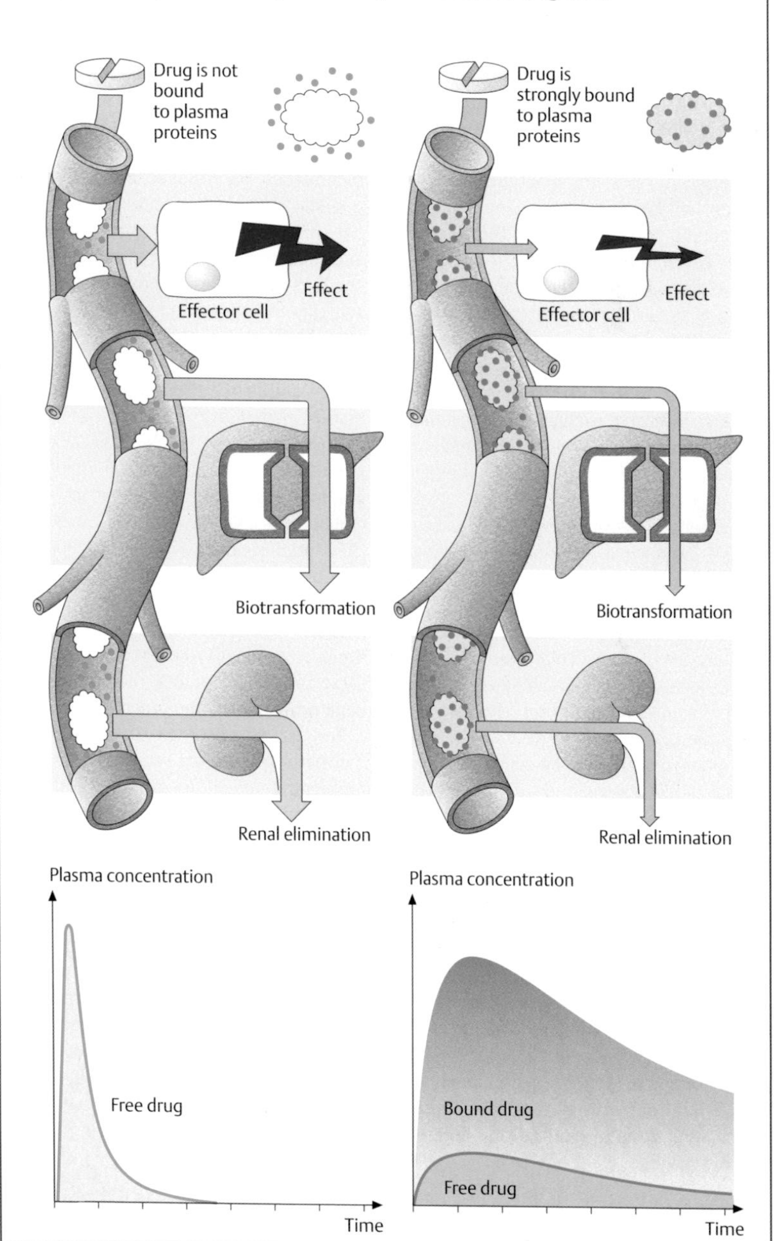

Drug is not bound to plasma proteins

Effector cell — Effect

Biotransformation

Renal elimination

Plasma concentration

Free drug

Time

Drug is strongly bound to plasma proteins

Effector cell — Effect

Biotransformation

Renal elimination

Plasma concentration

Bound drug

Free drug

Time

☐ The Liver as an Excretory Organ

As the major organ of drug biotransformation, the liver is richly supplied with blood, of which 1100 ml is received each minute from the intestines through the portal vein and 350 ml through the hepatic artery, comprising nearly 1/3 of cardiac output. The blood content of hepatic vessels and sinusoids amounts to 500 ml. Owing to the widening of the portal lumen, intrahepatic blood flow decelerates (**A**). Moreover, the endothelial lining of hepatic sinusoids (p. 24) contains pores large enough to permit rapid exit of plasma proteins. Thus, blood and hepatic parenchyma are able to maintain intimate contact and intensive exchange of substances, which is further facilitated by microvilli covering the hepatocyte surfaces abutting Disse's spaces.

The hepatocyte secretes biliary fluid into the bile canaliculi (dark green), tubular intercellular clefts that are sealed off the blood spaces by tight junctions. Secretory activity in the hepatocytes results in movement of fluid toward the canalicular space (**A**).

The hepatocyte is endowed with numerous metabolically important enzymes that are localized in part in mitochondria and in part on membranes of the *rough* (rER) and *smooth* (sER) *endoplasmic reticulum*. Enzymes of the sER play a most important role in drug biotransformation. At this site, direct consumption of molecular oxygen (O_2) takes place in oxidative reactions. Because these enzymes can catalyze either hydroxylation or oxidative cleavage of –N–C– or –O–C– bonds, they are referred to as "*mixed-function*" *oxidases or hydroxylases.* The integral component of this enzyme system is the iron-containing cytochrome P450 (see p. 38). Many P450 isozymes are known and they exhibit different patterns of substrate specificity. Interindividual genetic differences in isozyme make-up (e.g., CYP2D6) underlie subject-to-subject variations in drug biotransformation. The same holds for other enzyme systems; hence, the phenomenon is generally referred to as *genetic polymorphism of biotransformation.*

Compared with hydrophilic drugs not undergoing transport, lipophilic drugs are more rapidly taken up from the blood into hepatocytes and more readily gain access to mixed-function oxidases embedded in sER membranes. For instance, a drug having lipophilicity by virtue of an aromatic substituent (phenyl ring) (**B**) can be hydroxylated and thus become more hydrophilic (phase I reaction, p. 36). Besides oxidases, sER also contains reductases and glucuronyltransferases. The latter conjugate glucuronic acid with hydroxyl, carboxyl, amine, and amide groups and hence also phenolic products of phase I metabolism (phase II conjugation). Phase I and phase II metabolites can be transported back into the blood—probably via a gradient-dependent carrier—or actively secreted into bile via the ABC transporter (ATP-binding cassette transporter). Different transport proteins are available: for instance, MRP2 (the multidrug resistance associated protein 2) transports anionic conjugates into the bile canaliculi, whereas MRP3 can route these via the basolateral membrane of the hepatocyte toward the general circulation.

Prolonged exposure to substrates of one of the membrane-bound enzymes results in a proliferation of sER membranes in the liver (cf. **C** and **D**). The molecular mechanism of this sER "hypertrophy" has been elucidated for some drugs: thus, phenobarbital binds to a nuclear receptor (constitutive androstane receptor) that regulates the expression of cytochromes CYP2C9 and CYP2D6. Enzyme induction leads to accelerated biotransformation, not only of the inducing agent but also of other drugs (a form of **drug interaction**). With continued exposure, it develops in a few days, resulting in an increase in reaction velocity, maximally 2–3-fold, that disappears after removal of the inducing agent.

A. Flow patterns in portal vein, Disse's space, and hepatocyte

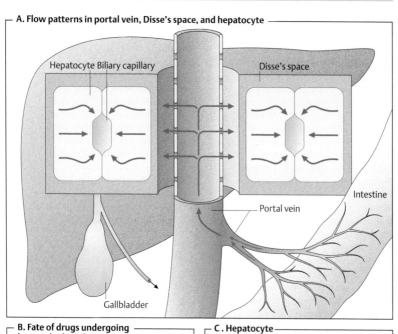

Hepatocyte Biliary capillary

Disse's space

Intestine

Portal vein

Gallbladder

B. Fate of drugs undergoing hepatic hydroxylation

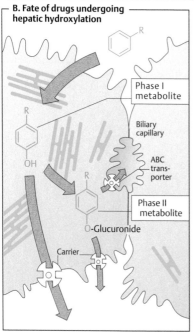

R

Phase I metabolite

R

OH

Biliary capillary

ABC trans-porter

R

Phase II metabolite

O-Glucuronide

Carrier

C. Hepatocyte

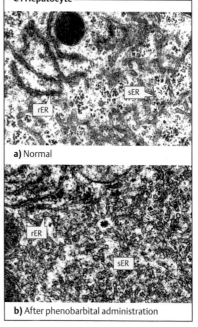

sER

rER

a) Normal

rER

sER

b) After phenobarbital administration

□ Biotransformation of Drugs

Many drugs undergo chemical modification in the body (**biotransformation**). Most often this process entails a loss of biological activity and an increase in hydrophilicity (water solubility), thereby promoting elimination via the renal route (p. 40). Since rapid drug elimination improves accuracy in titrating the therapeutic concentration, drugs are often designed with built-in weak links. Ester bonds are such links, being subject to *hydrolysis* by the ubiquitous esterases.

Hydrolytic cleavages, along with *oxidations*, *reductions*, *alkylations*, and *dealkylations*, constitute **phase I reactions** of drug metabolism. These reactions subsume all metabolic processes apt to alter drug molecules chemically and take place chiefly in the liver. In **phase II (synthetic) reactions**, *conjugation products* of either the drug itself or its phase I metabolites are formed, for instance, with glucuronic or sulfuric acid

The special case of the endogenous transmitter acetylcholine illustrates well the high velocity of ester hydrolysis. Acetylcholine is broken down so rapidly at its sites of release and action by acetylcholinesterase (p. 106) as to negate its therapeutic use. Hydrolysis of other esters catalyzed by various esterases is slower; though relatively fast in comparison with other biotransformations. The local anesthetic procaine is a case in point; it exerts its action at the site of application while being largely devoid of undesirable effects at other locations because it is inactivated by hydrolysis during absorption from the site of application.

Ester hydrolysis does not invariably lead to inactive metabolites, as exemplified by acetylsalicylic acid. The cleavage product, salicylic acid, retains pharmacological activity. In certain cases, drugs are administered in the form of esters in order to facilitate uptake into the body (enalapril–enalaprilat, p. 128; testosterone decanoate–testosterone, p. 248) or to reduce irritation of the gastric or intestinal mucosa (acetylsalicylic acid–salicylic acid; erythromycin succinate–erythromycin). In these cases the ester itself is not active but its hydrolytic product is. Thus, an inactive precursor or **prodrug** is administered and formation of the active molecule occurs only after hydrolysis in the blood.

Some drugs possessing amide bonds, such as prilocaine and of course peptides, can be hydrolyzed by peptidases and inactivated in this manner. Peptidases are also of pharmacological interest because they are responsible for the formation of highly reactive cleavage products (fibrin, p. 150) and potent mediators (angiotensin II, p. 128; bradykinin, enkephalin, p. 208) from biologically inactive peptides.

Peptidases exhibit some substrate selectivity and can be selectively inhibited, as exemplified by the formation of angiotensin II, whose actions inter alia include vasoconstriction. Angiotensin II is formed from angiotensin I by cleavage of the C-terminal dipeptide histidylleucine. Hydrolysis is catalyzed by "angiotensin-converting enzyme" (ACE). Peptide analogues such as captopril (p. 128) block this enzyme. Angiotensin II is degraded by angiotensinase A, which cleaves off the N-terminal asparagine residue. The product angiotensin III lacks vasoconstrictor activity.

A. Examples of chemical reactions in drug biotransformation (hydrolysis)

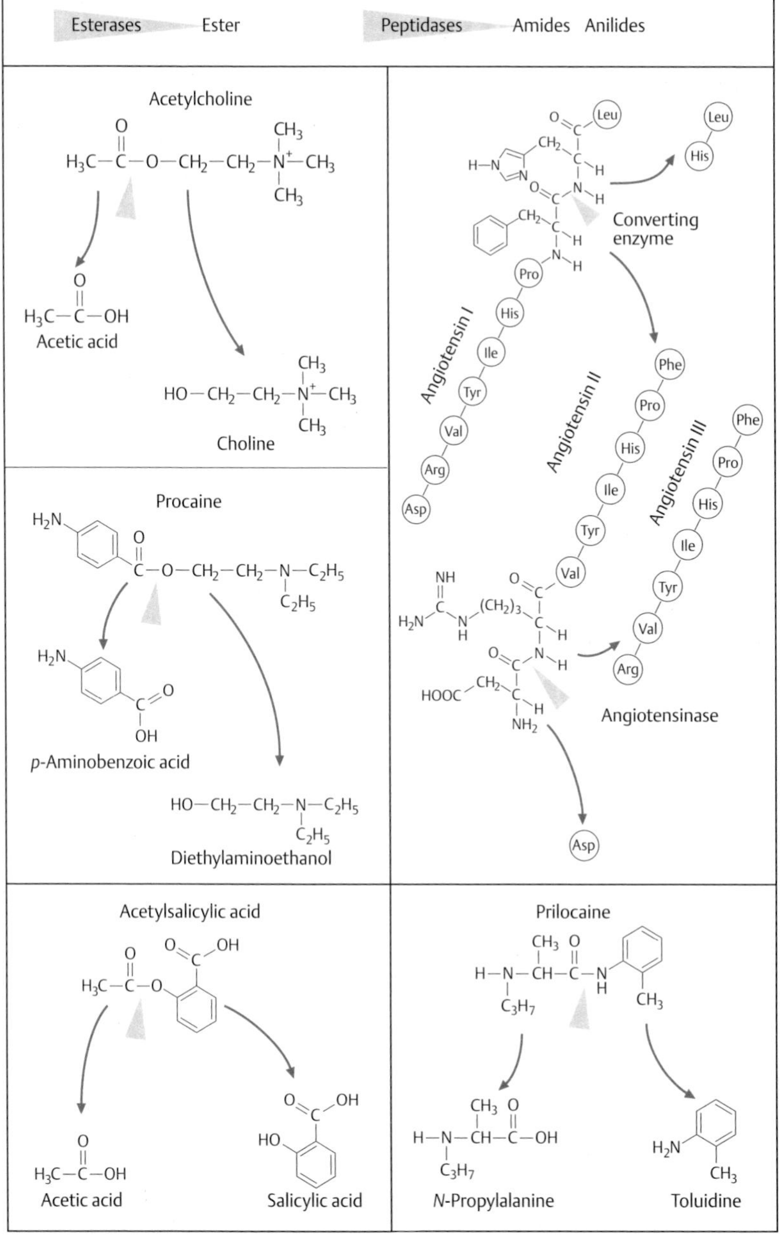

| Esterases | Ester | | Peptidases | Amides Anilides |

Acetylcholine

$$H_3C-\overset{\overset{\displaystyle O}{\|}}{C}-O-CH_2-CH_2-\overset{+}{N}\begin{array}{l}CH_3\\CH_3\\CH_3\end{array}$$

$$H_3C-\overset{\overset{\displaystyle O}{\|}}{C}-OH$$
Acetic acid

$$HO-CH_2-CH_2-\overset{+}{N}\begin{array}{l}CH_3\\CH_3\\CH_3\end{array}$$
Choline

Procaine

$$H_2N-\langle\rangle-\overset{\overset{\displaystyle O}{\|}}{C}-O-CH_2-CH_2-N\begin{array}{l}C_2H_5\\C_2H_5\end{array}$$

$$H_2N-\langle\rangle-\overset{\overset{\displaystyle O}{\|}}{C}-OH$$
p-Aminobenzoic acid

$$HO-CH_2-CH_2-N\begin{array}{l}C_2H_5\\C_2H_5\end{array}$$
Diethylaminoethanol

Acetylsalicylic acid

$$H_3C-\overset{\overset{\displaystyle O}{\|}}{C}-O$$

$$H_3C-\overset{\overset{\displaystyle O}{\|}}{C}-OH$$
Acetic acid

Salicylic acid

Angiotensin I

Converting enzyme

Angiotensin II

Angiotensin III

Angiotensinase

Leu
His
Pro
His
Ile
Tyr
Val
Arg
Asp

Phe
Pro
His
Ile
Tyr
Val
Arg

Phe
Pro
His
Ile
Tyr
Val

Asp

Prilocaine

$$H-N-CH-\overset{\overset{\displaystyle O}{\|}}{C}-N-\langle\rangle-CH_3$$
with CH_3, C_3H_7

$$H-N-CH-\overset{\overset{\displaystyle O}{\|}}{C}-OH$$
with CH_3, C_3H_7
N-Propylalanine

$$H_2N-\langle\rangle-CH_3$$
Toluidine

Oxidation reactions can be divided into two kinds: those in which oxygen is incorporated into the drug molecule, and those in which primary oxidation causes part of the molecule to be lost. The former include **hydroxylations**, **epoxidations**, and **sulfoxidations**. Hydroxylations may involve alkyl substituents (e.g., pentobarbital) or aromatic ring systems (e.g., propranolol). In both cases, products are formed that are conjugated to an organic acid residue, e.g., glucuronic acid, in a subsequent phase II reaction.

Hydroxylation may also take place at nitrogens, resulting in hydroxylamines (e.g., acetaminophen). Benzene, polycyclic aromatic compounds, (e.g., benzopyrene), and unsaturated cyclic carbohydrates can be converted by monooxygenases to **epoxides**, highly reactive electrophiles that are hepatotoxic and possibly carcinogenic.

The second type of oxidative biotransformation comprises **dealkylations**. In the case of primary or secondary amines, dealkylation of an alkyl group starts at the carbon adjacent to the nitrogen; in the case of tertiary amines, with hydroxylation of the nitrogen (e.g., lidocaine). The intermediary products are labile and break up into the dealkylated amine and aldehyde of the alkyl group removed. O-dealkylation and S-dearylation proceed via an analogous mechanism (e.g., phenacetin and azathioprine, respectively).

Oxidative **deamination** basically resembles the dealkylation of tertiary amines, beginning with the formation of a hydroxylamine that then decomposes into ammonia and the corresponding aldehyde. The latter is partly reduced to an alcohol and partly oxidized to a carboxylic acid.

Reduction reactions may occur at oxygen or nitrogen atoms. Keto oxygens are converted into a hydroxyl group, as in the reduction of the prodrugs cortisone and prednisone to the active glucocorticoids cortisol and prednisolone, respectively. N-reductions occur in azo or nitro compounds (e.g., nitrazepam). Nitro groups can be reduced to amine groups via nitroso and hydroxylamino intermediates. Likewise, dehalogenation is a reductive process involving a carbon atom (e.g., halothane, p. 216).

Methylations are catalyzed by a family of relatively specific methyltransferases involving the transfer of methyl groups to hydroxyl groups (O-methylation as in norepinephrine [noradrenaline]) or to amino groups (N-methylation of norepinephrine, histamine, or serotonin).

In thio compounds, **desulfuration** results from substitution of sulfur by oxygen (e.g., parathion). This example again illustrates that biotransformation is not always to be equated with bioinactivation. Thus, paraoxon (E600) formed in the organism from parathion (E605) is the actual active agent (bioactivation, "toxification", p. 106)

$$R^1{-}N{-}CH_2{-}CH_3 \xrightarrow{\;O\;} R^1{-}N{-}CH{-}CH_3$$

with R^2 on the nitrogen and OH below:

$$R^1{-}\underset{\underset{}{\overset{|}{N}}}{\overset{\overset{R^2}{|}}{}}{-}CH_2{-}CH_3 \xrightarrow{\;O\;} R^1{-}\underset{}{\overset{\overset{R^2}{|}}{N}}{-}\underset{\overset{|}{OH}}{\overset{|}{CH}}{-}CH_3$$

$$\downarrow$$

$$R^1{-}\overset{\overset{R^2}{|}}{N}{-}H \;+\; H{-}\overset{\overset{O}{\parallel}}{C}{-}CH_3$$

Dealkylation

A. Examples of chemical reactions in drug biotransformation

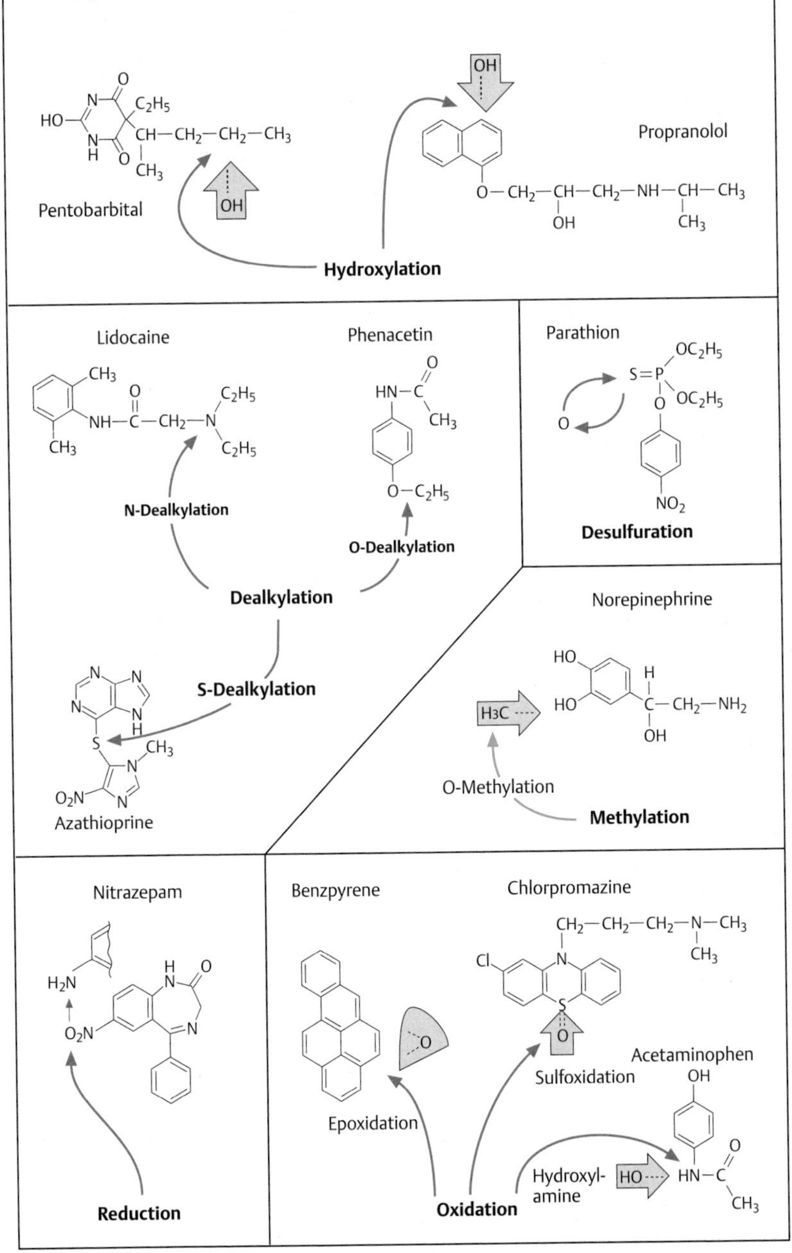

Pentobarbital

Propranolol

Hydroxylation

Lidocaine

Phenacetin

Parathion

N-Dealkylation

O-Dealkylation

Desulfuration

Dealkylation

S-Dealkylation

Azathioprine

Norepinephrine

O-Methylation

Methylation

Nitrazepam

Benzpyrene

Chlorpromazine

Acetaminophen

Epoxidation

Sulfoxidation

Hydroxyl-
amine

Reduction

Oxidation

□ Drug Metabolism by Cytochrome P450

Cytochrome P450 enzyme. A major part of phase I reactions is catalyzed by hemoproteins, the so-called cytochrome P450 (CYP) enzymes (**A**). To date about 40 genes for cytochrome P450 proteins have been identified in the human; among these, the protein families CYP1, CYP2, and CYP3 are important in drug metabolism (**B**). The bulk of CYP enzymes are located in the liver and the intestinal wall, which explains why these organs are responsible for the major part of drug metabolism.

Substrates, inhibitors, and inducers. Cytochromes are enzymes with broad substrate specificities. Accordingly, pharmaceuticals of diverse chemical structure can be metabolized by a given enzyme protein. When several drugs are metabolized by the same isozyme, clinically important interactions may result. In these, **substrates** (drugs metabolized by CYP) can be distinguished from **inhibitors** (drugs that are bound to CYP with high affinity, interfere with the breakdown of substrates, and are themselves metabolized slowly) (**A**). The amount of hepatic CYP enzymes is a major determinant of metabolic capacity. An increase in enzyme concentration usually leads to accelerated drug metabolism. Numerous endogenous and exogenous substances, such as drugs, can augment the expression of CYP enzymes and thus act as **CYP inducers** (p. 32). Many of these inducers activate specific transcription factors in the nucleus of hepatocytes, leading to activation of mRNA synthesis and subsequent production of CYP isozyme protein. Some inducers also increase the expression of P-glycoprotein transporters; as a result, enhanced metabolism by CYP and increased membrane transport by P-glycoprotein can act in concert to render a drug ineffective.

The table in (**B**) provides an overview of different CYP isozymes along with their substrates, inhibitors, and inducers. Obviously, when a patient is to be exposed to polypharmaceutic regimens (especially multimorbid subjects), it would be imprudent to start therapy without checking whether the drugs being contemplated include CYP inducers or inhibitors, some of which may dramatically alter pharmacokinetics.

Drug interaction due to CYP induction or inhibition. Life-threatening interactions have been observed in patients taking inducers of CYP3A4 isozyme during treatment with ciclosporin for the prevention of kidney and liver transplant rejection. Intake of rifampin [rifampicin] and also of St. John's wort preparations (available without prescription) may increase expression of CYP3A4 to such an extent as to lower plasma levels of ciclosporin below the therapeutic range (**C**). As immunosuppression becomes inadequate, the risk of transplant rejection will be enhanced. In the presence of rifampin, other drugs that are substrates of CYP3A4 may become ineffective. For this reason, the intake of rifampin is contraindicated in HIV patients being treated with protease inhibitors. As a rule, inhibitors of CYP enzymes elevate plasma levels of drugs that are substrates of the same CYP enzymes; in this manner, they raise the risk of undesirable toxic effects. The antifungal agent ketoconazole enhances the nephrotoxicity of ciclosporin by such a mechanism (**C**).

A. Cytochrome P450 in the liver

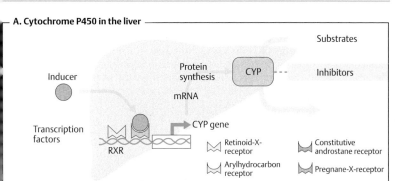

Substrates

Protein synthesis

CYP - - - Inhibitors

Inducer

mRNA

Transcription factors

RXR — CYP gene

Retinoid-X-receptor

Arylhydrocarbon receptor

Constitutive androstane receptor

Pregnane-X-receptor

B. Cytochrome P450 isozymes

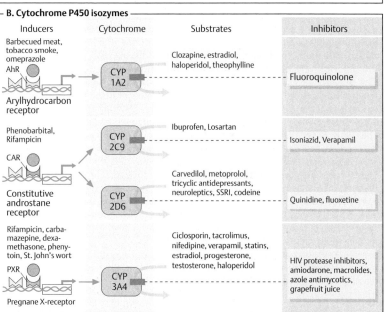

Inducers	Cytochrome	Substrates	Inhibitors
Barbecued meat, tobacco smoke, omeprazole AhR Arylhydrocarbon receptor	CYP 1A2	Clozapine, estradiol, haloperidol, theophylline	Fluoroquinolone
Phenobarbital, Rifampicin CAR Constitutive androstane receptor	CYP 2C9	Ibuprofen, Losartan	Isoniazid, Verapamil
	CYP 2D6	Carvedilol, metoprolol, tricyclic antidepressants, neuroleptics, SSRI, codeine	Quinidine, fluoxetine
Rifampicin, carba-mazepine, dexa-methasone, pheny-toin, St. John's wort PXR Pregnane X-receptor	CYP 3A4	Ciclosporin, tacrolimus, nifedipine, verapamil, statins, estradiol, progesterone, testosterone, haloperidol	HIV protease inhibitors, amiodarone, macrolides, azole antimycotics, grapefruit juice

C. Drug interactions and cytochrome P450

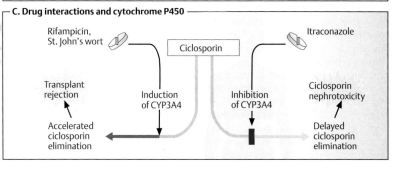

Rifampicin, St. John's wort

Ciclosporin

Itraconazole

Transplant rejection

Induction of CYP3A4

Inhibition of CYP3A4

Ciclosporin nephrotoxicity

Accelerated ciclosporin elimination

Delayed ciclosporin elimination

□ The Kidney as an Excretory Organ

Most drugs are eliminated in urine either chemically unchanged or as metabolites. The kidney permits elimination because the vascular wall structure in the region of the glomerular capillaries (**B**) allows unimpeded passage into urine of blood solutes having molecular weights (MW) < 5000. Filtration is restricted at MW < 50 000 and ceases at MW > 70 000. With few exceptions, therapeutically used drugs and their metabolites have much smaller molecular weights and can therefore undergo **glomerular filtration**, i. e., pass from blood into primary urine. Separating the **capillary endothelium** from the **tubular epithelium**, the **basal membrane** contains negatively charged macromolecules and acts as a filtration barrier for high-molecular-weight substances. The relative density of this barrier depends on the electric charge of molecules that attempt to permeate it. In addition, the diaphragmatic slits between podophyte processes play a part in glomerular filtration.

Apart from **glomerular filtration** (**B**), drugs present in blood may pass into urine by **active secretion** (**C**). Certain cations and anions are secreted by the epithelium of the proximal tubules into the tubular fluid via special energy-consuming transport systems. These transport systems have a limited capacity. When several substrates are present simultaneously, competition for the carrier may occur (see p. 326).

During passage down the renal tubule, primary urinary volume shrinks to about 1%; accordingly, there is a corresponding concentration of filtered drug or drug metabolites (**A**). The resulting concentration gradient between urine and interstitial fluid is preserved in the case of drugs incapable of permeating the tubular epithelium. However, with lipophilic drugs the concentration gradient will favor **reabsorption** of the filtered molecules. In this case, reabsorption is not based on an active process but results instead from passive diffusion. Accordingly,

for protonated substances, the extent of reabsorption is dependent upon urinary pH or the degree of dissociation. The degree of dissociation varies as a function of the urinary pH and the pK_a, which represents the pH value at which half of the substance exists in protonated (or unprotonated) form. This relationship is illustrated graphically (**D**) with the example of a protonated amine having a pK_a of 7. In this case, at urinary pH 7, 50% of the amine will be present in the protonated, hydrophilic, membrane-impermeant form (blue dots), whereas the other half, representing the uncharged amine (red dots), can leave the tubular lumen in accordance with the resulting concentration gradient. If the pK_a of an amine is higher (pK_a = 7.5) or lower (pK_a = 6.5), a correspondingly smaller or larger proportion of the amine will be present in the uncharged, reabsorbable form. Lowering or raising urinary pH by half a pH unit would result in analogous changes.

The same considerations hold for acidic molecules, with the important difference that alkalinization of the urine (increased pH) will promote the deprotonization of –COOH groups and thus impede reabsorption. Intentional alteration of urinary pH can be used in intoxications with proton-acceptor substances in order to hasten elimination of the toxin (e. g., alkalinization → phenobarbital; acidification → methamphetamine).

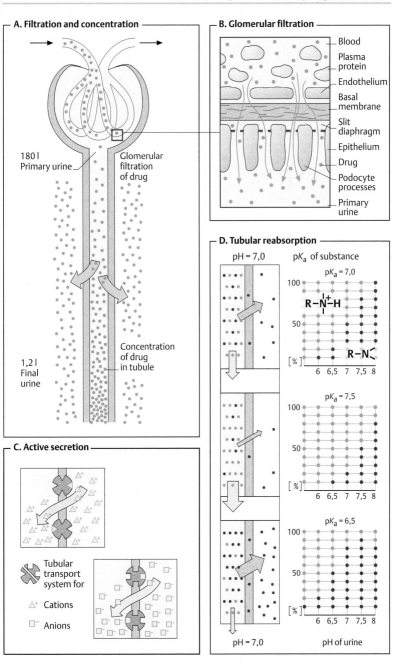

A. Filtration and concentration

180 l Primary urine

Glomerular filtration of drug

1,2 l Final urine

Concentration of drug in tubule

B. Glomerular filtration

Blood

Plasma protein

Endothelium

Basal membrane

Slit diaphragm

Epithelium

Drug

Podocyte processes

Primary urine

C. Active secretion

Tubular transport system for

△⁺ Cations

□⁻ Anions

D. Tubular reabsorption

pH = 7,0

pK_a of substance

pK_a = 7,0

100

50

[%]

$R-\overset{|}{\underset{|}{N}}-H$

$R-N$

6 6,5 7 7,5 8

pK_a = 7,5

100

50

[%]

6 6,5 7 7,5 8

pK_a = 6,5

100

50

[%]

6 6,5 7 7,5 8

pH = 7,0

pH of urine

□ Presystemic Elimination

The morphological barriers of the body are illustrated on pp. 22–25. Depending on the physicochemical properties of drugs, intended targets on the surface or the inside of cells, or of bacterial organisms, may be reached to varying degrees or not at all. Whenever a drug cannot be applied locally but must be given by the systemic route, its pharmacokinetics will be subject to yet another process. This becomes very obvious if we follow the route of an orally administered drug from its site of absorption to the general circulation. Any of the following may occur.

1. The drug permeates through the epithelial barrier of the gut into the enterocyte; however, a **P-glycoprotein** transports it back into the intestinal lumen. As a result, the amount actually absorbed can be greatly diminished. This counter-transport can vary interindividually for an identical substance and moreover may be altered by other drugs.

2. En route from the intestinal lumen to the general circulation, the ingested substance is broken down enzymatically, e. g., by **cytochrome P450 oxidases**.

   (a) Degradation may start already in the intestinal mucosa. Other drugs or agents may inhibit or stimulate the activity of enteral cytochrome oxidases. A peculiar example is grapefruit juice, which inhibits CYP3A4 oxidase in the gut wall and thereby causes blood concentrations of other important drugs to rise to toxic levels.

   (b) Metabolism in the liver, through which the drug must pass, plays the biggest role. Here, many enzymes are at work to alter endogenous and exogenous substances chemically so as to promote their elimination. Examples of different metabolic reactions are presented on pp. 34–39. Depending on the quantity of drug being taken up and metabolized by the hepato-cytes, only a fraction of the amount absorbed may reach the blood in the hepatic vein. Importantly, an increase in enzyme activity (increase in smooth endoplasmic reticulum) can be induced by other drugs.

The processes referred to under (2a, b) above are subsumed under the term "**presystemic elimination**."

3. Parenteral administration of a drug of course circumvents presystemic elimination. After i.v., s.c., or i.m. injection, the drug travels via the vena cava, the right heart ventricle, and the lungs to the left ventricle and, thence, to the systemic circulation and the coronary system. As a lipid-rich organ with a large surface, the lungs can take up lipophilic or amphiphilic agents to a considerable extent and release them slowly after blood levels fall again. During fast delivery of drug, the lungs act as a buffer and protect the heart against excessive concentrations after rapid i.v. injection.

In certain therapeutic situations, rapid presystemic elimination may be desirable. An important example is the use of glucocorticoids in the treatment of asthma. Because a significant portion of inhaled drug is swallowed, glucocorticoids with complete presystemic elimination entail only a minimal systemic load for the organism (p. 340). The use of acetylsalicylic acid for inhibition of thrombocyte aggregation (see p. 155) provides an example of a desirable presystemic conversion.

A. Presystemic elimination

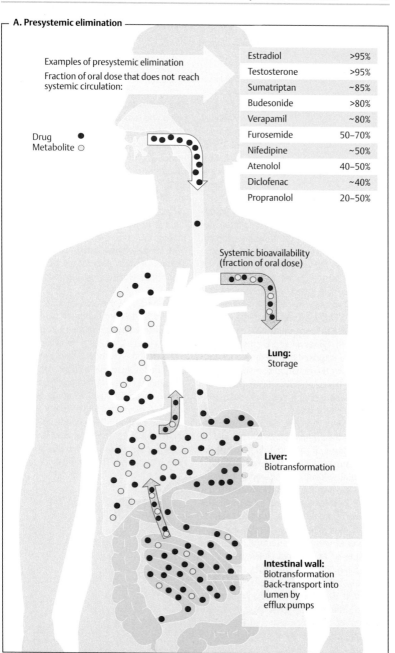

Examples of presystemic elimination
Fraction of oral dose that does not reach
systemic circulation:

Estradiol	>95%
Testosterone	>95%
Sumatriptan	~85%
Budesonide	>80%
Verapamil	~80%
Furosemide	50–70%
Nifedipine	~50%
Atenolol	40–50%
Diclofenac	~40%
Propranolol	20–50%

Drug ●
Metabolite ○

Systemic bioavailability
(fraction of oral dose)

Lung:
Storage

Liver:
Biotransformation

Intestinal wall:
Biotransformation
Back-transport into
lumen by
efflux pumps

☐ Drug Concentration in the Body as a Function of Time—First Order (Exponential) Rate Processes

Processes such as drug absorption and elimination display exponential characteristics. For absorption, this follows from the simple fact that the amount of drug being moved per unit of time depends on the concentration difference (gradient) between two body compartments (Fick's law). In drug absorption from the alimentary tract, the intestinal content and blood would represent the compartments containing initially high and low concentrations, respectively. In drug elimination via the kidney, excretion often depends on glomerular filtration, i.e., the filtered amount of drug present in primary urine. As the blood concentration falls, the amount of drug filtered per unit of time diminishes. The resulting exponential decline is illustrated in (**A**). The exponential time course implies constancy of the interval during which the concentration decreases by one-half. This interval represents the half-life ($t_{1/2}$) and is related to the elimination rate constant k by the equation $t_{1/2} = (\ln 2)/k$. The two parameters, together with the initial concentration c_0, describe a first-order (exponential) rate process.

The constancy of the process permits calculation of the plasma volume that would be cleared of drug, if the remaining drug were not to assume a homogeneous distribution in the total volume (a condition not met in reality). The **notional plasma volume freed of drug per unit of time** is termed the **clearance**. Depending on whether plasma concentration falls as a result of urinary excretion or of metabolic alteration, clearance is considered to be renal or hepatic. Renal and hepatic clearances add up to total clearance (Cl_{tot}) in the case of drugs that are eliminated unchanged via the kidney and biotransformed in the liver. Cl_{tot} represents the sum of all processes contributing to elimination; it is related to the half-life ($t_{1/2}$)

and the apparent volume of distribution V_{app} (p. 28) by the equation:

$$t_{1/2} = \ln 2 \, \frac{V_{app}}{Cl_{tot}}$$

The smaller the volume of distribution or the larger the total clearance, the shorter is the half-life.

In the case of drugs renally eliminated in unchanged form, the half-life of elimination can be calculated from the cumulative excretion in urine; the final total amount eliminated corresponds to the amount absorbed.

Hepatic elimination obeys exponential kinetics because metabolizing enzymes operate in the quasi-linear region of their concentration–activity curve, and hence the amount of drug metabolized per unit time diminishes with decreasing blood concentration.

The best-known exception to exponential kinetics is the elimination of alcohol (ethanol), which obeys a *linear* time course (zero-order kinetics), at least at blood concentrations > 0.02%. It does so because the rate-limiting enzyme, alcohol dehydrogenase, achieves half-saturation at very low substrate concentrations, i.e., at about 80 mg/l (0.008%). Thus, reaction velocity reaches a plateau at blood ethanol concentrations of about 0.02%, and the amount of drug eliminated per unit time remains constant at concentrations above this level.

A. Exponential elimination of drug

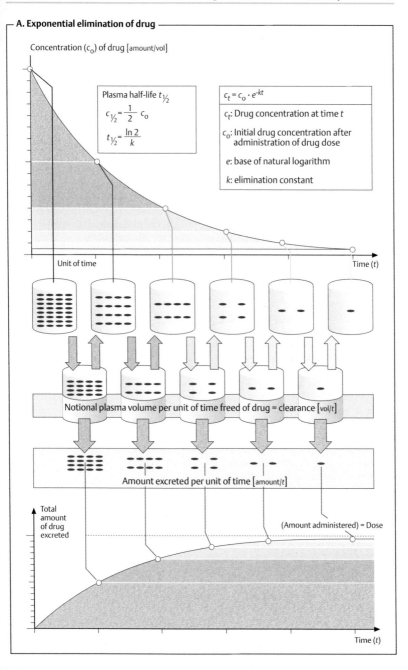

Concentration (c_0) of drug [amount/vol]

Plasma half-life $t_{1/2}$

$$c_{1/2} = \frac{1}{2} c_0$$

$$t_{1/2} = \frac{\ln 2}{k}$$

$$c_t = c_0 \cdot e^{-kt}$$

c_t: Drug concentration at time t

c_0: Initial drug concentration after administration of drug dose

e: base of natural logarithm

k: elimination constant

Unit of time

Time (t)

Notional plasma volume per unit of time freed of drug = clearance [vol/t]

Amount excreted per unit of time [amount/t]

Total amount of drug excreted

(Amount administered) = Dose

Time (t)

☐ Time Course of Drug Concentration in Plasma

(A). Drugs are taken up into and eliminated from the body by various routes. The body thus represents an open system wherein the actual drug concentration reflects the interplay of intake (ingestion) and egress (elimination). When orally administered drug is absorbed from the stomach and intestine, speed of uptake depends on many factors, including the speed of drug dissolution (in the case of solid dosage forms) and of gastrointestinal transit; the membrane penetrability of the drug; its concentration gradient across the mucosa–blood barrier; and mucosal blood flow. **Absorption** from the intestine causes the drug concentration in blood to increase. Transport in blood conveys the drug to different organs (**distribution**), into which it is taken up to a degree compatible with its chemical properties and rate of blood flow through the organ. For instance, well-perfused organs such as the brain receive a greater proportion than do less well-perfused ones. Uptake into tissue causes the blood concentration to fall. Absorption from the gut diminishes as the mucosa–blood gradient decreases. Plasma concentration reaches a peak when the amount of drug leaving the blood per unit of time equals that being absorbed.

Drug entry into hepatic and renal tissue constitutes movement into the **organs of elimination**. The characteristic phasic time course of drug concentration in plasma represents the sum of the constituent processes of **absorption**, **distribution**, and **elimination**, which overlap in time. When distribution takes place significantly faster than elimination, there is an initial rapid and then a greatly retarded fall in the plasma level, the former being designated the α-phase (distribution phase), the latter the β-phase (elimination phase). When the drug is distributed faster than it is absorbed, the time course of the plasma level can be described in mathematically simplified form by the Bateman function (k_1 and k_2 represent the rate constants for absorption and elimination, respectively).

(B). The velocity of absorption depends on the route of administration. The more rapid the absorption, the shorter will be the time (t_{max}) required to reach the peak plasma level (c_{max}), the higher will be the c_{max}, and the earlier will the plasma level begin to fall again.

The *area under the plasma level–time curve* (AUC) is independent of the route of administration, provided the doses and bioavailability are the same (law of corresponding areas). The AUC can thus be used to determine the **bioavailability F** of a drug. The ratio of AUC values determined after oral and intravenous administrations of a given dose of a particular drug corresponds to the proportion of drug entering the systemic circulation after oral administration. Thus,

$$F = \frac{AUC_{\text{oral administration}}}{AUC_{\text{iv administration}}}$$

The determination of plasma levels affords a comparison of different proprietary preparations containing the same drug in the same dosage. Identical plasma level–time curves of different manufacturers' products with reference to a standard preparation indicate **bioequivalence** with the standard of the preparation under investigation.

A. Time course of drug concentration

Absorption
Uptake from stomach and intestines into blood

Distribution
into body tissues:
α-phase

Elimination
from body by biotransformation (chemical alteration) excretion via kidney:
β-phase

Drug concentration in blood (c)

Bateman function

$$c = \frac{Dose}{V_{app}} \times \frac{k_1}{k_2 - k_1} \times (e^{-k_1 t} - e^{-k_2 t})$$

Time (t)

B. Mode of application and time course of drug concentration

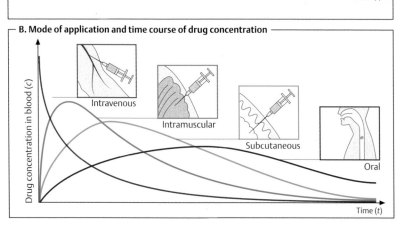

Drug concentration in blood (c)

Intravenous

Intramuscular

Subcutaneous

Oral

Time (t)

□ Time Course of Drug Plasma Levels during Repeated Dosing (A)

When a drug is administered at regular intervals over a prolonged period, the rise and fall of drug concentration in blood will be determined by the relationship between the half-life of elimination and the time interval between doses. If the amount of drug administered in each dose has been eliminated before the next dose is applied, repeated intake at constant intervals will result in similar plasma levels. If intake occurs before the preceding dose is eliminated completely, the next dose will add to the residual amount still present in the body—i.e., the drug **accumulates**. The shorter the dosing interval relative to the elimination half-life, the larger will be the residual amount of drug to which the next dose is added and the more extensively will the drug accumulate in the body. However, at a given dosing frequency, the drug does not accumulate infinitely and a **steady state** (concentration C_{ss} or **accumulation equilibrium** is eventually reached. This is so because the activity of elimination processes is concentration-dependent. The higher the drug concentration rises, the greater is the amount eliminated per unit time. After several doses, the concentration will have climbed to a level at which the amounts eliminated and taken in per unit of time become equal, i.e., a steady-state is reached. Within this concentration range, the plasma level will continue to rise (peak) and fall (trough) as dosing is continued at regular intervals. The height of the steady state (C_{ss}) depends upon the amount (D) administered per dosing interval (τ) and the clearance (Cl):

$$C_{ss} = \frac{D}{\tau \; Cl}$$

The speed at which the steady state is reached corresponds to the speed of elimination of the drug. The time needed to reach 90% of the concentration plateau is about 3 times the $t_{1/2}$ of elimination.

□ Time Course of Drug Plasma Levels during Irregular Intake (B)

In practice, it proves difficult to achieve a plasma level that undulates evenly around the desired effective concentration. For instance, if two successive doses are omitted ("?" in **B**), the plasma level will drop below the therapeutic range and a longer period will be required to regain the desired plasma level. In everyday life, patients will be apt to neglect to take drugs at the scheduled time. **Patient compliance** means strict adherence to the prescribed regimen. Apart from poor compliance, the same problem may occur when the total daily dose is divided into three individual doses (t.i.d.) and the first dose is taken at breakfast, the second at lunch, and the third at supper. Under these conditions, the nocturnal dosing interval will be twice the diurnal one. Consequently, plasma levels during the early morning hours may have fallen far below the desired, or possibly urgently needed, range.

A. Time course of drug concentration in blood during regular intake

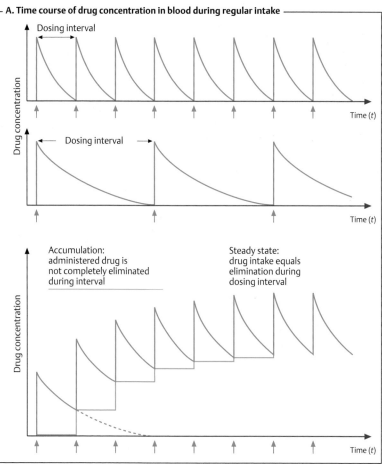

Dosing interval

Dosing interval

Accumulation:
administered drug is
not completely eliminated
during interval

Steady state:
drug intake equals
elimination during
dosing interval

B. Time course of drug concentration with irregular intake

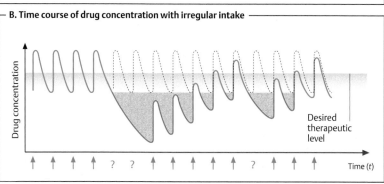

Desired
therapeutic
level

☐ Accumulation: Dose, Dose Interval, and Plasma Level Fluctuation (A)

Successful drug therapy in many illnesses is accomplished only if the drug concentration is maintained at a steady high level. This requirement necessitates regular drug intake and a dosage schedule that ensures that the plasma concentration neither falls below the therapeutically effective range nor exceeds the minimal toxic concentration. A constant plasma level would, however, be undesirable if it accelerated a loss of effectiveness (development of tolerance), or if the drug were required to be present at specified times only.

A steady plasma level can be achieved by giving the drug in a constant intravenous infusion, the height of the steady state plasma level being determined by the infusion rate. This procedure is routinely used in hospital settings, but is generally impracticable. With oral administration, dividing the total daily dosage into several individual doses, e.g., four, three, or two, offers a practical compromise. When the daily dose is given in several divided doses, the mean plasma level shows little fluctuation.

In practice, it is found that a regimen of frequent regular drug ingestion is not well adhered to by patients (unreliability or lack of "compliance" by patients). The degree of fluctuation in plasma level over a given dosing interval can be reduced by a dosage form permitting slow (sustained) release (p. 12).

The time required to reach steady-state accumulation during multiple constant dosing depends on the rate of elimination. As a rule of thumb, a plateau is reached after approximately three elimination half-lives ($t_{1/2}$).

For slowly eliminated drugs, which tend to accumulate extensively (phenprocoumon, digitoxin, methadone), the optimal plasma level is attained only after a long period. Here, increasing the initial doses (loading dose) will speed up the attainment of equilibrium, which is subsequently maintained with a lower dose (maintenance dose). For slowly eliminated substances, single daily dosing may suffice to maintain a steady plasma level.

☐ Change in Elimination Characteristics during Drug Therapy (B)

With any drug taken regularly and accumulating to the desired plasma level, it is important to consider that conditions for biotransformation and excretion do not necessarily remain constant. Elimination may be hastened due to enzyme induction (p. 38) or to a change in urinary pH (p. 40). Consequently, the steady-state plasma level declines to a new value corresponding to the new rate of elimination. The drug effect may diminish or disappear. Conversely, when elimination is impaired (e. g., in progressive renal insufficiency), the mean plasma level of renally eliminated drugs rises and may enter a toxic concentration range.

A. Accumulation: dose, dose interval, and fluctuation of plasma level

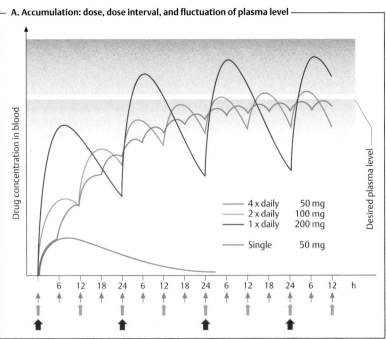

B. Changes in elimination kinetics in the course of drug therapy

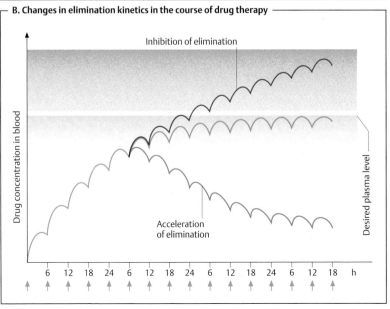

□ Dose–Response Relationship

The effect of a substance depends on the amount administered, i.e., the dose. If the dose chosen is below the critical threshold (subliminal dosing), an effect will be absent. Depending on the nature of the effect to be measured, increasing doses may cause the effect to increase in intensity. Thus, the effect of an antipyretic or hypotensive drug can be quantified in a graded fashion, in that the extent of fall in body temperature or blood pressure is being measured. A dose–effect relationship is then encountered, as discussed on p. 54.

The dose–effect relationship may vary depending on the sensitivity of the individual person receiving the drug: i.e., for the same effect, different doses may be required in different individuals. The interindividual variation in sensitivity is especially obvious with effects of the "all-or-none" kind.

To illustrate this point, we consider an experiment in which the subjects individually respond in all-or-none fashion, as in the Straub tail phenomenon (**A**). Mice react to morphine with excitation, evident in the form of an abnormal posture of the tail and limbs. The dose dependence of this phenomenon is observed in groups of animals (e.g., 10 mice per group) injected with increasing doses of morphine. At the low dose only the most sensitive, at increasing doses a growing proportion, and at the highest dose all of the animals are affected (**B**). There is a relationship between the frequency of responding animals and the dose given. At 2 mg/kg, 1 out of 10 animals reacts; at 10 mg/kg, 5 out of 10 respond. The **dose–frequency relationship** results from the different sensitivity of individuals, which, as a rule, exhibits a log-normal distribution (**C**, graph at right, linear scale). If the cumulative frequency (total number of animals responding at a given dose) is plotted against the logarithm of the dose (abscissa), a *sigmoidal* curve results (**C**, graph at left, semi-logarithmic scale). The inflection point of the curve lies at the dose at which one half of the group has responded. The dose range encompassing the dose–frequency relationship reflects the variation in individual sensitivity to the drug. Although similar in shape, a dose–frequency relationship has, thus, a meaning different from that of a **dose–effect relationship**. The latter can be evaluated in one individual and results from an intraindividual dependency of the effect on drug concentration.

The evaluation of a dose–effect-relationship within a group of human subjects is made more difficult by interindividual differences in sensitivity. To account for the biological variation, measurements have to be carried out on a representative sample and the results averaged. Thus, recommended therapeutic doses will be appropriate for the majority of patients, but not necessarily for each individual.

The variation in sensitivity may be based on pharmacokinetic differences (same dose → different plasma levels) or on differences in target organ sensitivity (same plasma level → different effects).

To enhance therapeutic safety, clinical pharmacology has led efforts to discover the causes responsible for interindividual drug responsiveness in patients. This field of research is called *pharmacogenetics.* Often the underlying reason is a difference in enzyme property or activity. Ethnic variations are additionally observed. Prudent physicians will attempt to determine the metabolic status of a patient before prescribing a particular drug.

A. Abnormal posture in mouse given morphine

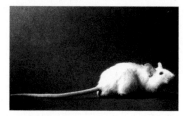

B. Incidence of effect as a function of dose

Dose = 0   = 2 mg/kg   = 10 mg/kg

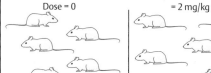

= 20 mg/kg   = 100 mg/kg   = 140 mg/kg

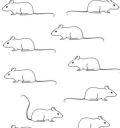
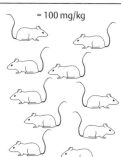
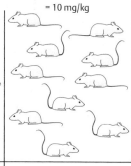
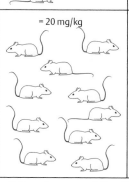
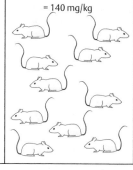

C. Dose–frequency relationship

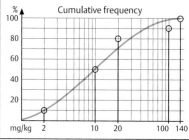
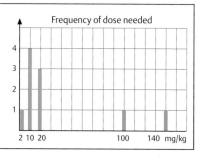

Cumulative frequency

Frequency of dose needed

☐ Concentration–Effect Relationship (A)

As a rule, the therapeutic effect or toxic action of a drug depends critically on the response of a single organ or a limited number of organs; for example, blood flow is affected by a change in vascular luminal width. By isolating critical organs or tissues from a larger functional system, these actions can be studied with more accuracy; for instance, vasoconstrictor agents can be examined in isolated preparations from different regions of the vascular tree, e. g., the portal or saphenous veins, or the mesentery, coronary, or basilar arteries. In many cases, isolated organs or organ parts can be kept viable for hours in an appropriate nutrient medium sufficiently supplied with oxygen and held at a suitable temperature. Responses of the preparation to a physiological or pharmacological stimulus can be determined by a suitable recording apparatus. Thus, narrowing of a blood vessel is recorded with the help of two wire loops by which the vessel is suspended under tension.

Experimentation on isolated organs offers several *advantages*:

1. The drug concentration in the tissue is usually known.
2. Reduced complexity and ease of relating stimulus and effect.
3. It is possible to circumvent compensatory responses that may partially cancel the primary effect in the intact organism; for example, the heart rate-increasing action of norepinephrine cannot be demonstrated in the intact organism because a simultaneous rise in blood pressure elicits a counterregulatory reflex that slows cardiac rate.
4. The ability to examine a drug effect over its full range of intensities; for example, it would be impossible in the intact organism to follow negative chronotropic effects to the point of cardiac arrest.

Disadvantages are:

1. Unavoidable tissue injury during dissection.
2. Loss of physiological regulation of function in the isolated tissue.
3. The artificial milieu imposed on the tissue.

These drawbacks are less important if isolated organ systems are used merely for comparing the potency of different substances. The use of isolated cells offers a further simplification of the test system. Thus, quantitation of certain drug effects can be achieved with particular ease in cell cultures. A more marked "reduction" consists in the use of isolated subcellular structures, such as plasma membranes, endoplasmic reticulum, or lysosomes. With increasing reduction, extrapolation to the intact organism becomes more difficult and less certain.

☐ Concentration–Effect Curves (B)

As the concentration is raised by a constant factor, the *increment in effect* diminishes steadily and tends asymptotically toward zero the closer one comes to the maximally effective concentration. The concentration at which a maximal effect occurs cannot be measured accurately; however, that eliciting a half-maximal effect (EC_{50}) is readily determined. This typically corresponds to the inflection point of the concentration–response curve in a semi-logarithmic plot (log concentration on abscissa). Full characterization of a concentration–effect relationship requires determination of the EC_{50}, the maximally possible effect (E_{max}), and the slope at the point of inflection.

A. Measurement of effect as a function of concentration

Portal vein
Mesenteric artery

Coronary artery

Basilar artery

Saphenous vein

Vasoconstriction
Active tension

1 min

1   2   5   10   20   30   40   50   100

Drug concentration

B. Concentration–effect relationship

Effect
(in mm of registration unit, e.g., tension developed)

Concentration (linear)

Effect
(% of maximum effect)

Concentration (logarithmic)

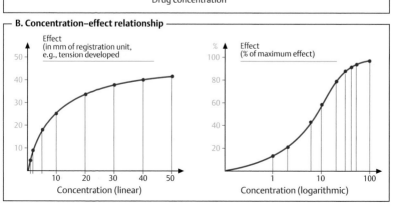

☐ Concentration–Binding Curves

In order to elicit their effect, drug molecules must be bound to the cells of the effector organ. Binding commonly occurs at specific cell structures, namely, the receptors. The analysis of drug binding to receptors aims to determine the affinity of ligands, the kinetics of interaction, and the characteristics of the binding site itself.

In studying the affinity and number of such binding sites, use is made of membrane suspensions of different tissues. This approach is based on the expectation that binding sites will retain their characteristic properties during cell homogenization.

Provided that binding sites are freely accessible in the medium in which membrane fragments are suspended, drug concentration at the "site of action" will equal that in the medium. The drug under study is radiolabeled (enabling low concentrations to be measured quantitatively), added to the membrane suspension, and allowed to bind to receptors. Membrane fragments and medium are then separated, e.g., by filtration, and the amount of bound drug (ligand) is measured. Binding increases in proportion to concentration as long as there is a negligible reduction in the number of free binding sites ($c \approx 1$ and $B \approx 10\%$ of maximum binding; $c \approx 2$ and $B \approx 20\%$). As binding sites approach saturation, the number of free sites decreases and the increment in binding is no longer proportional to the increase in concentration (in the example illustrated, an increase in concentration by 1 is needed to increase binding from 10% to 20%; however, an increase by 20 is needed to raise it from 70% to 80%).

The **law of mass action** describes the hyperbolic relationship between binding (B) and ligand concentration (c). This relationship is characterized by the drug's affinity ($1/K_D$) and the maximum binding (B_{max}), i.e., the total number of binding sites per unit of weight of membrane homogenate.

$$B = B_{max} \frac{c}{c + K_D}$$

K_D is the equilibrium dissociation constant and corresponds to that ligand concentration at which 50% of binding sites are occupied. The values given in (**A**) and used for plotting the concentration–binding graph (**B**) result when $K_D = 10$.

The differing affinity of different ligands for a binding site can be demonstrated elegantly by binding assays. Although simple to perform, these binding assays pose the difficulty of correlating unequivocally the binding sites concerned with the pharmacological effect; this is particularly difficult when more than one population of binding sites is present. Therefore, receptor binding must not be assumed until it can be shown that:

- Binding is saturable (*saturability*).
- The only substances bound are those possessing the same pharmacological mechanism of action (*specificity*).
- Binding *affinity* of different substances is *correlated* with their pharmacological potency.

Binding assays provide information about the affinity of ligands, but they do not give any clue as to whether a ligand is an agonist or antagonist (p. 60).

Radiolabeled drugs bound to their receptors may be of help in purifying and analyzing further the receptor protein.

A. Measurement of binding (*B*) as a function of concentration (*c*)

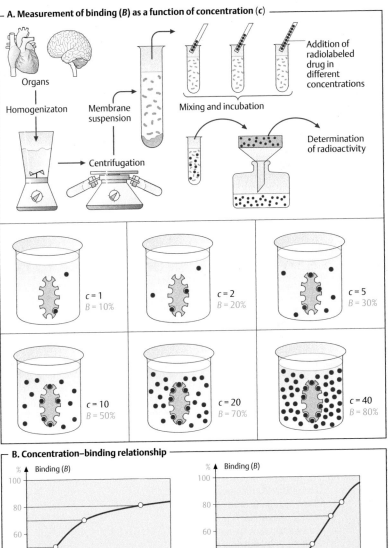

Organs

Homogenizaton

Membrane suspension

Centrifugation

Addition of radiolabeled drug in different concentrations

Mixing and incubation

Determination of radioactivity

$c = 1$ $B = 10\%$

$c = 2$ $B = 20\%$

$c = 5$ $B = 30\%$

$c = 10$ $B = 50\%$

$c = 20$ $B = 70\%$

$c = 40$ $B = 80\%$

B. Concentration–binding relationship

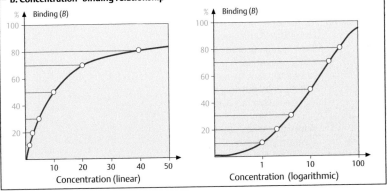

% Binding (*B*)

Concentration (linear)

% Binding (*B*)

Concentration (logarithmic)

☐ Types of Binding Forces

Unless a drug comes into contact with intrinsic structures of the body, it cannot affect body function.

Covalent Bonding

Two atoms enter a covalent bond if each donates an electron to a shared electron pair (cloud). This state is depicted in structural formulas by a dash. The covalent bond is "firm," that is, not reversible or poorly so. Few drugs are covalently bound to biological structures. The bond, and possibly the effect, persist for a long time after intake of a drug has been discontinued, making therapy difficult to control. Examples include alkylating cytostatics (p. 300) or organophosphates (p. 311). Conjugation reactions occurring in biotransformation also represent covalent linkages (e. g., to glucuronic acid).

Noncovalent Bonding

In noncovalent bonding there is no formation of a shared electron pair. The bond is reversible and is typical of most drug–receptor interactions. Since a drug usually attaches to its site of action by multiple contacts, several of the types of bonds described below may participate.

Electrostatic attraction (A). A positive and a negative charge attract each other.

Ionic interaction: An ion is a particle charged either positively (cation) or negatively (anion), i.e., the atom is deficient in electrons or has surplus electrons, respectively. Attraction between ions of opposite charge is inversely proportional to the square of the distance between them; it is the initial force drawing a charged drug to its binding site. Ionic bonds have a relatively high stability.

Dipole–ion interaction: When bonding electrons are asymmetrically distributed over the atomic nuclei involved, one atom will bear a negative (δ^-), and its partner a positive (δ^+) partial charge. The molecule thus presents a positive and a negative pole, i.e., it has polarity or is a dipole. A partial charge can interact electrostatically with an ion of opposite charge.

Dipole-dipole interaction is the electrostatic attraction between opposite partial charges. When a hydrogen atom bearing a partial positive charge bridges two atoms bearing partial negative charges, a hydrogen bond is created.

van der Waals bonds (B) are formed between apolar molecular groups that have come into close proximity. Spontaneous transient distortion of electron clouds (momentary faint dipole, $\delta\delta$) may induce an opposite dipole in the neighboring molecule. The van der Waals bond, therefore, is also a form of electrostatic attraction, albeit of very low strength (inversely proportional to 7th power of distance).

Hydrophobic interaction (C). The attraction between the water dipoles is strong enough to hinder intercalation of any apolar (uncharged) molecules. By tending toward each other, H_2O molecules squeeze apolar particles from their midst. Accordingly, in the organism, apolar particles such as fatty acid chains of cell membranes or apolar regions of a receptor have an increased probability of remaining in nonaqueous, apolar surroundings.

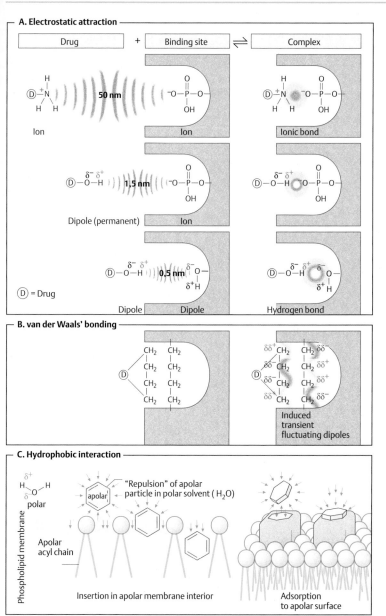

A. Electrostatic attraction

| Drug | + | Binding site | ⇌ | Complex |

Ion — 50 nm — Ion → Ionic bond

Dipole (permanent) — 1.5 nm — Ion → Hydrogen bond

D = Drug

Dipole — 0.5 nm — Dipole → Hydrogen bond

B. van der Waals' bonding

Induced transient fluctuating dipoles

C. Hydrophobic interaction

polar

"Repulsion" of apolar particle in polar solvent (H_2O)

Phospholipid membrane

Apolar acyl chain

Insertion in apolar membrane interior

Adsorption to apolar surface

☐ Agonists—Antagonists

An **agonist** (**A**) has affinity (tendency to adhere) for a receptor and affects the receptor protein in such a manner as to cause a change in cell function—"**intrinsic activity.**" The biological effect of the agonist (i.e., the change in cell function) depends on the effectiveness of signal transduction steps (p. 66) associated with receptor activation. The maximal effect of an agonist may already occur when only a fraction of the available receptors is occupied (**B**, agonist A). Another agonist (agonist B), possessing equal affinity but less ability to activate the receptor and the associated signal transduction steps (i.e., less intrinsic activity), will produce a smaller maximal effect even if all receptors are occupied—smaller **efficacy**. Agonist B is a *partial agonist*. The **potency** of an agonist is characterized by the concentration (EC_{50}) at which a half-maximal effect is attained.

Antagonists (**A**) attenuate the effect of agonists: they act "antiagonistically." **Competitive antagonists** possess affinity for the receptors, but their binding does not elicit a change in cell function. In other words, they are devoid of intrinsic activity. When present simultaneously, an agonist and a competitive antagonist vie for occupancy of the receptor. The affinities and concentrations of both competitors determine whether binding of agonist or antagonist predominates. By increasing the concentration of the agonist, blockade induced by an antagonist can be surmounted (**C**): that is, the concentration–effect curve of the agonist is shifted "right"—to higher concentrations—with preservation of the maximal effect.

☐ Models of the Molecular Mechanism of Agonist/Antagonist Action (A)

Agonist induces an active conformation. The *agonist* binds to the inactive receptor and thereby causes the resting conformation to change into the active state. The *antagonist* attaches to the inactive receptor without altering its conformation.

Agonist stabilizes spontaneously occurring active conformation. The receptor may spontaneously "flip" into the active conformation. Usually, however, the statistical probability of such an event is so small that a spontaneous excitation of the cells remains undetectable. Selective binding of the *agonist* can occur only to the active conformation and thus favors the existence of this state. The *antagonist* shows affinity only for the inactive state, promoting existence of the latter. If the system has little spontaneous activity, no measurable effect will result from adding an antagonist. However, if the system displays high spontaneous activity, the antagonist is liable to produce an effect opposite to that of an agonist: *inverse agonist*. A "true" antagonist without intrinsic activity ("neutral antagonist") displays equal affinity for the active and inactive conformations of the receptor and does not interfere with the basal activity of the cell. According to this model, a *partial agonist* has less selectivity for the active state; however, to a certain extent it binds also to the inactive state.

☐ Other Forms of Antagonism

Allosteric antagonism. The antagonist is bound outside the agonist's site of attachment at the receptor and induces a decrease in agonist affinity. The latter is increased in the case of **allosteric synergism**.

Functional antagonism. Two agonists acting via different receptors affect the same variable (e.g., luminal diameter of bronchi) in opposite directions (epinephrine → dilation; histamine → constriction).

A. Molecular mechanisms of drug–receptor interaction

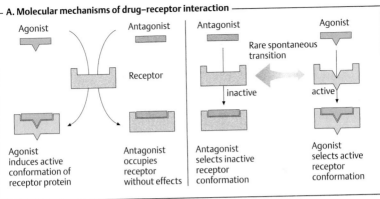

Agonist

Antagonist

Receptor

Agonist
induces active
conformation of
receptor protein

Antagonist
occupies
receptor
without effects

Antagonist

Rare spontaneous
transition

Agonist

inactive

active

Antagonist
selects inactive
receptor
conformation

Agonist
selects active
receptor
conformation

B. Potency and efficacy of agonists

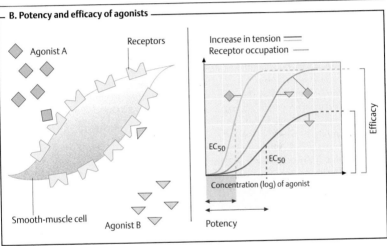

Agonist A

Receptors

Increase in tension
Receptor occupation

EC_{50}

EC_{50}

Efficacy

Concentration (log) of agonist

Smooth-muscle cell

Agonist B

Potency

C. Competitive antagonism

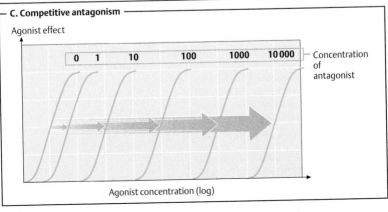

Agonist effect

0   1   10   100   1000   10 000

Concentration
of
antagonist

Agonist concentration (log)

☐ Enantioselectivity of Drug Action

Many drugs are racemates, including β-blockers, nonsteroidal anti-inflammatory agents, as well as the anticholinergic *benzetimide* (**A**). A **racemate** consists of a molecule and its corresponding mirror image which, like the left and right hands, cannot be superimposed. Such **chiral** ("handed") pairs of molecules are referred to as **enantiomers**. Typically, chirality is due to a single carbon (C) atom bonded to four different substituents (*asymmetric carbon atom*). Enantiomerism is a special case of stereoisomerism. Nonchiral stereoisomers are called **diastereomers** (e. g., quinidine/quinine).

Bond lengths in enantiomers, but not necessarily diastereomers, are the same. Therefore, enantiomers possess **similar physicochemical properties** (e. g., solubility, melting point) and both forms are usually obtained in equal amounts by chemical synthesis. As a result of enzymatic activity, however, only one of the enantiomers is usually found in nature.

In solution, enantiomers **rotate the plane of oscillation of linearly polarized light in opposite directions**; hence they are referred to as "*dextro-rotatory*" or "*levo-rotatory*," designated by the prefixes *d*- or (+)- and *l*- or (−)-, respectively. The direction of rotation gives no clue concerning the spatial structure of enantiomers. The *absolute* configuration, as determined by certain rules, is described by the prefixes (*S*)- and (*R*)-. In some compounds, designation as the D- and L-forms is possible by reference to the structure of D- and L-glyceraldehyde.

For drugs to exert biological actions, contact with reaction partners in the body is required. When the reaction favors one of the enantiomers, *enantioselectivity* is observed.

Enantioselectivity of affinity. If a receptor has sites for three of the substituents (symbolized in **B** by a cone, sphere, and cube) on the asymmetric carbon to attach to, only one of the enantiomers will have optimal fit. Its affinity will then be higher. Thus, *dexetimide* displays an affinity at the muscarinic ACh receptors almost 10 000 times (p. 104) that of *levetimide*; and at β-adrenoceptors (*S*)-(−)-propranolol has an affinity 100 times that of the (*R*)-(+) form.

Enantioselectivity of intrinsic activity. The mode of attachment at the receptor also determines whether an effect is elicited; and whether or not a substance has intrinsic activity, i. e., acts as an agonist. For instance, (−)-*dobutamine* is an agonist at β-adrenoceptors, whereas the (+)-enantiomer is an antagonist.

Inverse enantioselectivity at another receptor. An enantiomer may possess an unfavorable configuration at one receptor that may, however, be optimal for interaction with another receptor. In the case of *dobutamine*, the (+)-enantiomer has affinity at β-adrenoceptors that is 10 times higher than that of the (−)-enantiomer, both having agonist activity. However, the α-adrenoceptor stimulant action is due to the (−)-form (see above).

As described for receptor interactions, enantioselectivity may also be manifested in drug interactions with **enzymes** and **transport proteins**. Enantiomers may display different affinities and reaction velocities.

Conclusion. The enantiomers of a racemate can differ sufficiently in their pharmacodynamic and pharmacokinetic properties to constitute two distinct drugs.

A. Example of an enantiomeric pair with different affinities for a stereoselective receptor

RACEMATE
Benzetimide

ENANTIOMER
Dexetimide

Ratio
1 : 1

ENANTIOMER
Levetimide

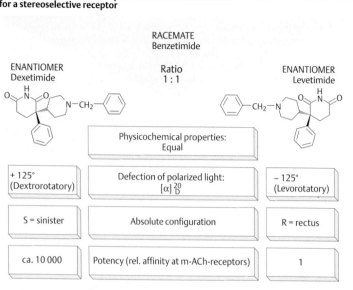

	Physicochemical properties: Equal	
+ 125° (Dextrorotatory)	Defection of polarized light: $[\alpha]_D^{20}$	− 125° (Levorotatory)
S = sinister	Absolute configuration	R = rectus
ca. 10 000	Potency (rel. affinity at m-ACh-receptors)	1

B. Reasons for different pharmacological properties of enantiomers

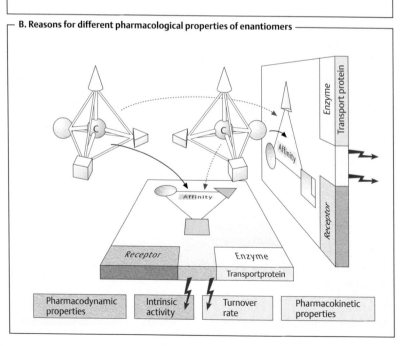

| Pharmacodynamic properties | Intrinsic activity | Turnover rate | Pharmacokinetic properties |

□ Receptor Types

Receptors are macromolecules that operate to bind mediator substances and transduce this binding into an effect, i.e., a change in cell function. Receptors differ in terms of their structure and the manner in which they translate occupancy by a ligand into a cellular response (**signal transduction**).

G-Protein coupled receptors (**A**) consist of an amino acid chain that weaves in and out of the membrane in serpentine fashion. The extramembranal loop regions of the molecule may possess sugar residues at different N-glycosylation sites. The seven α-helical membrane-spanning domains probably form a circle around a central pocket that carries the attachment sites for the mediator substance. Binding of the mediator molecule or of a structurally related agonist molecule induces a change in the conformation of the receptor protein, enabling the latter to interact with a G-protein (= guanyl nucleotide-binding protein). G-proteins lie at the inner leaf of the plasmalemma and consist of three subunits designated α, β, and γ. There are various G-proteins that differ mainly with regard to their α-unit. Association with the receptor activates the G-protein, leading in turn to activation of another protein (enzyme, ion channel). A large number of mediator substances act via G-protein-coupled receptors (see p. 66 for more details).

An example of a **ligand-gated ion channel** (**B**) is the nicotinic cholinoceptor of the motor end plate. The receptor complex consists of five subunits, each of which contains four transmembrane domains. Simultaneous binding of two acetylcholine (ACh) molecules to the two α-subunits results in opening of the ion channel with entry of Na^+ (and exit of some K^+), membrane depolarization, and triggering of an action potential (p. 186). The neuronal *N*-cholinoceptors apparently consist only of α- and β-subunits. Some of the receptors for the transmitter γ-aminobutyric acid (GABA) belong to this receptor family: the $GABA_A$ subtype is linked to a chloride channel (and also to a benzodiazepine binding site, see p. 223). Glutamate and glycine both act via ligand-gated ion channels.

The insulin receptor protein represents a **ligand-operated enzyme** (**C**), a catalytic receptor. When insulin binds to the extracellular attachment site, a tyrosine kinase activity is "switched on" at the intracellular portion. Protein phosphorylation leads to altered cell function via the assembly of other signal proteins. Receptors for growth hormones also belong to the catalytic receptor class.

Protein synthesis regulating receptors (**D**) for steroids and thyroid hormone are found in the cytosol and in the cell nucleus, respectively. The receptor proteins are located intracellularly; depending on the hormone, either in the cytosol (e.g., glucocorticoids, mineralocorticoids, androgens, and gestagens) or in the cell nucleus (e.g., estrogens, thyroid hormone). Binding of hormone exposes a normally hidden domain of the receptor protein, thereby permitting the latter to bind to a particular DNA nucleotide sequence on a gene and to regulate its transcription. The ligand–receptor complexes thus function as transcription regulating factors. Transcription is usually initiated or enhanced, rarely blocked.

The hormone–receptor complexes interact pairwise with DNA. These pairs (dimers) may consist of two identical hormone–receptor complexes (homodimeric form, e.g., with adrenal or gonadal hormones). The thyroid hormone–receptor complex occurs in heterodimeric form and combines with a *cis*-retinoic acid-receptor complex.

A. G-Protein-coupled receptor

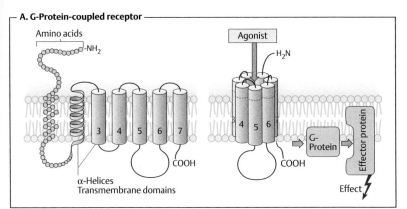

Amino acids
-NH₂

Agonist

H₂N

3 4 5 6 7

COOH

α-Helices
Transmembrane domains

3 4 5 6

COOH

G-Protein → Effector protein

Effect

B. Ligand-gated ion channel

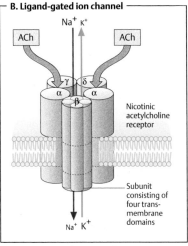

Na⁺ K⁺

ACh

ACh

γ δ

α β α

Nicotinic
acetylcholine
receptor

Subunit
consisting of
four trans-
membrane
domains

Na⁺ K⁺

C. Ligand-regulated enzyme

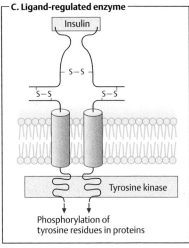

Insulin

S—S

S—S   S—S

Tyrosine kinase

Phosphorylation of
tyrosine residues in proteins

D. Protein synthesis-regulating receptor

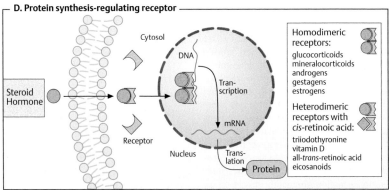

Cytosol

DNA

Tran-
scription

mRNA

Steroid
Hormone

Receptor

Nucleus

Trans-
lation

Protein

Homodimeric
receptors:

glucocorticoids
mineralocorticoids
androgens
gestagens
estrogens

Heterodimeric
receptors with
cis-retinoic acid:

triiodothyronine
vitamin D
all-*trans*-retinoic acid
eicosanoids

☐ Mode of Operation of G-Protein-coupled Receptors

Signal transduction at G-protein coupled receptors uses essentially the same basic mechanism (**A**). Agonist binding to the receptor leads to a change in receptor protein conformation. This change propagates to the G-protein: the α-subunit exchanges GDP for GTP, then dissociates from the two other subunits, associates with an effector protein and alters its functional state. In principle, the β- and γ-subunits are also able to interact with effector proteins. The α-subunit slowly hydrolyses bound GTP to GDP. G_α-GDP has no affinity for the effector protein and reassociates with the β- and γ-subunits (**A**). G-proteins can undergo lateral diffusion in the membrane; they are not assigned to individual receptor proteins. However, a relation exists between receptor types and G-protein types (**B**). Furthermore, the α-subunits of individual G-proteins are distinct in terms of their affinity for different effector proteins, as well as the kind of influence exerted on the effector protein. G_α-GTP of the G_s-protein stimulates adenylate cyclase, while G_α-GTP of the G_i-protein is inhibitory. The G-protein-coupled receptor family includes muscarinic cholinoceptors, adrenoceptors for norepinephrine and epinephrine, as well as receptors for dopamine, histamine, serotonin, glutamate, GABA, morphine, prostaglandins, leukotrienes, and many other mediators and hormones.

Major effector proteins for G-protein-coupled receptors include **adenylate cyclase** (ATP → intracellular messenger **cAMP**), **phospholipase C** (phosphatidylinositol → intracellular messengers **inositol trisphosphate** and **diacylglycerol**) as well as ion channel proteins (**B**). Numerous cell functions are regulated by cellular cAMP concentration, because cAMP enhances activity of protein kinase A, which catalyzes the transfer of phosphate groups onto functional proteins. Elevation of cAMP levels leads inter alia to relaxation of smooth muscle tonus,

enhanced contractility of cardiac muscle, as well as increased glycogenolysis and lipolysis (p. 88). Phosphorylation of cardiac calcium channel proteins increases the probability of channel opening during membrane depolarization. It should be noted that cAMP is inactivated by phosphodiesterase. Inhibitors of this enzyme elevate intracellular cAMP concentration and elicit effects resembling those of epinephrine.

The receptor protein itself may undergo phosphorylation, with a resultant loss of its ability to activate the associated G-protein. This is one of the mechanisms that contribute to a decrease in sensitivity of a cell during prolonged receptor stimulation by an agonist (*desensitization*).

Activation of phospholipase C leads to cleavage of the membrane phospholipid phosphatidylinositol 4,5-bisphosphate into **inositol trisphosphate** (IP_3) and **diacylglycerol** (DAG). IP_3 promotes release of Ca^{2+} from storage organelles, whereby contraction of smooth muscle cells, breakdown of glycogen, or exocytosis may be initiated. DAG stimulates protein kinase C, which phosphorylates certain serine- or threonine-containing enzymes.

Certain G-proteins can induce opening of **channel proteins**. In this way, potassium channels can be activated (e. g., acetylcholine effect on sinus node, p. 104; opioid effect on neural impulse transmission, p. 208).

A. G-Protein-mediated effect of an agonist

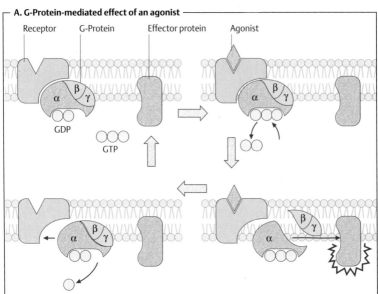

B. G-Proteins, cellular messenger substances, and effects

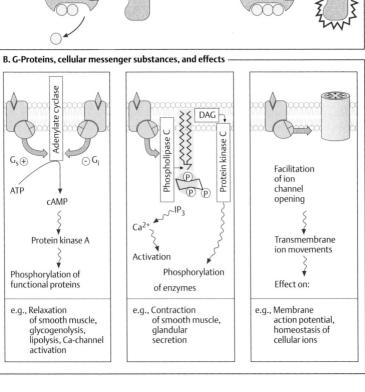

□ Time Course of Plasma Concentration and Effect

After the administration of a drug, its concentration in plasma rises, reaches a peak, and then declines gradually to the starting level, owing to the processes of distribution and elimination (p. 46). Plasma concentration at a given point in time depends on the dose administered. Many drugs exhibit a linear relationship between plasma concentration and dose within the therapeutic range (**dose-linear kinetics [A]**; note different scales on ordinate). However, the same does not apply to drugs whose elimination processes are already sufficiently activated at therapeutic plasma levels so as to preclude further proportional increases in the rate of elimination when the concentration is increased further. Under these conditions, a smaller proportion of the dose administered is eliminated per unit time.

A model example of this behavior is the elimination of ethanol (p. 44). Because the metabolizing enzyme, alcohol dehydrogenase, is already saturated at low ethanol concentrations, only the same amount per unit time is broken down despite rising concentrations.

The time courses of the *effect* and of the *concentration* in plasma are not identical, because the concentration–effect relationship is complex (e. g., with a threshold phenomenon) and often obeys a hyperbolic function (**B**; cf. p. 54). This means that the time course of the effect exhibits dose dependence also in the presence of dose-linear kinetics (**C**).

In the lower dose range (example 1), the plasma level passes through a concentration range (0–0.9) in which the change in concentration still correlates quasi-linearly with the change in effect. The time courses of the concentration in plasma and the effect (**A** and **C**, left graphs) are very similar. However, after a high dose (100), the plasma level will remain in a concentration range (between 90 and 20) where changes in concentration

do not evoke significant changes in effect. Accordingly, the time–effect curve displays a kind of plateau after high doses (100). The effect only begins to wane after the plasma level has fallen to a range (below 20) in which changes in plasma level are reflected in the intensity of the effect.

The dose-dependence of the time course of the drug effect is exploited when the duration of the effect is to be prolonged by administration of a dose in excess of that required for the effect. This is done in the case of penicillin G (p. 270), when a dosing interval of 8 hours is recommended although the drug is eliminated with a half-life of 30 minutes. This procedure is, of course, feasible only if supramaximal dosing is not associated with toxic effects.

It follows that a nearly constant effect can be achieved, although the plasma level may fluctuate greatly during the interval between doses.

The hyperbolic relationship between plasma concentration and effect explains why the time course of the effect, unlike that of the plasma concentration, cannot be described in terms of a simple exponential function. A half-life can only be given for the processes of drug absorption and elimination, hence the change in plasma levels, but generally not for the onset or decline of the effect.

A. Dose-linear kinetics (note different ordinates)

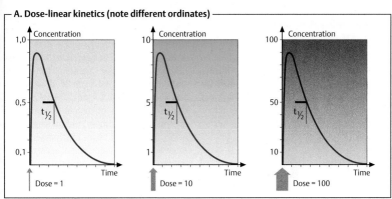

B. Concentration–effect relationship

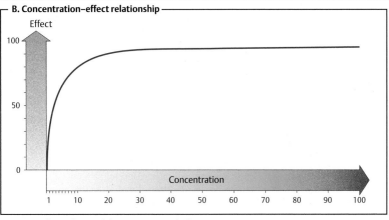

C. Dose dependence of the time course of effect

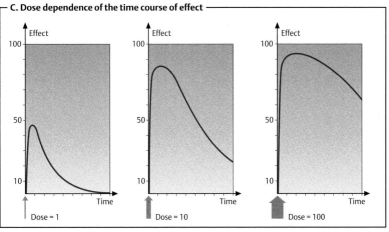

□ Undesirable Drug Effects, Side Effects

The desired (or intended) principal effect of any drug is to modify body function in such a manner as to alleviate symptoms caused by the patient's illness. In addition, a drug may also elicit unwanted effects that in turn may cause complaints, provoke illness, or even lead to death.

Causes of Adverse Effects

Overdosage (A). The drug is administered in a higher dose than is required for the principal effect; this directly or indirectly affects other body functions.

For instance, **morphine** (p. 208), given in the appropriate dose, affords excellent pain relief by influencing nociceptive pathways in the CNS. In excessive doses, it inhibits the respiratory center and makes apnea imminent. The dose-dependence of both effects can be graphed in the form of dose–response curves (DRCs). The distance between the two DRCs indicates the difference between the therapeutic and toxic doses. This *margin of safety* ("therapeutic index") indicates the risk of toxicity when standard doses are exceeded.

It should be noted that, apart from the amount administered, the rate of drug delivery is important. The faster blood levels rise, the higher concentrations will climb (p. 49). Rather than being required therapeutically, the initial concentration peak following i.v. injection of morphinelike agents causes side effects (intoxication and respiratory depression, p. 208).

"The dose alone makes the poison" (Paracelsus). This holds true for both medicines and environmental poisons. *No substance as such is toxic!* In order to assess the risk of toxicity, knowledge is required of: (1) the effective dose during exposure; (2) the dose level at which damage is likely to occur.

Increased sensitivity (B). If certain body functions develop hyperreactivity, unwanted effects can occur even at normal dose levels. Increased sensitivity of the respiratory center to morphine is found in patients with chronic lung disease, in neonates, or during concurrent exposure to other respiratory depressant agents. The DRC is shifted to the left and a smaller dose of morphine is sufficient to paralyze respiration. Genetic anomalies of metabolism may also lead to hypersensitivity (pharmacogenetics, p. 78). The above forms of hypersensitivity must be distinguished from allergies involving the immune system (p. 72).

Lack of selectivity (C). Despite appropriate dosing and normal sensitivity, undesired effects can occur because the drug does not specifically act on the targeted (diseased) tissue or organ. For instance, the anticholinergic atropine is bound only to acetylcholine receptors of the muscarinic type; however, these are present in many different organs. Moreover, the neuroleptic chlorpromazine is able to interact with several different receptor types. Thus, its action is neither organ-specific nor receptor-specific.

The consequences of lack of selectivity can often be avoided if the drug does not require the blood route to reach the target organ but is, instead, applied locally, as in the administration of parasympatholytics in the form of eye drops or in an aerosol for inhalation.

Side effects that arise as a consequence of a known mechanism of action are plausible and the connection with drug ingestion is simple to recognize. It is more difficult to detect unwanted effects that arise from an unknown action. Some compelling examples of these include fetal damage after intake of a hypnotic (thalidomide), pulmonary hypertension after appetite depressants, and fibrosis after antimigraine drugs.

With every drug use, unwanted effects must be taken into account. Before prescribing a drug, the physician should therefore do a **risk–benefit analysis**.

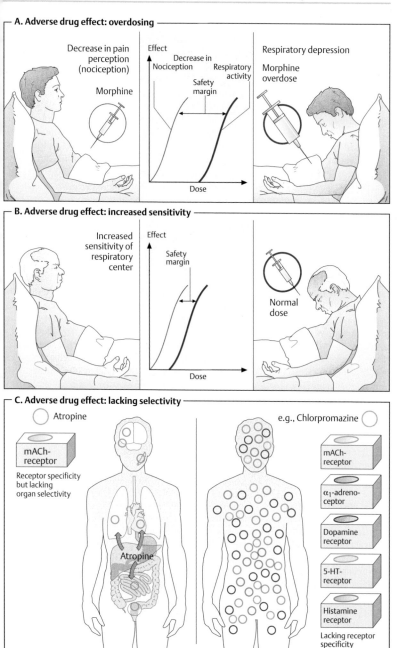

A. Adverse drug effect: overdosing

Decrease in pain perception (nociception)

Morphine

Effect

Decrease in Nociception   Respiratory activity

Safety margin

Dose

Respiratory depression

Morphine overdose

B. Adverse drug effect: increased sensitivity

Increased sensitivity of respiratory center

Effect

Safety margin

Dose

Normal dose

C. Adverse drug effect: lacking selectivity

Atropine

mACh-receptor

Receptor specificity but lacking organ selectivity

Atropine

e.g., Chlorpromazine

mACh-receptor

α_1-adreno-ceptor

Dopamine receptor

5-HT-receptor

Histamine receptor

Lacking receptor specificity

☐ **Drug Allergy**

The immune system normally functions to inactivate and remove high-molecular-weight "foreign" matter taken up by the organism. Immune responses can, however, occur without appropriate cause or with exaggerated intensity and may harm the organism; for instance, when allergic reactions are caused by drugs (active ingredient or pharmaceutical excipients). Only a few drugs, e. g., (heterologous) proteins, have a molecular weight large enough to act as effective **antigens** or **immunogens**, capable by themselves of initiating an immune response. Most drugs or their metabolites (so-called **haptens**) must first be converted to an antigen by linkage to a body protein. In the case of penicillin G, a cleavage product (penicilloyl residue) probably undergoes covalent binding to protein.

During **initial contact** with the drug, the immune system is sensitized: antigen-specific lymphocytes of the T-type and B-type (antibody formation) proliferate in lymphatic tissue and some of them remain as so-called memory cells. Usually, these processes remain clinically silent.

During the **second contact**, antibodies are already present and memory cells proliferate rapidly. A detectable immune response—the allergic reaction—occurs. This can be of severe intensity, even at a low dose of the antigen. Four types of reactions can be distinguished:

Type 1, anaphylactic reaction. Drug-specific antibodies of the *IgE type* combine via their Fc moiety with receptors on the surface of *mast cells*. Binding of the drug provides the stimulus for the release of histamine and other mediators. In the most severe form, a life-threatening anaphylactic shock develops, accompanied by hypotension, bronchospasm (asthma attack), laryngeal edema, urticaria, stimulation of gut musculature, and spontaneous bowel movements (p. 118).

Type 2, cytotoxic reaction. *Drug–antibody (IgG) complexes* adhere to the surface of *blood cells*, where either circulating drug molecules or complexes already formed in blood accumulate. These complexes mediate the *activation of complement*, a family of proteins that circulate in the blood in an inactive form, but can be activated in a cascadelike succession by an appropriate stimulus. "Activated complement," normally directed against microorganisms, can *destroy the cell membranes* and thereby cause cell death; it also promotes phagocytosis, attracts neutrophil granulocytes (chemotaxis), and stimulates other inflammatory responses. Activation of complement on blood cells results in their destruction, evidenced by hemolytic anemia, agranulocytosis, and thrombocytopenia.

Type 3, immune-complex vasculitis (serum sickness, Arthus reaction). *Drug–antibody complexes* precipitate on *vascular walls, complement* is activated, and an *inflammatory reaction* is triggered. Attracted neutrophils, in a futile attempt to phagocytose the complexes, liberate lysosomal enzymes that damage the vascular walls (inflammation, vasculitis). Symptoms may include fever, exanthema, swelling of lymph nodes, arthritis, nephritis, and neuropathy.

Type 4, contact dermatitis. A cutaneously applied drug is bound to the surface of *T-lymphocytes* directed specifically against it. The lymphocytes release signal molecules (*lymphokines*) into their vicinity that activate macrophages and provoke an inflammatory reaction.

Remarkably, virtually no drug group is completely free of allergic side effects. However, some chemical structures are prone to cause allergic reactions.

A. Adverse drug effect: allergic reaction

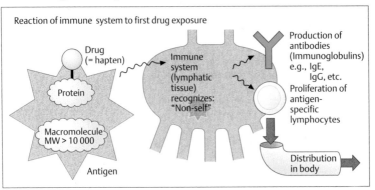

Reaction of immune system to first drug exposure

Drug (= hapten)

Protein

Macromolecule MW > 10 000

Antigen

Immune system (lymphatic tissue) recognizes: "Non-self"

Production of antibodies (Immunoglobulins) e.g., IgE, IgG, etc.

Proliferation of antigen-specific lymphocytes

Distribution in body

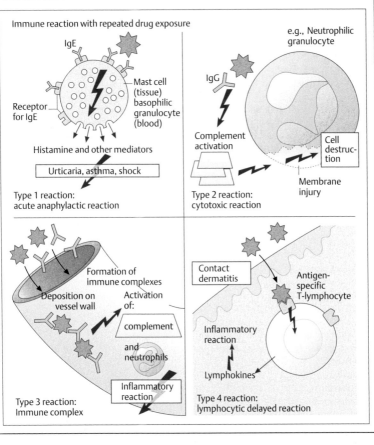

Immune reaction with repeated drug exposure

IgE

Receptor for IgE

Mast cell (tissue) basophilic granulocyte (blood)

Histamine and other mediators

Urticaria, asthma, shock

Type 1 reaction: acute anaphylactic reaction

e.g., Neutrophilic granulocyte

IgG

Complement activation

Cell destruction

Membrane injury

Type 2 reaction: cytotoxic reaction

Formation of immune complexes

Deposition on vessel wall

Activation of:

complement

and neutrophils

Inflammatory reaction

Type 3 reaction: Immune complex

Contact dermatitis

Antigen-specific T-lymphocyte

Inflammatory reaction

Lymphokines

Type 4 reaction: lymphocytic delayed reaction

□ Cutaneous Reactions

Upon systemic distribution, many drugs evoke skin reactions that are caused on an immunological basis. Moreover, cutaneous injury can also arise from nonimmunological mechanisms. Cutaneous side effects vary in severity from harmless to lethal. Cutaneous reactions are a common form of drug adverse reaction. Nearly half of them are attributed to antibiotics or sulfonamides, and one-third to nonsteroidal anti-inflammatory agents, with many other pharmaceuticals joining the list.

The following clinical pictures are noted:

- **Toxic erythema** with a maculopapular rash similar to that of measles and scarlet fever (**B**, left). **Urticaria** with itchy swellings as part of a Type 1 reaction including anaphylactic shock.
- **Fixed eruptions** (drug exanthemas) with mostly few demarcated, painful lesions, usually located in intertriginous skin regions (genital area, mucous membranes). With repeated exposure, these typically recur at the same sites.
- **Steven–Johnson syndrome** (SJS, erythema multiforme) and **toxic epidermal necrolysis** (TEN or **Lyell syndrome**) with apoptosis of keratinocytes and bullous detachment of the epidermis from the dermis. When more than 30% of the body surface is affected, TEN is present. Its course is dramatic and the outcome not rarely fatal.

The aforementioned reactions are thought to involve the following pathogenetic mechanisms.

- With penicillins, opening of the β-lactam bond is possible. The resulting penicilloyl group binds as a hapten to a protein. This may lead to an Ig-E mediated **anaphylactic reaction**, manifested on the skin as urticaria.
- **Biotransformation** via cytochrome oxidase may yield reactive products. Presumably keratinocytes are capable of such metabolic reactions. In this way, the

para-amino group of sulfonamides can be converted into a hydroxyl amine group, which then acts as a hapten to induce a Type 4 reaction in the skin. Fixed maculopapular lesions are thought to arise on this basis.

- **Pemphiguslike** manifestations with formation of blisters. The development of cutaneous manifestations is not as ominous as in SJS or TEN, the blisters being located intraepidermally. This condition involves the formation of autoantibodies directed against adhesion proteins (desmogelin) of desmosomes, which link keratinocytes to each other. D-Penicillamine and rifampin are inducers of the rare drug-associated pemphigus (p. 308).
- **Photosensitivity** reactions result from exposure to sunlight, in particular the UVA component. In **phototoxic** reactions, drug molecules absorb photic energy and turn into reactive compounds that damage skin cells at their site of production. In **photoallergic** reactions, photoreaction products bind covalently to proteins as haptens and trigger Type 4 allergic responses. The type and localization are difficult to predict.

A. Adverse drug effect: cutaneous reaction

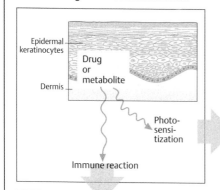

Epidermal keratinocytes
Dermis

Drug or metabolite

Photo-sensitization

Immune reaction

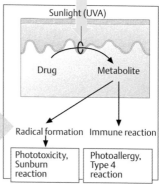

Sunlight (UVA)

Drug → Metabolite

Radical formation   Immune reaction

Phototoxicity, Sunburn reaction

Photoallergy, Type 4 reaction

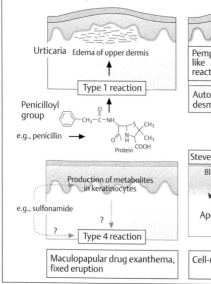

Urticaria   Edema of upper dermis

Type 1 reaction

Penicilloyl group

e.g., penicillin →

Protein

Production of metabolites in keratinocytes

e.g., sulfonamide

Type 4 reaction

Maculopapular drug exanthema, fixed eruption

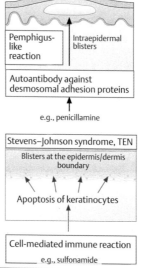

Pemphigus-like reaction   Intraepidermal blisters

Autoantibody against desmosomal adhesion proteins

e.g., penicillamine

Stevens–Johnson syndrome, TEN

Blisters at the epidermis/dermis boundary

Apoptosis of keratinocytes

Cell-mediated immune reaction
e.g., sulfonamide

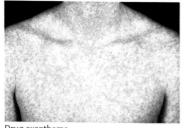

Drug exanthema

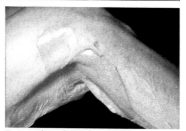

Toxic epidermal necrolysis (TEN)

□ Drug Toxicity in Pregnancy and Lactation

Drugs taken by the mother can be passed on transplacentally or via breast milk and can adversely affect the unborn or the neonate.

Pregnancy (A). Limb malformations induced by the hypnotic thalidomide (Contergan) first focused attention on the potential of drugs to cause malformations (*teratogenicity*). Drug effects on the unborn fall into two basic categories:

1. Predictable effects that derive from the known pharmacological drug properties. Examples include masculinization of the female fetus by androgenic hormones; brain hemorrhage due to oral anticoagulants; bradycardia due to β-blockers.
2. Effects that specifically affect the developing organism and that cannot be predicted on the basis of the known pharmacological activity profile.

In assessing the risks attending drug use during pregnancy, the following points have to be considered:

a *Time of drug use.* The possible sequelae of exposure to a drug depend on the stage of fetal development, as shown in (**A**). Thus, the hazard posed by a drug with a specific action is limited in time, as illustrated by the tetracyclines, which produce effects on teeth and bones only after the third month of gestation, when mineralization begins.

b *Transplacental passage.* Most drugs can pass in the placenta from the maternal into the fetal circulation. The syncytiotrophoblast formed by the fusion of cytotrophoblast cells represents the major diffusion barrier. It possesses a higher permeability to drugs than suggested by the term "placental barrier." Accordingly, all centrally-acting drugs administered to a pregnant woman can easily reach the fetal organism. Relevant examples include antiepileptics, anxiolytics, hypnotics, antidepressants, and neuroleptics.

c *Teratogenicity.* Statistical risk estimates are available for familiar, frequently used drugs. For many drugs, teratogenic potency cannot be demonstrated; however, in the case of novel drugs it is usually not yet possible to define their teratogenic hazard.

Drugs with established human teratogenicity include derivatives of vitamin A (etretinate, isotretinoic acid [used internally in skin diseases]). A peculiar type of damage results from the synthetic estrogenic agent diethylstilbestrol following its use during pregnancy: daughters of treated mothers have an increased incidence of cervical and vaginal carcinoma at the age of about 20 years. Use of this substance in pregnancy was banned in the United States in 1971.

In assessing the risk–benefit ratio, it is also necessary to consider the benefit for the child resulting from adequate therapeutic treatment of its mother. For instance, therapy with antiepileptic drugs is indispensable, because untreated epilepsy endangers the unborn child at least as much as does administration of anticonvulsants.

Drug withdrawal reactions are liable to occur in neonates whose mothers are ingesting drugs of abuse or antidepressants of the SSRI type (p. 228).

Lactation (B). Drugs present in the maternal organism can be secreted in breast milk and thus be ingested by the infant. Evaluation of risks should be based on factors listed in **B**. In case of doubt, potential danger to the infant can be averted only by weaning.

A. Pregnancy: fetal damage due to drugs

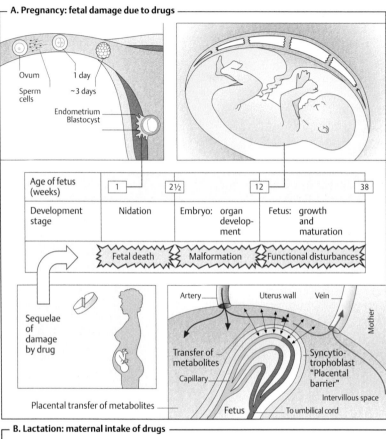

Ovum
Sperm cells
1 day
~3 days
Endometrium
Blastocyst

Age of fetus (weeks)	1	2½	12	38
Development stage	Nidation	Embryo: organ development	Fetus: growth and maturation	

Fetal death   Malformation   Functional disturbances

Sequelae of damage by drug

Artery   Uterus wall   Vein

Transfer of metabolites

Capillary

Syncytiotrophoblast "Placental barrier"

Intervillous space

Mother

Placental transfer of metabolites   Fetus   To umbilical cord

B. Lactation: maternal intake of drugs

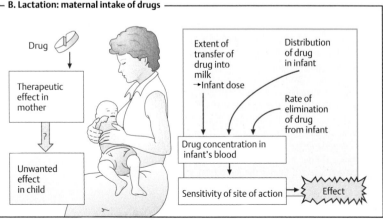

Drug

Therapeutic effect in mother

Unwanted effect in child

Extent of transfer of drug into milk → Infant dose

Distribution of drug in infant

Rate of elimination of drug from infant

Drug concentration in infant's blood

Sensitivity of site of action   Effect

□ Pharmacogenetics

Pharmacogenetics is concerned with the genetic variability of drug effects. Differences in genetic sequences that occur at a frequency of at least 1% are designated as **polymorphisms**. **Rare variants** are observed in less than 1% of a population. Polymorphisms may either influence the pharmacokinetics of a drug (**A**) or occur in the target genes that mediate the therapeutic effect of drugs (**B**).

Genetic variants of pharmacokinetics. Polymorphisms can occur in all genes that participate in the absorption, distribution, biotransformation, and elimination of drugs. Subjects who break down a drug more slowly owing to a genetic defect are classified as "slow metabolizers" or poor metabolizers" in contrast to "normal metabolizers." When delayed biotransformation causes an excessive rise in plasma levels, the incidence of toxic effects increases, as evidenced by the example of the immunosuppressants azathioprine and mercaptopurine. Both substances are converted to inactive methylthiopurines by the enzyme **thiopurine methyltransferase** (TMPT). About 10% of patients carry a genetic polymorphism that leads to reduced TMPT activity and in < 1% enzyme activity is undetectable. As a result of the diminished purine methylation, the plasma level of active drug rises and, hence, the risk of toxic bone marrow damage rises. To avoid unwanted toxic effects, TMPT activity can be determined in erythrocytes before therapy with mercaptopurine is started. In fact, TMPT polymorphism is the first pharmacogenetic test to be introduced into clinical practice. In patients with complete TMPT deficiency, the dose of azathioprine should be reduced by 90%.

Other genetic variants of drug metabolism may have a similar impact: a defect of **N-acetyltransferase 2** impedes the N-acetylation of diverse drugs, including isoniazid, hydralazine, sulfonamides, clonazepam, and nitrazepam. "Slow acetylators" (50–60% of the population) are more likely than "fast acetylators" to develop toxic reactions and neuropathy. A genetic defect of the **cytochrome P450 isozyme CYP2D6** (originally described as debrisoquine–sparteine polymorphism) occurs in ~8% of Europeans and results in delayed elimination of a various drugs, including metoprolol, flecainide, nortriptyline, desipramine, and amitriptyline.

Genetic variants of pharmacodynamics. Genetic polymorphisms can also involve genes that directly or indirectly mediate the effects of drugs and, hence, alter pharmacodynamics (**B**). In these cases, the biological effects of a drug are changed, rather than its plasma levels. The genetic variants of β-adrenoceptors provide an example. For instance, hypertensive patients carrying an arginine at amino acid position 389 of the $β_1$-receptor respond to metoprolol with a more marked fall in blood pressure than do patients carrying a glycine residue at this position. Since $β_1$-blockers have a relatively large margin of safety and, as a rule, dosage is determined by the observed effect, genotyping of patients prior to administration of β-blockers would appear unnecessary.

Future research may be expected to identify numerous genetic polymorphisms in the target molecules of drugs. A genetic examination **before the start of drug therapy** will be a sensible precaution, particularly when drugs with a narrow margin of safety or a long half-life are to be used on a fixed dosage regimen.

A. Genetic variants of pharmacokinetics

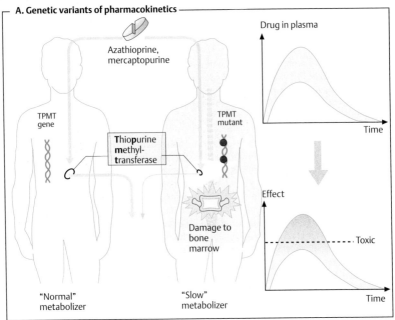

Azathioprine, mercaptopurine

Drug in plasma

Time

TPMT gene

TPMT mutant

Thiopurine methyltransferase

Damage to bone marrow

Effect

Toxic

Time

"Normal" metabolizer

"Slow" metabolizer

B. Genetic variants of pharmacodynamics

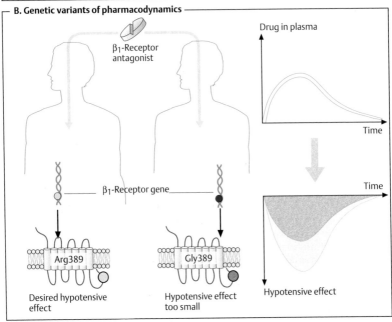

β₁-Receptor antagonist

Drug in plasma

Time

β₁-Receptor gene

Time

Arg389

Gly389

Desired hypotensive effect

Hypotensive effect too small

Hypotensive effect

☐ Placebo (A)

A **placebo** is a dosage form devoid of an active ingredient—a dummy medication. Administration of a placebo may elicit the desired effect (relief of symptoms) or undesired effects that reflect a change in the patient's psychological situation brought about by the therapeutic setting.

Physicians may consciously or unconsciously communicate to the patient whether or not they are concerned about the patient's problem, or are certain about the diagnosis and about the value of prescribed therapeutic measures. In the care of a physician who projects personal warmth, competence, and confidence, the patient in turn feels comfort and less anxiety and optimistically anticipates recovery. The physical condition determines the psychic disposition and vice versa. Consider gravely wounded combatants in war, oblivious to their injuries while fighting to survive, only to experience severe pain in the safety of the field hospital; or the patient with a peptic ulcer caused by emotional stress.

Clinical trials. In the individual case, it may be impossible to decide whether therapeutic success is attributable to the drug or to the therapeutic situation. What is therefore required is a comparison of the effects of a drug and of a placebo in matched groups of patients by means of statistical procedures, i.e., a placebo-controlled trial. For serious diseases, the comparison group has to be treated with the best therapy known to date, rather than a placebo. To be acceptable, the test group receiving the new medicine must show a result superior to that of the comparison group.

A prospective trial is planned in advance. A retrospective (case–control) study follows patients backward in time, the decision to analyze being made only after completion of therapy. Patients are randomly allotted to two groups, namely, the placebo and the active or test drug group. In a double-blind

trial, neither the patients nor the treating physicians know which patient is given drug and which placebo. Finally, a switch from drug to placebo and vice versa can be made in a successive phase of treatment, the crossover trial. In this fashion, drug vs. placebo comparisons can be made not only between two patient groups but also within either group.

Homeopathy (B) is an alternative method of therapy, developed in the 1800s by Samuel Hahnemann. His idea was this: when given in normal (allopathic) dosage, a drug (in the sense of medicament) will produce a constellation of symptoms; however, in a patient whose disease symptoms resemble just this mosaic of symptoms, the same drug (*simile principle*) would effect a cure when given in a very low dosage ("*potentiation*"). The body's self-healing powers were to be properly activated only by minimal doses of the medicinal substance. The homeopath's task is not to diagnose the causes of morbidity, but to find the drug with a "symptom profile" most closely resembling that of the patient's illness. This requires in-depth probing into the patient's complaints. With the accompaniment of a prescribed ("ritualized") shaking procedure, the drug is then highly diluted (in 10-fold or 100-fold series).

No direct action or effect on body functions can be demonstrated for homeopathic medicines. Therapeutic success is due to the suggestive powers of the homeopath and the expectancy of the patient. When an illness is strongly influenced by emotional (psychic) factors and cannot be treated well by allopathic means, a case can be made in favor of exploiting suggestion as a therapeutic tool. Homeopathy is one of several possible methods of doing so.

A. Therapeutic effects resulting from physician's power of suggestion

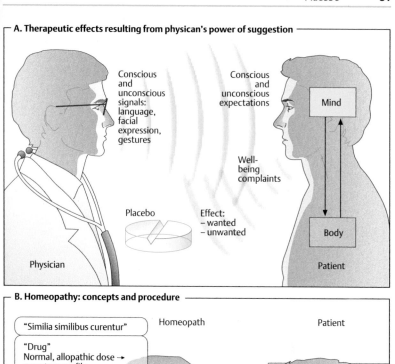

Conscious and unconscious signals: language, facial expression, gestures

Conscious and unconscious expectations

Mind

Well-being complaints

Placebo

Effect:
– wanted
– unwanted

Body

Physician

Patient

B. Homeopathy: concepts and procedure

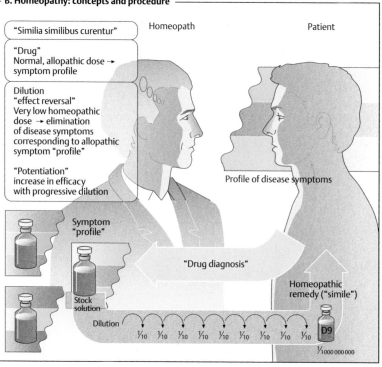

Homeopath

Patient

"Similia similibus curentur"

"Drug"
Normal, allopathic dose → symptom profile

Dilution
"effect reversal"
Very low homeopathic dose → elimination of disease symptoms corresponding to allopathic symptom "profile"

"Potentiation"
increase in efficacy with progressive dilution

Profile of disease symptoms

Symptom "profile"

"Drug diagnosis"

Stock solution

Homeopathic remedy ("simile")

Dilution $\frac{1}{10}$ $\frac{1}{10}$ $\frac{1}{10}$ $\frac{1}{10}$ $\frac{1}{10}$ $\frac{1}{10}$ $\frac{1}{10}$ $\frac{1}{10}$ $\frac{1}{10}$ D9

$\frac{1}{1\,000\,000\,000}$

Systems Pharmacology

□ Sympathetic Nervous System

In the course of phylogeny an efficient control system evolved that enabled the functions of individual organs to be orchestrated in increasingly complex life forms and permitted rapid adaptation to changing environmental conditions. This regulatory system consists of the central nervous system (CNS) (brain plus spinal cord) and two separate pathways for two-way communication with peripheral organs, namely, the somatic and the autonomic nervous systems. The **somatic nervous system**, comprising exteroceptive and interoceptive afferents, special sense organs, and motor efferents, serves to perceive *external* states and to target appropriate body movement (sensory perception: threat → response: flight or attack). The **autonomic** (**vegetative**) **nervous system** (ANS) together with the endocrine system controls the *milieu interieur*. It adjusts internal organ functions to the changing needs of the organism. Neural control permits very quick adaptation, whereas the endocrine system provides for a long-term regulation of functional states. The ANS operates largely beyond voluntary control: it functions autonomously. Its central components reside in the hypothalamus, brainstem, and spinal cord. The ANS also participates in the regulation of endocrine functions.

The ANS has **sympathetic** and **parasympathetic** (p. 102) branches. Both are made up of centrifugal (efferent) and centripetal (afferent) nerves. In many organs innervated by both branches, respective activation of the sympathetic and parasympathetic input evokes opposing responses.

In various disease states (organ malfunctions), drugs are employed with the intention of normalizing susceptible organ functions. To understand the biological effects of substances capable of inhibiting or exciting sympathetic or parasympathetic nerves, one must first envisage the functions subserved by the sympathetic and parasympathetic divisions (**A**, Response to sympathetic activation). In simplistic terms, activation of the sympathetic division can be considered a means by which the body achieves a state of maximal work capacity as required in fight-or-flight situations.

In both cases, there is a need for vigorous activity of skeletal musculature. To ensure adequate supply of oxygen and nutrients, blood flow in skeletal muscle is increased; cardiac rate and contractility are enhanced, resulting in a larger blood volume being pumped into the circulation. Narrowing of splanchnic blood vessels diverts blood into vascular beds in muscle.

Because digestion of food in the intestinal tract is dispensable and essentially counterproductive, the propulsion of intestinal contents is slowed to the extent that peristalsis diminishes and sphincters are narrowed. However, in order to increase nutrient supply to heart and musculature, glucose from the liver and free fatty acids from adipose tissue must be released into the blood. The bronchi are dilated, enabling tidal volume and alveolar oxygen uptake to be increased.

Sweat glands are also innervated by sympathetic fibers (wet palms due to excitement); however, these are exceptional as regards their neurotransmitter (ACh, p. 110).

The lifestyles of modern humans are different from those of our hominid ancestors, but biological functions have remained the same: a "stress"-induced state of maximal work capacity, albeit without energy-consuming muscle activity.

A. Response to sympathetic activation

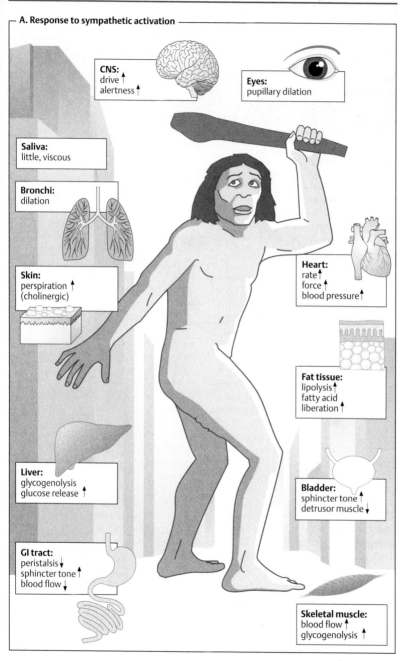

CNS:
drive ↑
alertness ↑

Eyes:
pupillary dilation

Saliva:
little, viscous

Bronchi:
dilation

Skin:
perspiration ↑
(cholinergic)

Heart:
rate ↑
force ↑
blood pressure ↑

Fat tissue:
lipolysis ↑
fatty acid
liberation ↑

Liver:
glycogenolysis
glucose release ↑

Bladder:
sphincter tone ↑
detrusor muscle ↓

GI tract:
peristalsis ↓
sphincter tone ↑
blood flow ↓

Skeletal muscle:
blood flow ↑
glycogenolysis ↑

□ Structure of the Sympathetic Nervous System

The sympathetic preganglionic neurons (first neurons) project from the intermediolateral column of the spinal gray matter to the *paired paravertebral ganglionic chain* lying alongside the vertebral column and to *unpaired prevertebral ganglia*. These **ganglia** represent sites of synaptic contact between **preganglionic axons** (1st neurons) and **nerve cells** (2nd neurons or sympathocytes) that emit axons terminating at **postganglionic synapses** (or contacts) on cells in various end organs. In addition, there are preganglionic neurons that project either to peripheral ganglia in end organs or to the adrenal medulla.

Sympathetic transmitter substances. Whereas **acetylcholine** (see p.104) serves as the chemical transmitter at ganglionic synapses between **first and second neurons**, **norepinephrine** (noradrenaline) is the mediator at synapses of the second neuron (**B**). This second neuron does not synapse with only a single cell in the effector organ; rather it branches out, each branch making *en passant* contacts with several cells. At these junctions the nerve axons form enlargements (**varicosities**) resembling beads on a string. Thus, excitation of the neuron leads to activation of a larger aggregate of effector cells, although the action of released norepinephrine may be confined to the region of each junction. Excitation of preganglionic neurons innervating the adrenal medulla causes liberation of acetylcholine. This, in turn, elicits secretion of **epinephrine** (adrenaline) into the blood, by which it is distributed to body tissues as a hormone (**A**).

□ Adrenergic Synapse

Within the varicosities, norepinephrine is stored in small membrane-enclosed vesicles (granules, 0.05–0.2 μm in diameter). In the axoplasm, norepinephrine is formed by stepwise enzymatic synthesis from L-tyrosine, which is converted by tyrosine hydroxylase to L-Dopa (see p.188). L-Dopa in turn is decarboxylated to dopamine, which is taken up into storage vesicles by the vesicular monoamine transporter (VMAT). In the vesicle, dopamine is converted to norepinephrine by dopamine β-hydroxylase. In the adrenal medulla, the major portion of norepinephrine undergoes enzymatic methylation to epinephrine.

When stimulated electrically, the sympathetic nerve discharges the contents of part of its vesicles, including norepinephrine, into the extracellular space. Liberated **norepinephrine** reacts with **adrenoceptors** located postjunctionally on the membrane of effector cells or prejunctionally on the membrane of varicosities. Activation of pre-synaptic α_2-receptors inhibits norepinephrine release. Through this negative feedback, release can be regulated.

The effect of released norepinephrine wanes quickly, because ~90% is transported back into the axoplasm by a specific transport mechanism (norepinephrine transporter, NAT) and then into storage vesicles by the vesicular transporter (neuronal reuptake). The NAT can be inhibited by tricyclic antidepressants and cocaine. Moreover, norepinephrine is taken up by transporters into the effector cells (extraneuronal monoamine transporter, EMT). Part of the norepinephrine undergoing reuptake is enzymatically inactivated to normetanephrine via **c**atecholamine **O**-**m**ethyl**t**ransferase (COMT, present in the cytoplasm of postjunctional cells) and to dihydroxymandelic acid via **m**ono**a**mine **o**xidase (MAO, present in mitochondria of nerve cells and postjunctional cells).

The liver is richly endowed with COMT and MAO; it therefore contributes significantly to the degradation of circulating norepinephrine and epinephrine. The end product of the combined actions of MAO and COMT is vanillylmandelic acid.

A. Epinephrine as hormone, norepinephrine as transmitter

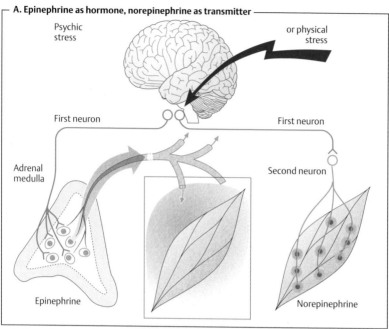

Psychic stress

or physical stress

First neuron

First neuron

Adrenal medulla

Second neuron

Epinephrine

Norepinephrine

B. Second neuron of sympathetic system, varicosity, norepinephrine release

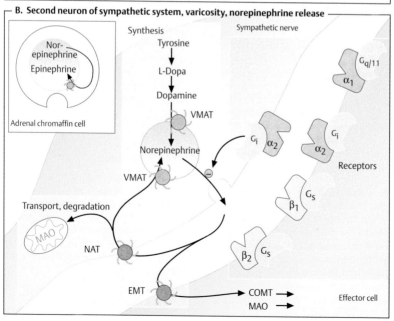

Nor-epinephrine

Epinephrine

Adrenal chromaffin cell

Synthesis

Sympathetic nerve

Tyrosine

L-Dopa

Dopamine

VMAT

$G_{q/11}$

α_1

Norepinephrine

G_i α_2

VMAT

G_i α_2

Receptors

Transport, degradation

G_s β_1

MAO

NAT

β_2 G_s

EMT

COMT

MAO

Effector cell

□ Adrenoceptor Subtypes and Catecholamine Actions

The biological effects of epinephrine and norepinephrine are mediated by nine different adrenoceptors ($\alpha_{1A,B,D}$, $\alpha_{2A,B,C}$, β_1, β_2, β_3). To date, only the classification into α_1, α_2, β_1 and β_2 receptors has therapeutic relevance.

□ Smooth Muscle Effects

The opposing effects on smooth muscle (**A**) of α- and β-adrenoceptor activation are due to differences in signal transduction. α_1-Receptor stimulation leads to intracellular release of Ca^{2+} via activation of the inositol trisphosphate (IP_3) pathway. In concert with the protein calmodulin, Ca^{2+} can activate myosin kinase, leading to a rise in tonus via phosphorylation of the contractile protein myosin ($\rightarrow$ vasoconstriction). α_2-Adrenoceptors can also elicit a contraction of smooth muscle cells by activating phospholipase C (PLC) via the βγ-subunits of G_1 proteins.

cAMP inhibits activation of myosin kinase. Via stimulatory G-proteins (G_s), β_2-receptors mediate an increase in cAMP production ($\rightarrow$ vasodilation).

Vasoconstriction induced by local application of α-sympathomimetics can be employed in infiltration anesthesia (p. 204) or for nasal decongestion (naphazoline, tetrahydrozoline, xylometazoline; p. 94, 336, 338). Systemically administered epinephrine is important in the treatment of anaphylactic shock and cardiac arrest.

Bronchodilation. β_2-Adrenoceptor-mediated *bronchodilation* plays an essential part in the treatment of bronchial asthma and chronic obstructive lung disease (p. 340). For this purpose, β_2-agonists are usually given by inhalation; preferred agents being those with low oral bioavailability and low risk of systemic unwanted effects (e. g., fenoterol, salbutamol, terbutaline).

Tocolysis. The uterine relaxant effect of β_2-adrenoceptor agonists, such as fenoterol, can be used to prevent *premature labor*. β_2-Vasodilation in the mother with an imminent drop in systemic blood pressure results in reflex tachycardia, which is also due in part to the β_1-stimulant action of these drugs.

□ Cardiostimulation

By stimulating β-receptors, and hence **cAMP** production, catecholamines augment all heart functions including systolic force, velocity of myocyte shortening, sinoatrial rate, conduction velocity, and excitability. In pacemaker fibers, cAMP-gated channels ("pacemaker channels") are activated, whereby *diastolic depolarization* is hastened and the firing threshold for the action potential is reached sooner (**B**). cAMP activates protein kinase A, which phosphorylates different Ca^{2+} transport proteins. In this way, contraction of heart muscle cells is accelerated, as more Ca^{2+} enters the cell from the extracellular space via L-type Ca^{2+} channels and release of Ca^{2+} from the sarcoplasmic reticulum (via ryanodine receptors, RyR) is augmented. Faster relaxation of heart muscle cells is effected by phosphorylation of troponin and phospholamban.

In acute heart failure or cardiac arrest, β-mimetics are used as a short-term emergency measure; in chronic failure they are not indicated.

□ Metabolic Effects

Via cAMP, β_2-receptors mediate increased conversion of glycogen to glucose (*glycogenolysis*) in both liver and skeletal muscle. From the liver, glucose is released into the blood. In adipose tissue, triglycerides are hydrolyzed to fatty acids (*lipolysis* mediated by β_2- and β_3-receptors), which then enter the blood.

A. Effects of catecholamines on vascular smooth muscle

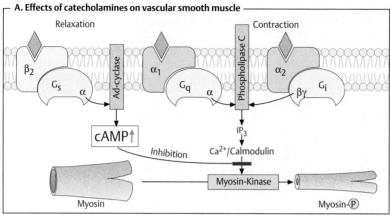

B. Cardiac effects of catecholamines

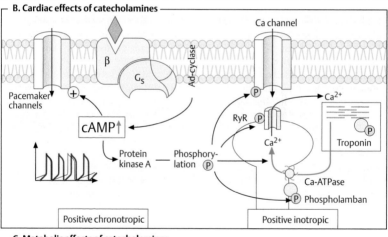

C. Metabolic effects of catecholamines

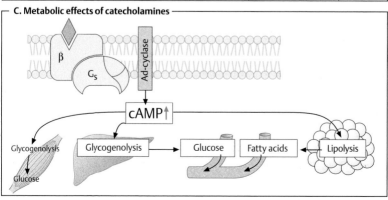

□ Structure–Activity Relationships of Sympathomimetics

Owing to its equally high affinity for all α- and β-receptors, epinephrine does not permit selective activation of a particular receptor subtype. Like most catecholamines, it is also unsuitable for oral administration (catechole is a trivial name for *o*-hydroxyphenol). Norepinephrine differs from epinephrine by its high affinity for α-receptors and low affinity for $β_2$-receptors. The converse holds true for the synthetic substance, isoproterenol (isoprenaline) (**A**).

Norepinephrine   →   α, $β_1$
Epinephrine   →   α, $β_1$ $β_2$
Isoproterenol   → $β_1$, $β_2$

Knowledge of **structure–activity relationships** has permitted the synthesis of sympathomimetics that display a high degree of selectivity at adrenoceptor subtypes.

Direct-acting sympathomimetics (i.e. adrenoceptor agonists) typically share a *phenlethylamine* structure. The *side chain β-hydroxyl group* confers affinity for α- and β-receptors. *Substitution on the amino group* reduces affinity for α-receptors, but increases it for β-receptors (exception: α-agonist phenylephrine), with optimal affinity being seen after the introduction of only one isopropyl group. Increasing the bulk of amino substituents favors affinity for $β_2$-receptors (e.g., fenoterol, salbutamol). Both *hydroxyl groups* on the aromatic nucleus contribute to affinity; high activity at α-receptors is associated with hydroxyl groups at the 3 and 4 positions. Affinity for β-receptors is preserved in congeners bearing hydroxyl groups at positions 3 and 5 (orciprenaline, terbutaline, fenoterol).

The hydroxyl groups of catecholamines are responsible for the very low lipophilicity of these substances. Polarity is increased at physiological pH owing to protonation of the amino group. Deletion of one or all hydroxyl groups improves the membrane penetrability at the intestinal mucosa–blood barrier and the blood–brain barrier. Accordingly, these noncatecholamine congeners can be given orally and can exert CNS actions; however, this structural change entails a loss in affinity.

Absence of one or both aromatic hydroxyl groups is associated with an increase in **indirect sympathomimetic activity**, denoting the ability of a substance to release norepinephrine from its neuronal stores without exerting an agonist action at the adrenoceptor (p. 92).

A change in position of aromatic hydroxyl groups (e.g., in orciprenaline, fenoterol, or terbutaline) or their substitution (e.g., salbutamol) protects against *inactivation by COMT* (p. 87). Introduction of a small alkyl residue at the carbon atom adjacent to the amino group (ephedrine, methamphetamine) confers resistance to *degradation by MAO* (p. 87); replacement on the amino groups of the methyl residue with larger substituents (e.g., ethyl in etilefrine) impedes deamination by MAO. Accordingly, the congeners are less subject to presystemic inactivation.

Since structural requirements for high affinity on the one hand and oral applicability on the other do not match, choosing a sympathomimetic is a matter of compromise. If the high affinity of epinephrine is to be exploited, absorbability from the intestine must be foregone (epinephrine, isoprenaline). If good bioavailability with oral administration is desired, losses in receptor affinity must be accepted (etilefrine).

A. Interaction between epinephrine and the β_2-adrenoceptor

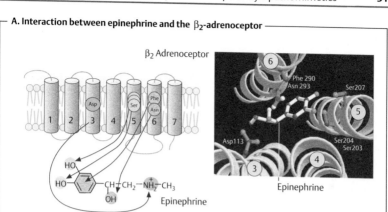

β_2 Adrenoceptor

Epinephrine

B. Structure–activity relationship of epinephrine

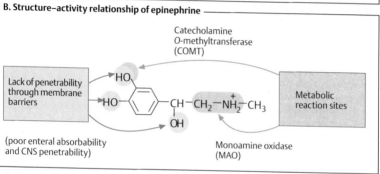

Catecholamine
O-methyltransferase
(COMT)

Lack of penetrability
through membrane
barriers

Metabolic
reaction sites

(poor enteral absorbability
and CNS penetrability)

Monoamine oxidase
(MAO)

C. Direct sympathomimetics

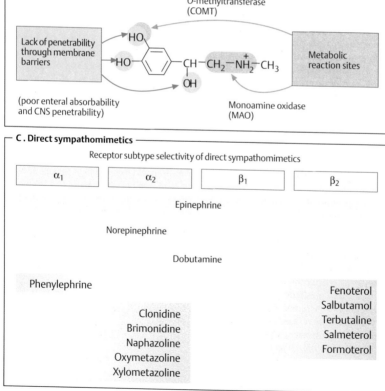

Receptor subtype selectivity of direct sympathomimetics

α_1	α_2	β_1	β_2

Epinephrine

Norepinephrine

Dobutamine

Phenylephrine

Clonidine
Brimonidine
Naphazoline
Oxymetazoline
Xylometazoline

Fenoterol
Salbutamol
Terbutaline
Salmeterol
Formoterol

□ Indirect Sympathomimetics

Raising the concentration of norepinephrine in the synaptic space intensifies the stimulation of adrenoceptors. In principle, this can be achieved by:

- Promoting the neuronal release of norepinephrine
- Inhibiting processes operating to lower its intrasynaptic concentration, in particular neuronal reuptake with subsequent vesicular storage or breakdown by monoamine oxidase (MAO)

Chemically altered derivatives differ from norepinephrine with regard to the relative affinity for these systems and affect these functions differentially.

Inhibitors of MAO (A) block enzyme located in mitochondria, which serves to scavenge axoplasmic free norepinephrine (NE). Inhibition of the enzyme causes free NE concentrations to rise. Likewise, dopamine catabolism is impaired, making more of it available for NE synthesis. In the CNS, inhibition of MAO affects neuronal storage not only of NE but also of dopamine and serotonin. The functional sequelae of these changes include a general increase in psychomotor drive (thymeretic effect) and mood elevation (**A**). *Moclobemide* reversibly inhibits MAO_A and is used as an antidepressant. The MAO_B inhibitor *selegiline* (deprenyl) retards the catabolism of dopamine, an effect used in the treatment of Parkinsonism (p. 188).

Indirect sympathomimetics (B) in the narrow sense comprise amphetamine-like substances and cocaine. Cocaine blocks the norepinephrine transporter (NAT), besides acting as a local anesthetic. Amphetamine is taken up into varicosities via NAT, and from there into storage vesicles (via the vesicular monoamine transporter), where it displaces NE into the cytosol. In addition, amphetamine blocks MAO, allowing cytosolic NE concentration to rise unimpeded. This induces the plasmalemmal NAT to transport NE in the opposite direction, that is, to liberate it into the extracellular space. Thus, amphetamine promotes a nonexocytotic release of NE. The effectiveness of such indirect sympathomimetics diminishes quickly or disappears (**tachyphylaxis**) with repeated administration.

Indirect sympathomimetics can penetrate the blood–brain barrier and evoke such CNS effects as a feeling of well-being, enhanced physical activity and mood (**euphoria**), and decreased sense of hunger or fatigue. Subsequently, the user may feel tired and depressed. These after-effects are partly responsible for the urge to readminister the drug (high abuse potential). To prevent their misuse, these substances are subject to governmental regulations (e. g., Food and Drugs Act, Canada; Controlled Drugs Act, USA) restricting their prescription and distribution.

When amphetamine-like substances are misused to enhance athletic performance ("*doping*"), there is a risk of dangerous physical overexertion. Because of the absence of a sense of fatigue, a drugged athlete may be able to mobilize ultimate energy reserves. In extreme situations, cardiovascular failure may result (**B**).

Closely related chemically to amphetamine are the so-called appetite suppressants or anorexiants (p. 329). These may also cause dependence and their therapeutic value and safety are questionable. Some of these (D-norpseudoephedrine, amfepramone) have been withdrawn.

Sibutramine inhibits neuronal reuptake of NE and serotonin (similarly to antidepressants, p. 226). It diminishes appetite and is classified as an antiobesity agent (p. 328).

A. Monoamine oxidase inhibitor

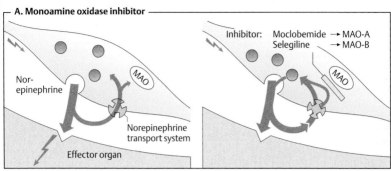

Nor-epinephrine

Norepinephrine transport system

Effector organ

Inhibitor: Moclobemide → MAO-A
Seleglinie → MAO-B

MAO

B. Indirect sympathomimetics with central stimulant activity and abuse potential

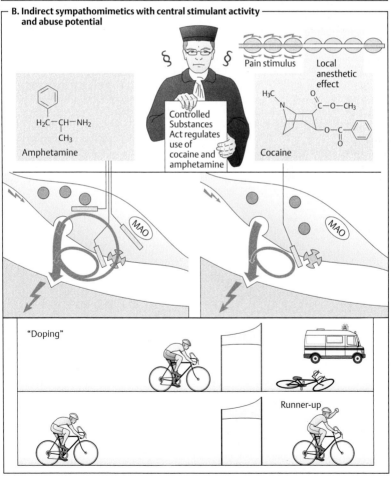

Pain stimulus

Local anesthetic effect

$H_2C-CH-NH_2$
CH_3

Amphetamine

Controlled Substances Act regulates use of cocaine and amphetamine

H_3C

Cocaine

MAO

MAO

"Doping"

Runner-up

□ α-Sympathomimetics, α-Sympatholytics

α-**Sympathomimetics** can be used *systemically* in certain types of hypotension (p. 324) and *locally* for nasal or conjunctival decongestion (p. 336) or as adjuncts in infiltration anesthesia (p. 204) for the purpose of delaying the removal of local anesthetic. With local use, underperfusion of the vasoconstricted area results in a lack of oxygen (**A**). In the extreme case, local hypoxia can lead to tissue necrosis. The appendages (e. g., digits, toes, ears) are particularly vulnerable in this regard, thus precluding vasoconstrictor adjuncts in infiltration anesthesia at these sites.

Vasoconstriction induced by an α-sympathomimetic is followed by a phase of enhanced blood flow (**reactive hyperemia, A**). This reaction can be observed after applying α-sympathomimetics (naphazoline, tetrahydrozoline, xylometazoline) to the nasal mucosa. Initially, vasoconstriction reduces mucosal blood flow and, hence, capillary pressure. Fluid exuded into the interstitial space is drained through the veins, thus shrinking the nasal mucosa. Owing to the reduced supply of fluid, secretion of nasal mucus decreases. In coryza, nasal patency is restored. However, after vasoconstriction subsides, reactive hyperemia causes renewed exudation of plasma fluid into the interstitial space, the nose is "stuffy" again, and the patient feels a need to reapply decongestant. In this way, a vicious cycle threatens. Besides rebound congestion, persistent use of a decongestant entails the risk of atrophic damage caused by the prolonged hypoxia of the nasal mucosa.

α-**Sympatholytics (B).** The interaction of norepinephrine with α-adrenoceptors can be inhibited by α-sympatholytics (α-adrenoceptor antagonists, α-blockers). This inhibition can be put to therapeutic use in antihypertensive treatment (vasodilation → peripheral resistance ↓, blood pressure ↓, p. 122). The first α-sympatholytics blocked the action of norepinephrine not only at *postsynaptic* α_1-adrenoceptors but also at *presynaptic* α_2-receptors (**nonselective α-blockers**, e. g., phenoxybenzamine, phentolamine).

Presynaptic α_2-adrenoceptors function like sensors that enable norepinephrine concentration outside the axolemma to be monitored, thus regulating its release via a local feedback mechanism. When presynaptic α_2-receptors are stimulated, further release of norepinephrine is inhibited. Conversely, their blockade leads to uncontrolled release of norepinephrine with an overt enhancement of sympathetic effects at β_1-adrenoceptor-mediated myocardial neuroeffector junctions, resulting in tachycardia and tachyarrhythmia.

Selective α_1-Sympatholytics (α_1-**blockers**, e. g., prazosin, or the longer-acting terazosin and doxazosin) do not disinhibit norepinephrine release.

α_1-Blockers may be used in hypertension (p. 315). Because they prevent reflex vasoconstriction, they are likely to cause postural hypotension with pooling of blood in lower limb capacitance veins during change from the supine to the erect position (orthostatic collapse, p. 324).

In benign hyperplasia of the prostate, α_1-blockers (terazosin, alfuzosin, tamsulosin) may serve to lower tonus of smooth musculature in the prostatic region and thereby improve micturition. Tamsulosin shows enhanced affinity for the α_{1A} subtype; the risk of hypotension is therefore supposedly diminished.

A. Reactive hyperemia due to α-sympathomimetics, e.g., following decongestion of nasal mucosa

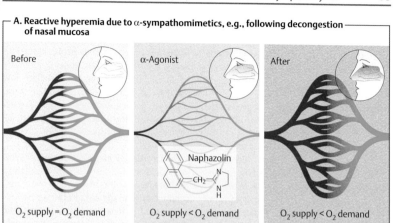

Before

α-Agonist

Naphazolin

After

O₂ supply = O₂ demand

O₂ supply < O₂ demand

O₂ supply < O₂ demand

B. Autoinhibition of norepinephrine release and α-sympatholytics

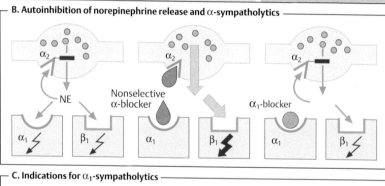

NE

Nonselective α-blocker

α₁-blocker

C. Indications for α₁-sympatholytics

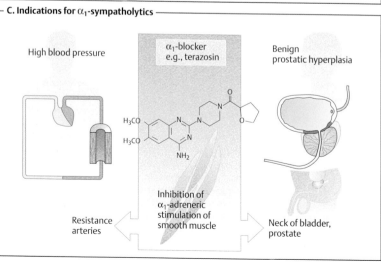

High blood pressure

α₁-blocker e.g., terazosin

Benign prostatic hyperplasia

Resistance arteries

Inhibition of α₁-adreneric stimulation of smooth muscle

Neck of bladder, prostate

□ β-Sympatholytics (β-Blockers)

β-Sympatholytics are antagonists of norepinephrine and epinephrine at β-adrenoceptors; they lack affinity for α-receptors.

Therapeutic effects. β-Blockers protect the heart from the oxygen-wasting effect of sympathetic inotropism by blocking cardiac β-receptors; thus, cardiac work can no longer be augmented above basal levels (the heart is "coasting"). This effect is utilized *prophylactically in angina pectoris* to prevent a myocardial stress that could trigger an ischemic attack (p. 316). β-Blockers also serve to *lower cardiac rate* (sinus tachycardia, p. 136) and *protect the failing heart* against excessive sympathetic drive (p. 322). β-Blockers lower *elevated blood pressure.* The mechanism underlying their *antihypertensive action* is unclear. Applied topically to the eye, β-blockers are used in the management of *glaucoma*; they lower production of aqueous humor (p. 346).

Undesired effects. β-Blockers are used very frequently and are mostly well tolerated if risk constellations are taken into account. The hazards of treatment with β-blockers become apparent particularly when continuous activation of β-receptors is needed in order to maintain the function of an organ.

Congestive heart failure. For a long time, β-blockers were considered generally contraindicated in heart failure. Increased release of norepinephrine gives rise to an increase in heart rate and systolic muscle tension, enabling cardiac output to be maintained despite progressive cardiac disease. When sympathetic drive is eliminated during β-receptor-blockade, stroke volume and cardiac rate decline, a latent myocardial insufficiency is unmasked, and overt insufficiency is exacerbated. Sympathoactivation not only helps for some time to maintain pump function in chronic congestive failure but itself also contributes to the progression of insufficiency: triggering of arrhythmias, increased O_2-consumption, enhanced cardiac hypertrophy (**A**).

On the other hand, convincing clinical evidence demonstrates that, under appropriate conditions (prior testing of tolerability, low dosage), β-blockers are able to improve prognosis in congestive heart failure. Protection against heart rate increases and arrhythmias may be important underlying factors.

Bradycardia, AV block. Elimination of sympathetic drive can lead to a marked fall in cardiac rate as well as to disorders of impulse conduction from the atria to the ventricles.

Bronchial asthma. Increased sympathetic activity prevents bronchospasm in patients disposed to paroxysmal constriction of the bronchial tree (bronchial asthma, bronchitis in smokers). In this condition, β_2-receptor blockade may precipitate acute respiratory distress (**B**).

Hypoglycemia in diabetes mellitus. When treatment with insulin or oral hypoglycemics in the diabetic patient lowers blood glucose below a critical level, epinephrine is released, which then stimulates hepatic glucose release via activation of β_2-receptors. β-Blockers suppress this counterregulation, besides masking other epinephrine-mediated warning signs of imminent hypoglycemia, such as tachycardia and anxiety. The danger of hypoglycemic shock is therefore aggravated.

Altered vascular responses: When β_2-receptors are blocked, the vasodilating effect of epinephrine is abolished, leaving the α-receptor-mediated vasoconstriction unaffected: "*cold hands and feet.*"

β-Blockers exert an "**anxiolytic**" action that may be due to the suppression of somatic responses (palpitations; trembling) to epinephrine release that is induced by emotional stress; in turn, these responses would exacerbate "anxiety" or "stage-fright." Because alertness is not impaired by β-blockers, these agents are occasionally taken by orators and musicians before a major performance (**C**).

A. β-Sympatholytics: effect on cardiac function

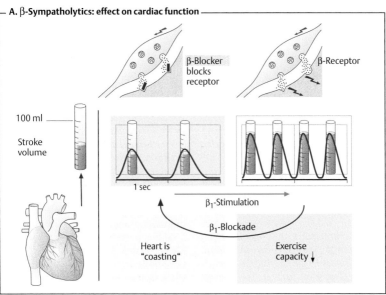

B. β-Sympatholytics: effect on bronchial and vascular tone

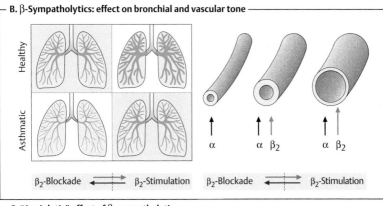

C. "Anxiolytic" effect of β-sympatholytics

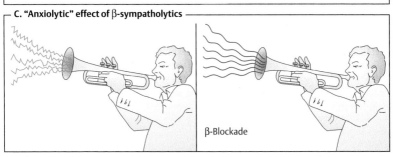

□ Types of β-Blockers

The basic structure shared by most β-sympatholytics (p. 11) is the side chain of β-sympathomimetics (cf. isoproterenol with the β-blockers propranolol, pindolol, atenolol). As a rule, this basic structure is linked to an aromatic nucleus by a methylene and oxygen bridge. The side chain C-atom bearing the hydroxyl group forms the chiral center. With some exceptions (e. g., timolol, penbutolol), all β-sympatholytics exist as racemates (p. 62).

Compared with the dextrorotatory form, the levorotatory enantiomer possesses a greater than 100-fold higher affinity for the β-receptor, and is, therefore, practically alone in contributing to the β-blocking effect of the racemate. The side chain and substituents on the amino group critically affect affinity for β-receptors, whereas the aromatic nucleus determines whether the compound possesses **intrinsic sympathomimetic activity** (**ISA**), that is, acts as a *partial* agonist or partial antagonist. A partial agonism or antagonism is present when the intrinsic activity of a drug is so small that, even with full occupancy of all available receptors, the effect obtained is only a fraction of that elicited by a full agonist. In the presence of a partial agonist (e. g., pindolol), the ability of a full agonist (e. g., isoprenaline) to elicit a maximal effect would be attenuated, because binding of the full agonist is impeded. Partial agonists thus also act antagonistically, although they maintain a certain degree of receptor stimulation. It remains an open question whether ISA confers a therapeutic advantage on a β-blocker. At any rate, patients with congestive heart failure should be treated with β-blockers devoid of ISA.

As cationic amphiphilic drugs, β-blockers can exert a **membrane-stabilizing effect**, as evidenced by the ability of the more lipophilic congeners to inhibit Na^+ channel function and impulse conduction in cardiac tissues. At the usual therapeutic dosage, the high concentration required for these effects will not be reached.

Some β-sympatholytics possess higher affinity for cardiac β_1-receptors than for β_2-receptors and thus display **cardioselectivity** (e. g., metoprolol, acebutolol, atenolol, bisoprolol, $\beta_1 : \beta_2$ selectivity 20–50-fold). None of these blockers is sufficiently selective to permit use in patients with bronchial asthma or diabetes mellitus (p. 96).

The chemical structure of β-blockers also determines their **pharmacokinetic properties**. Except for hydrophilic representatives (atenolol), β-sympatholytics are completely absorbed from the intestines and subsequently undergo **presystemic elimination** to a major extent (**A**).

All the above differences are of little clinical importance. The abundance of commercially available congeners would thus appear all the more curious (**B**). Propranolol was the first β-blocker to be introduced into therapy in 1965. Thirty years later, about 20 different congeners were marketed in different countries (analogue preparations). This questionable development is unfortunately typical of any drug group that combines therapeutic with commercial success, in addition to having a relatively fixed active structure. Variation of the molecule will create a new *patentable* chemical, not necessarily a drug with a novel action. Moreover, a drug no longer protected by patent is offered as a *generic* by different manufacturers under dozens of different proprietary names. Propranolol alone has been marketed in 2003 by 12 manufacturers in Germany under nine different names. In the USA, the drug is at present offered by ~40 manufacturers, mostly under its generic designation, and in Canada by six manufacturers, mostly under a hyphenated brand name containing its INN with a prefix.

A. Types of β-sympatholytics

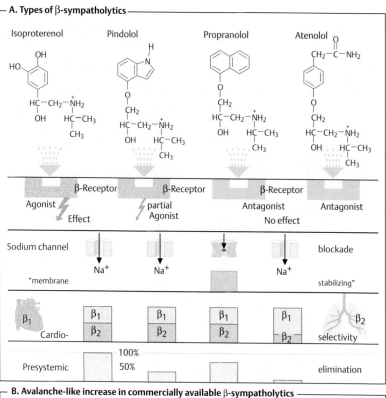

B. Avalanche-like increase in commercially available β-sympatholytics

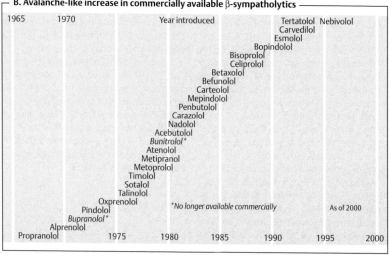

*No longer available commercially

As of 2000

□ Antiadrenergics

Antiadrenergics are drugs capable of lowering transmitter output from sympathetic neurons, i. e., the "sympathetic tone." Their action is hypotensive (indication: hypertension, p. 314); however, being poorly tolerated, they enjoy only limited therapeutic use.

Clonidine is an α_2-agonist whose high lipophilicity (dichlorophenyl ring) permits rapid penetration through the blood–brain barrier. The activation of *postsynaptic* α_2-receptors dampens the activity of vasomotor neurons in the medulla oblongata, resulting in a resetting of systemic arterial pressure at a lower level. In addition, activation of presynaptic α_2-receptors in the periphery (pp. 86, 94) leads to a decreased release of both norepinephrine (NE) and acetylcholine. Beside its main use as an antihypertensive, clonidine is also employed to manage withdrawal reactions in subjects being treated for opioid addiction.

Side effects. Lassitude, dry mouth; rebound hypertension after abrupt cessation of clonidine therapy.

Methyldopa (dopa = **d**ihydr**o**xy**p**henyl**a**lanine), being an amino acid, is transported across the blood–brain barrier, decarboxylated in the brain to α-methyldopamine, and then hydroxylated to α-methyl-NE. The decarboxylation of methyldopa competes for a portion of the available enzymatic activity so that the rate of conversion of L-dopa to NE (via dopamine) is decreased. The *false transmitter* α-methyl-NE can be stored; however, unlike the endogenous mediator, it has a higher affinity for α_2- than for α_1-receptors and therefore produces effects similar to those of clonidine. The same events take place in peripheral adrenergic neurons.

Adverse effects. Fatigue, orthostatic hypotension, extrapyramidal Parkinson-like symptoms (p. 188), cutaneous reactions, hepatic damage, immune-hemolytic anemia.

Reserpine, an alkaloid from the climbing shrub *Rauwolfia serpentina* (native to the Indian subcontinent), abolishes the vesicular storage of biogenic amines (NE, dopamine [DA], serotonin [5-HT]) by inhibiting the (nonselective) vesicular monoamine transporter located in the membrane of storage vesicles. Since the monoamines are not taken up into vesicles, they become subject to catabolism by MAO; the amount of NE released per nerve impulse is decreased. To a lesser degree, release of epinephrine from the adrenal medulla is also impaired. At higher doses, there is irreversible damage to storage vesicles ("pharmacological sympathectomy"), days to weeks being required for their re-synthesis. Reserpine readily enters the brain, where it also impairs vesicular storage of biogenic amines.

Adverse effects. Disorders of extrapyramidal motor function with development of pseudo-parkinsonism (p. 188), sedation, depression, stuffy nose, impaired libido, impotence; and increased appetite.

Guanethidine possesses high affinity for the axolemmal and vesicular amine transporters. It is stored instead of NE, but is unable to mimic functions of the latter. In addition, it stabilizes the axonal membrane, thereby impeding the propagation of impulses into the sympathetic nerve terminals. Storage and release of epinephrine from the adrenal medulla are not affected, owing to the absence of a reuptake process. The drug does not cross the blood–brain barrier.

Adverse effects. Cardiovascular crises are a possible risk: emotional stress of the patient may cause sympathoadrenal activation with epinephrine release from the adrenal medulla. The resulting rise in blood pressure can be all the more marked as persistent depression of sympathetic nerve activity induces supersensitivity of effector organs to circulating catecholamines.

A. Inhibitors of sympathetic tone

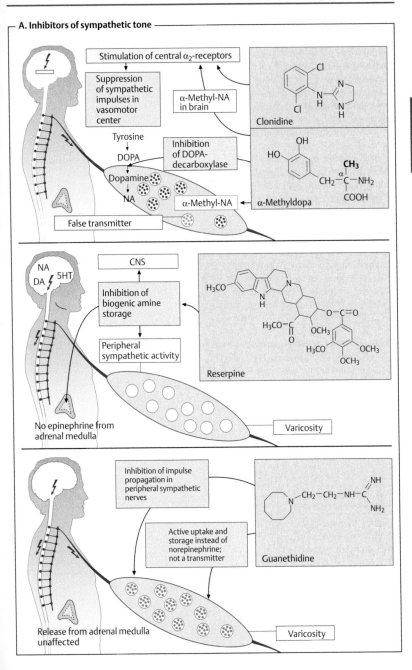

Stimulation of central α_2-receptors

Suppression of sympathetic impulses in vasomotor center

α-Methyl-NA in brain

Clonidine

Tyrosine
↓
DOPA

Inhibition of DOPA-decarboxylase

Dopamine
↓
NA

α-Methyl-NA ← α-Methyldopa

False transmitter

NA DA 5HT

CNS

Inhibition of biogenic amine storage

Peripheral sympathetic activity

Reserpine

No epinephrine from adrenal medulla

Varicosity

Inhibition of impulse propagation in peripheral sympathetic nerves

Active uptake and storage instead of norepinephrine; not a transmitter

Guanethidine

Release from adrenal medulla unaffected

Varicosity

□ Parasympathetic Nervous System

Responses to activation of the parasympathetic system. Parasympathetic nerves regulate processes connected with energy assimilation (food intake, digestion, absorption) and storage. These processes operate when the body is at rest, allowing a decreased tidal volume (increased bronchomotor tone) and decreased cardiac activity. Secretion of saliva and intestinal fluids promotes the digestion of food stuffs; transport of intestinal contents is speeded up because of enhanced peristaltic activity and lowered tone of sphincteric muscles. To empty the urinary bladder (micturition), wall tension is increased by detrusor activation with a concurrent relaxation of sphincter tonus.

Activation of ocular parasympathetic fibers (see below) results in narrowing of the pupil and increased curvature of the lens, enabling near objects to be brought into focus (accommodation).

Anatomy of the parasympathetic system. The cell bodies of parasympathetic preganglionic neurons are located in the brainstem and the sacral spinal cord. Parasympathetic outflow is channeled from the brainstem (1) through the third cranial nerve (oculomotor n.) via the ciliary ganglion to the eye; (2) through the seventh cranial nerve (facial n.) via the pterygopalatine and submaxillary ganglia to lachrymal glands and salivary glands (sublingual, submandibular), respectively; (3) through the ninth cranial nerve (glossopharyngeal n.) via the otic ganglion to the parotid gland; and (4) via the tenth cranial nerve (vagus n.) to intramural ganglia in thoracic and abdominal viscera. Approximately 75% of all parasympathetic fibers are contained within the vagus nerve. The neurons of the sacral division innervate the distal colon, rectum, bladder, the distal ureters, and the external genitalia.

Acetylcholine (ACh) as a transmitter. ACh serves as mediator at terminals of all postganglionic parasympathetic fibers, in addition to fulfilling its transmitter role at ganglionic synapses within both the sympathetic and parasympathetic divisions and the motor end plates on striated muscle (p. 182). However, different types of receptors are present at these synaptic junctions (see table). The existence of distinct cholinoceptors at different cholinergic synapses allows selective pharmacological interventions.

Localization of Receptors	Agonist	Antagonist	Receptor Type
Target tissues of 2nd parasympathetic neurons; e. g., smooth muscle, glands	ACh Muscarine	Atropine	Muscarinic (M) cholinoceptor; G-protein-coupled receptor protein with 7 transmembrane domains
Sympathetic & parasympathetic gangliocytes	ACh Nicotine	Trimethaphan	Ganglionic type
Motor end plate in skeletal muscle	ACh Nicotine	d-Tubocurarine	Nicotinic (N) cholinoceptor ligand-gated cation channel
			Muscle type

A. Responses to parasympathetic activation

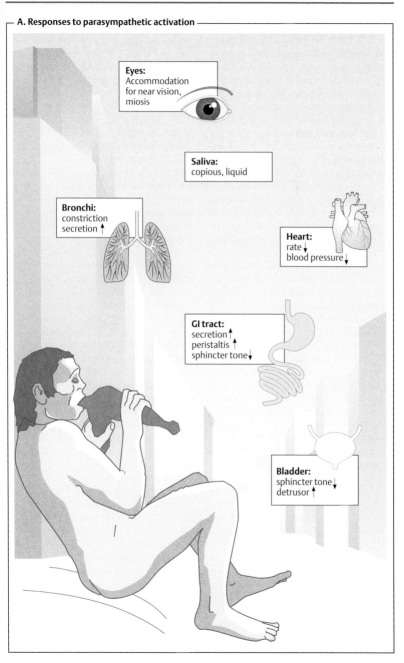

Eyes:
Accommodation for near vision, miosis

Saliva:
copious, liquid

Bronchi:
constriction
secretion ↑

Heart:
rate ↓
blood pressure ↓

GI tract:
secretion ↑
peristaltis ↑
sphincter tone ↓

Bladder:
sphincter tone ↓
detrusor ↑

□ Cholinergic Synapse

Acetylcholine (ACh) is the transmitter at postganglionic synapses of parasympathetic nerve endings. It is highly concentrated in synaptic storage vesicles densely present in the axoplasm of the presynaptic terminal. ACh is formed from **choline** and activated acetate (**acetylcoenzyme A**), a reaction catalyzed by the cytosolic enzyme **choline acetyltransferase**. The highly polar choline is taken up into the axoplasm by the specific choline-transporter (CHT) localized to membranes of cholinergic axons terminals and a subset of storage vesicles. During persistent or intensive stimulation, the CHT ensures that ACh synthesis and release are sustained. The newly formed ACh is loaded into storage vesicles by the vesicular ACh transporter (VAChT). The mechanism of transmitter release is not known in full detail. The vesicles are anchored via the protein synapsin to the cytoskeletal network. This arrangement permits clustering of vesicles near the presynaptic membrane while preventing fusion with it. During activation of the nerve membrane, Ca^{2+} is thought to enter the axoplasm through voltage-gated channels and to activate protein kinases that phosphorylate synapsin. As a result, vesicles close to the membrane are detached from their anchoring and allowed to fuse with the presynaptic membrane. During fusion, vesicles discharge their contents into the synaptic gap and simultaneously insert CHT into the plasma membrane. ACh quickly diffuses through the synaptic gap (the acetylcholine molecule is a little longer than 0.5 nm; the synaptic gap as narrow as 20–30 nm). At the postsynaptic effector cell membrane, ACh reacts with its **receptors**. As these receptors can also be activated by the alkaloid muscarine, they are referred to as **muscarinic (M-) ACh receptors**. In contrast, at ganglionic and motor end plate (p.182) ACh receptors, the action of ACh is mimicked by nicotine and, hence, mediated by **nicotinic ACh receptors**.

Released ACh is rapidly hydrolyzed and inactivated by a specific **acetylcholinesterase**, localized to pre- and postjunctional membranes (basal lamina of motor end plates), or by a less specific serum cholinesterase (butyrylcholinesterase), a soluble enzyme present in serum and interstitial fluid.

M-ACh receptors can be divided into five subtypes according to their molecular structure, signal transduction, and ligand affinity. Here, the M_1, M_2 and M_3 receptor subtypes are considered. M_1 receptors are present on nerve cells, e.g., in ganglia, where they enhance impulse transmission from preganglionic axon terminals to ganglion cells. M_2 receptors mediate acetylcholine effects on the heart: opening of K^+ channels leads to slowing of diastolic depolarization in sinoatrial pacemaker cells and a decrease in heart rate. M_3 receptors play a role in the regulation of smooth muscle tone, e.g., in the gut and bronchi, where their activation causes stimulation of phospholipase C, membrane depolarization, and increase in muscle tone. M_3 receptors are also found in glandular epithelia, which similarly respond with activation of phospholipase C and increased secretory activity. In the CNS, where all subtypes are present, ACh receptors serve diverse functions ranging from regulation of cortical excitability, memory and learning, pain processing, and brainstem motor control.

In blood vessels, the relaxant action of ACh on muscle tone is indirect, because it involves stimulation of M_3-cholinoceptors on endothelial cells that respond by liberating NO (nitrous oxid = endothelium-derived relaxing factor). The latter diffuses into the subjacent smooth musculature, where it causes a relaxation of active tonus (p.124).

— A. Acetylcholine: release, effects, and degradation

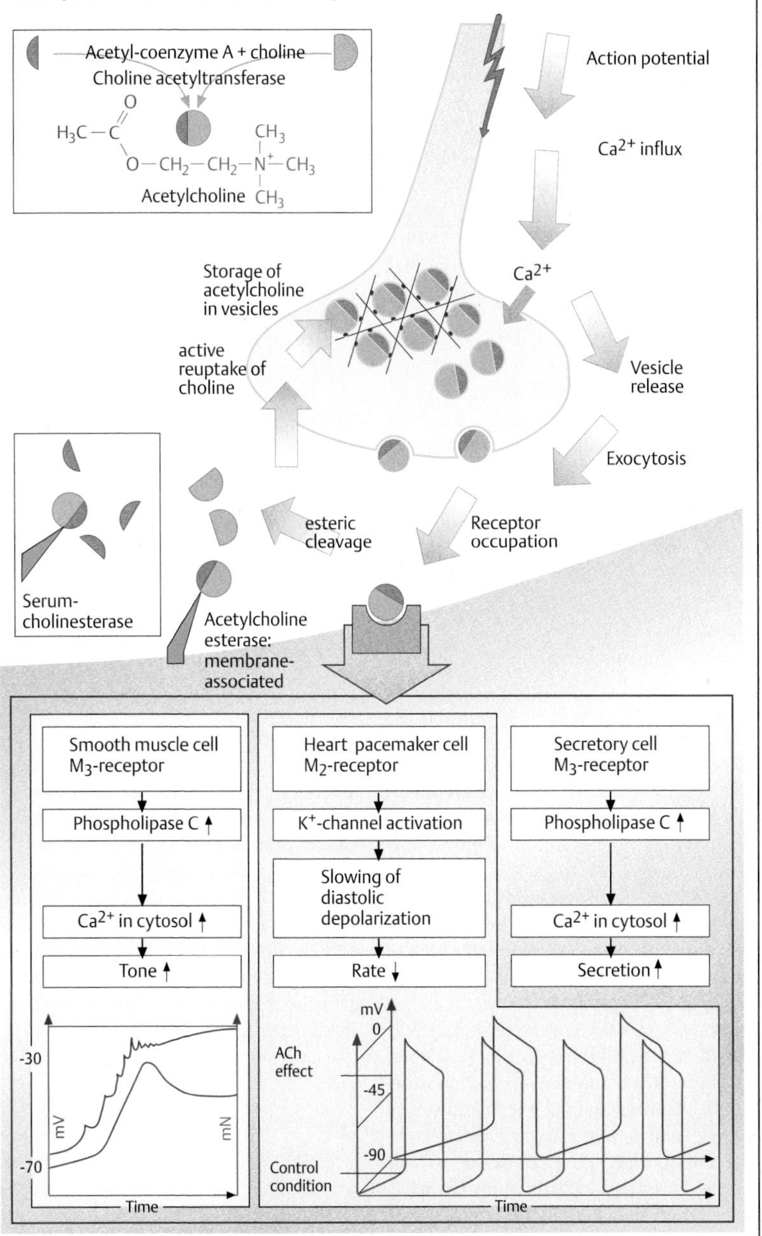

Acetyl-coenzyme A + choline
Choline acetyltransferase

$$H_3C-C\overset{O}{\Big\|}O-CH_2-CH_2-\overset{+}{N}\!\begin{matrix}CH_3\\CH_3\\CH_3\end{matrix}$$

Acetylcholine

Action potential

Ca^{2+} influx

Storage of acetylcholine in vesicles

active reuptake of choline

Ca^{2+}

Vesicle release

Exocytosis

esteric cleavage

Receptor occupation

Serum-cholinesterase

Acetylcholine esterase: membrane-associated

Smooth muscle cell M_3-receptor	Heart pacemaker cell M_2-receptor	Secretory cell M_3-receptor
Phospholipase C ↑	K^+-channel activation	Phospholipase C ↑
Ca^{2+} in cytosol ↑	Slowing of diastolic depolarization	Ca^{2+} in cytosol ↑
Tone ↑	Rate ↓	Secretion ↑

ACh effect

Control condition

☐ Parasympathomimetics

Acetylcholine (ACh) is too rapidly hydrolyzed and inactivated by acetylcholinesterase (AChE) to be of any therapeutic use; however, its action can be replicated by other substances, namely, direct or indirect parasympathomimetics.

Direct parasympathomimetics. The choline ester of carbamic acid, *carbachol*, activates M-cholinoceptors, but is not hydrolyzed by AChE. Carbachol can thus be effectively employed for local application to the eye (glaucoma) and systemic administration (bowel atonia, bladder atonia). The alkaloids *pilocarpine* (from *Pilocarpus jaborandi*) and *arecoline* (from *Areca catechu*; betel nut) also act as direct parasympathomimetics. As tertiary amines, they moreover exert central effects. The central effect of muscarine-like substances consists in an enlivening, mild stimulation that is probably the effect desired in betel chewing, a widespread habit in South Asia. Of this group, only pilocarpine enjoys therapeutic use, which is almost exclusively by local application to the eye in glaucoma (p. 346).

Indirect parasympathomimetics inhibit local AChE and raise the concentration of ACh at receptors of cholinergic synapses. This action is evident at all synapses where ACh is the mediator. Chemically, these agents include esters of carbamic acid (**carbamates** such as *physostigmine*, *neostigmine*) and of phosphoric acid (**organophosphates** such as *paraoxon* = E600, and *nitrostigmine* = parathion = E605, its prodrug).

Members of both groups react like ACh with AChE. The esters are hydrolyzed upon formation of a complex with the enzyme. The rate-limiting step in ACh hydrolysis is deacetylation of the enzyme, which takes only milliseconds, thus permitting a high turnover rate and activity of AChE. **Decarbaminoylation** following hydrolysis of a carbamate takes hours to days, the enzyme remaining inhibited as long as it is carbaminoylated. Cleavage of the phosphate residue. i.e., **dephosphorylation**, is practically impossible; enzyme inhibition is irreversible.

Uses. The quaternary carbamate neostigmine is employed as an indirect parasympathomimetic in *postoperative atonia of the bowel or bladder*. Applied topically to the eye, neostigmine is used in the treatment of glaucoma. Furthermore, it is needed to overcome the relative AChE-deficiency at the motor end plate in myasthenia gravis or to reverse the neuromuscular blockade (p. 184) caused by nondepolarizing muscle relaxants (decurarization before discontinuation of anaesthesia). Pyridostigmine has a similar use. The tertiary carbamate physostigmine can be used as an *antidote in poisoning with parasympatholytic drugs*, because it has access to AChE in the brain. Carbamates and organophosphates also serve as insecticides. Although they possess high acute toxicity in humans, they are more rapidly degraded than is DDT following their release into the environment.

In the early stages of **Alzheimer disease**, administration of centrally acting AChE inhibitors can bring about transient improvement in cognitive function or slow down deterioration in some patients. Suitable drugs include **rivastigmine**, **donepezil**, and **galantamine**, which require slowly increasing dosage. Peripheral side effects (inhibition of ACh breakdown) limit therapy. Donepezil and galantamine are not esters of carbamic acid and act by a different molecular action. Galantamine is also thought to promote the action of ACh at nicotinic cholinoceptors by an allosteric mechanism.

A. Direct and indirect parasympathomimetics

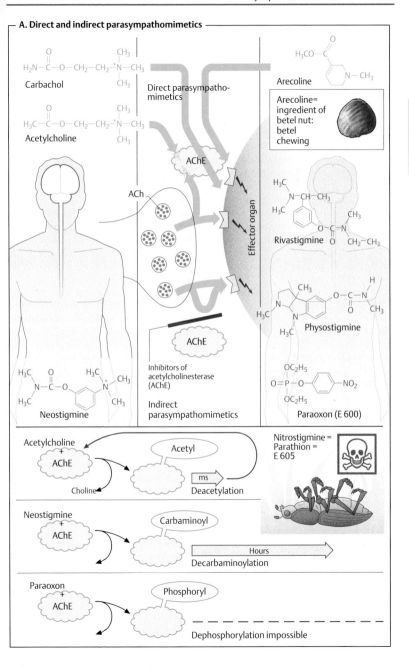

Carbachol

Acetylcholine

Direct parasympatho-mimetics

ACh

AChE

Effector organ

Inhibitors of acetylcholinesterase (AChE)

Indirect parasympathomimetics

Neostigmine

Arecoline

Arecoline= ingredient of betel nut: betel chewing

Rivastigmine

Physostigmine

Paraoxon (E 600)

Acetylcholine + AChE

Acetyl

Choline

ms

Deacetylation

Nitrostigmine = Parathion = E 605

Neostigmine + AChE

Carbaminoyl

Hours

Decarbaminoylation

Paraoxon + AChE

Phosphoryl

Dephosphorylation impossible

☐ Parasympatholytics

Excitation of the **parasympathetic** division causes release of acetylcholine at neuroeffector junctions in different target organs. The major effects are summarized in (**A**) (blue arrows). Some of these effects have therapeutic applications, as indicated by the clinical uses of parasympathomimetics (p. 106).

Substances acting antagonistically at the M-cholinoceptor are designated **parasympatholytics** (prototype: the alkaloid **atropine**; actions marked red in the panels). Therapeutic use of these agents is complicated by their low organ selectivity. Possibilities for a targeted action include:

- Local application
- Selection of drugs with favorable membrane penetrability
- Administration of drugs possessing receptor subtype selectivity.

Parasympatholytics are employed for the following purposes:

1. Inhibition of glandular secretion.

Bronchial secretion. **Premedication** with atropine before inhalation anesthesia prevents a possible hypersecretion of bronchial mucus, which cannot be expectorated by coughing during anesthesia.

Gastric secretion. Atropine displays about equally high affinity for all muscarinic cholinoceptor subtypes and thus lacks organ specificity. Pirenzepine has preferential affinity for the M_1 subtype and was used to inhibit production of HCl in the gastric mucosa, because vagally mediated stimulation of acid production involves M_1 receptors. This approach has proved inadequate because the required dosage of pirenzepine produced too many atropine-like side effects. Also, more effective pharmacological means are available to lower HCl production in a graded fashion (H_2-antihistaminics, proton pump inhibitors).

2. Relaxation of smooth musculature.

As a rule, administration of a parasympatholytic agent by inhalation is quite effective in **chronic obstructive pulmonary disease**. Ipratropium has a relatively short lasting effect; four aerosol puffs usually being required per day. The newly introduced substance tiotropium needs to be applied only once daily because of its "adhesiveness." Tiotropium is effective in chronic obstructive lung disease; however, it is not indicated in the treatment of bronchial asthma.

Spasmolysis by *N*-butylscopolamine in **biliary** or **renal colic** (p. 130). Because of its quaternary nitrogen atom, this drug does not enter the brain and requires parenteral administration. Its spasmolytic action is especially marked because of additional ganglionic blocking and direct muscle-relaxant actions.

Lowering of pupillary sphincter tonus and pupillary dilation by local administration of homatropine or tropicamide (**mydriatics**) allows observation of the ocular fundus. For diagnostic uses, only short-term pupillary dilation is needed. The effect of both agents subsides quickly in comparison with that of atropine (duration of several days).

3. Cardioacceleration.

Ipratropium is used in bradycardia and AV-block, respectively, to raise heart rate and to facilitate cardiac *impulse conduction*. As a quaternary substance, it does not penetrate into the brain, which greatly reduces the risk of CNS disturbances (see below). However, it is also poorly absorbed from the gut (absorption rate < 30%). To achieve adequate levels in the blood, it must be given in significantly higher dosage than needed parenterally.

Atropine may be given to prevent **cardiac arrest** resulting from vagal reflex activation, incidental to anaesthetic induction, gastric lavage, or endoscopic procedures.

A. Effects of parasympathetic stimulation and blockade

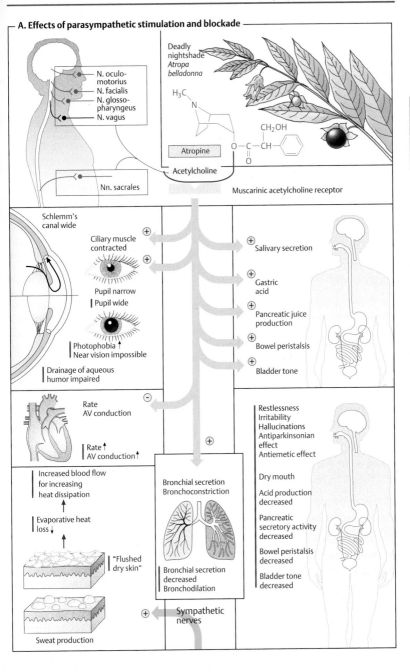

N. oculomotorius
N. facialis
N. glossopharyngeus
N. vagus

Nn. sacrales

Deadly nightshade *Atropa belladonna*

Atropine

Acetylcholine

Muscarinic acetylcholine receptor

Schlemm's canal wide

Ciliary muscle contracted ⊕

Pupil narrow
Pupil wide ⊕

Photophobia ↑
Near vision impossible

Drainage of aqueous humor impaired

⊕ Salivary secretion

⊕ Gastric acid

⊕ Pancreatic juice production

⊕ Bowel peristalsis

⊕ Bladder tone

Rate
AV conduction ⊖

Rate ↑
AV conduction ↑

⊕

Restlessness
Irritability
Hallucinations
Antiparkinsonian effect
Antiemetic effect

Dry mouth

Acid production decreased

Pancreatic secretory activity decreased

Bowel peristalsis decreased

Bladder tone decreased

Increased blood flow for increasing heat dissipation

Evaporative heat loss ↓

"Flushed dry skin"

Bronchial secretion
Bronchoconstriction

Bronchial secretion decreased
Bronchodilation

⊕ Sympathetic nerves

Sweat production

4. CNS damping effects. Scopolamine is effective in the *prophylaxis of kinetosis* (motion sickness, sea sickness, see p. 342); it is mostly applied by a transdermal patch. Scopolamine (pK_a = 7.2) penetrates the blood–brain barrier faster than does atropine (pK_a = 9), because at physiological pH a larger proportion is present in the neutral, membrane-permeant form.

In *psychotic excitement* (agitation), sedation can be achieved with scopolamine. Unlike atropine, scopolamine exerts a calming and amnesiogenic action that can also be used to advantage in anesthetic premedication.

Symptomatic treatment in parkinsonism for the purpose of restoring a dopaminergic-cholinergic balance in the corpus striatum. Antiparkinsonian agents, such as benztropine (p. 188) readily penetrate the blood–brain barrier. At centrally equieffective dosages, their peripheral effects are less marked than those of atropine.

Contraindications for parasympatholytics.
Closed angle glaucoma. Since drainage of aqueous humor is impeded during relaxation of the pupillary sphincter, intraocular pressure rises.

Prostatic hyperplasia with impaired micturition: loss of parasympathetic control of the detrusor muscle exacerbates difficulties in voiding urine.

Atropine poisoning. Parasympatholytics have a wide therapeutic margin. Rarely life-threatening, poisoning with atropine is characterized by the following peripheral and central effects.

Peripheral. **Tachycardia**; **dry mouth**; **hyperthermia** secondary to the inhibition of sweating. Although sweat glands are innervated by sympathetic fibers, these are cholinergic in nature. When sweat secretion is inhibited, the body loses the ability to dissipate metabolic heat by evaporation of sweat. There is a compensatory vasodilation in the skin, allowing increased heat exchange through increased cutaneous blood flow. Decreased peristaltic activity of the intestines leads to **constipation**.

Central. Motor restlessness, progressing to maniacal agitation, psychic disturbances, **disorientation** and **hallucinations**. It may be noted that scopolamine-containing herbal preparations (especially from *Datura stramonium*) served as hallucinogenic intoxicants in the Middle Ages. Accounts of witches' rides to satanic gatherings and similar excesses are likely the products of CNS poisoning. Recently, Western youths have been reported to make "recreational" use of Angel's Trumpet flowers (several *Brugmansia* species grown as ornamental shrubs). Plants of this genus are a source of scopolamine used by South American natives since pre-Columbian times.

Elderly subjects have an enhanced sensitivity, particularly toward the CNS toxic manifestations. In this context, the diversity of drugs producing atropine-like side effects should be borne in mind: e.g., tricyclic antidepressants, neuroleptics, antihistaminics, antiarrhythmics, antiparkinsonian agents.

Apart from symptomatic, general measures (gastric lavage, cooling with ice water), **therapy of severe atropine intoxication** includes the administration of the indirect parasympathomimetic physostigmine (p. 106). The most common instances of "atropine"-intoxication are observed after ingestion of the berrylike fruits of belladonna (in children). A similar picture may be seen after intentional overdosage with tricyclic antidepressants in attempted suicide.

A. Parasympatholytics

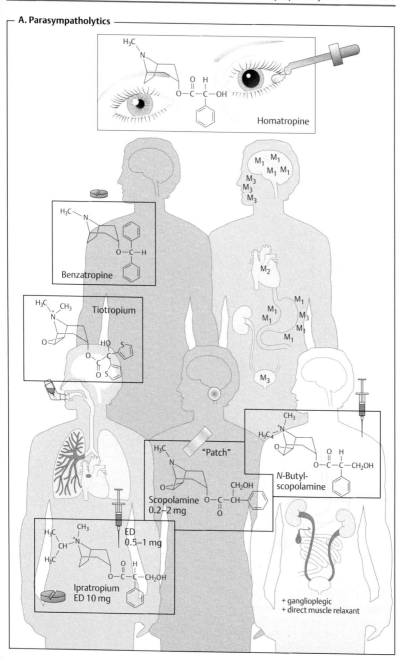

Homatropine

Benzatropine

Tiotropium

N-Butyl-scopolamine

"Patch"

Scopolamine 0.2–2 mg

ED 0.5–1 mg

Ipratropium ED 10 mg

+ ganglioplegic
+ direct muscle relaxant

□ Actions of Nicotine

Acetylcholine (ACh) is a mediator in the ganglia of the sympathetic and parasympathetic divisions of the autonomic nervous system. Here, ACh receptors are considered that are activated by nicotine (nicotinic receptors; NAChR, p. 102) and that play a leading part in fast ganglionic neurotransmission. These receptors represent ligand-gated ion channels with a structure and mode of operation as described on p. 64. Opening of the ion pore induces Na^+ influx followed by membrane depolarization and excitation of the cell. NAChR tend to desensitize rapidly; that is, during prolonged occupation by an agonist the ion pore closes spontaneously and cannot reopen until the agonist detaches itself.

□ Localization of Nicotinic ACh Receptors

Autonomic nervous system (**A**, middle). In analogy to autonomic ganglia, NAChR are found also on epinephrine-releasing cells of the adrenal medulla, which are innervated by spinal first neurons. At all these synapses, the receptor is located postsynaptically in the somatodendritic region of the gangliocyte.

Motor end plate. Here the ACh receptors are of the *motor type* (p. 182).

Central nervous system (CNS; **A**, top). NAChR are involved in various functions. They have a predominantly presynaptic location and promote transmitter release from innervated axon terminals by means of depolarization. Together with ganglionic NAChR they belong to the *neuronal type*, which differs from the motor type in terms of the composition of its five subunits.

□ Effects of Nicotine on Body Function

Nicotine served as an experimental tool for the classification of acetylcholine receptors. As a tobacco alkaloid, nicotine is employed daily by a vast part of the human race for the enjoyment of its central stimulant action. Nicotine activates the brain's reward system, thereby promoting dependence. Regular intake leads to habituation, which is advantageous in some respects (e. g., stimulation of the area postrema, p. 342). In habituated subjects, cessation of nicotine intake results in mainly psychological withdrawal symptoms (increased nervousness, lack of concentration). Prevention of these is an additional important incentive for continuing nicotine intake. Peripheral effects caused by stimulation of autonomic ganglia may be perceived as useful ("laxative" effect of the first morning cigarette). Sympathoactivation without corresponding physical exertion ("silent stress") may in the long term lead to grave cardiovascular damage (p. 114).

□ Aids for Smoking Cessation

Administration of *nicotine* by means of skin patch, chewing gum, or nasal spray is intended to eliminate craving for cigarette smoking. Breaking of the habit is to be achieved by stepwise reduction of the nicotine dose. Initially this may happen; however, the long-term relapse rate is disappointingly high.

Bupropion (amfebutamon) shows structural similarity with amphetamine (p. 329) and inhibits neuronal reuptake of dopamine and norepinephrine. It is supposed to aid smokers in "kicking the habit," possibly because it evokes CNS effects resembling those of nicotine. The high relapse rate after termination of the drug and substantial side effects put its therapeutic value in doubt.

A. Effects of nicotine in body

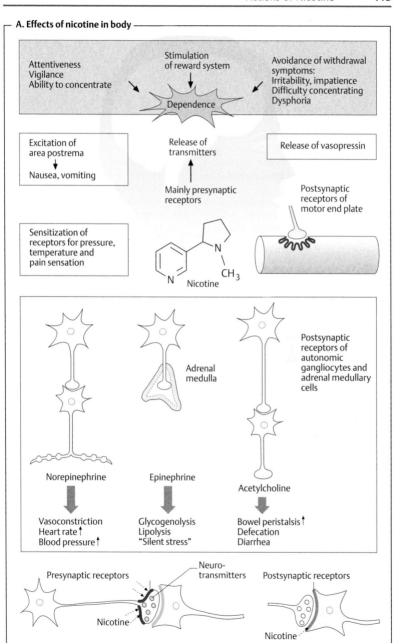

Attentiveness
Vigilance
Ability to concentrate

Stimulation
of reward system

Avoidance of withdrawal
symptoms:
Irritability, impatience
Difficulty concentrating
Dysphoria

Dependence

Excitation of
area postrema
↓
Nausea, vomiting

Release of
transmitters

Release of vasopressin

Mainly presynaptic
receptors

Postsynaptic
receptors of
motor end plate

Sensitization of
receptors for pressure,
temperature and
pain sensation

Nicotine

Adrenal
medulla

Postsynaptic
receptors of
autonomic
gangliocytes and
adrenal medullary
cells

Norepinephrine

Epinephrine

Acetylcholine

Vasoconstriction
Heart rate ↑
Blood pressure ↑

Glycogenolysis
Lipolysis
"Silent stress"

Bowel peristalsis ↑
Defecation
Diarrhea

Presynaptic receptors

Neuro-
transmitters

Postsynaptic receptors

Nicotine

Nicotine

□ Consequences of Tobacco Smoking

The dried and cured leaves of the nightshade plant *Nicotiana tabacum* are known as tobacco. Tobacco is mostly smoked, less frequently chewed or taken as dry snuff. Combustion of tobacco generates ~4000 chemical compounds in detectable quantities. The xenobiotic burden on the smoker depends on a range of parameters, including tobacco quality, presence of a filter, rate and temperature of combustion, depth of inhalation, and duration of breath holding.

Tobacco contains 0.2–5% nicotine. In tobacco smoke, nicotine is present as a constituent of small tar particles. The amount of nicotine absorbed during smoking depends on the nicotine content, the size of membrane area exposed to tobacco smoke (N.B.: inhalation), and the pH of the absorbing surface. It is rapidly absorbed through bronchi and lung alveoli when present in free base form. However, protonation of the pyrrolidine nitrogen renders the corresponding part of the molecule hydrophilic and absorption is impeded. To maximize the yield of nicotine, tobaccos of some manufacturers are made alkaline. Smoking of a single cigarette produces peak plasma levels in the range of 25–50 ng/ml. The effects described on p. 113 become evident. When intake stops, nicotine concentration in plasma shows an initial rapid fall, due to distribution into tissues, and a terminal elimination phase with a half-life of 2 hours. Nicotine is degraded by oxidation.

The enhanced risk of **vascular disease** (coronary stenosis, myocardial infarction, and central and peripheral ischemic disorders, such as stroke and intermittent claudication) is likely to be a consequence of chronic exposure to nicotine. At the least, nicotine is under discussion as a factor favoring the progression of atherosclerosis. By releasing epinephrine, it elevates plasma levels of glucose and free fatty acids in the absence of an immediate physiological need for these energy-rich metabolites. Furthermore, it promotes platelet aggregability, lowers fibrinolytic activity of blood, and enhances coagulability.

The health risks of tobacco smoking are, however, attributable not only to nicotine but also to various other ingredients of tobacco smoke. Some of these promote formation of thrombogenic plaques; others possess demonstrable carcinogenic properties (e.g., the tobacco-specific nitrosoketone).

Dust particles inhaled in tobacco smoke, together with bronchial mucus, must be removed by the ciliated epithelium from the airways. However, ciliary activity is depressed by tobacco smoke and mucociliary transport is impaired. This favors bacterial infection and contributes to the chronic bronchitis associated with regular smoking (smoker's cough). Chronic injury to the bronchial mucosa could be an important causative factor in increasing the risk in smokers of death from bronchial carcinoma.

Statistical surveys provide an impressive correlation between the numbers of cigarettes smoked per day and the risk of death from coronary disease or lung cancer. On the other hand, statistics also show that, on cessation of smoking, the increased risk of death from coronary infarction or other cardiovascular disease declines over 5–10 years almost to the level of nonsmokers. Similarly, the risk of developing bronchial carcinoma is reduced.

An association with tobacco use has also been established for cancers of the larynx, pharynx, esophagus, stomach, pancreas, kidney, and bladder.

A. Sequelae of tobacco smoking

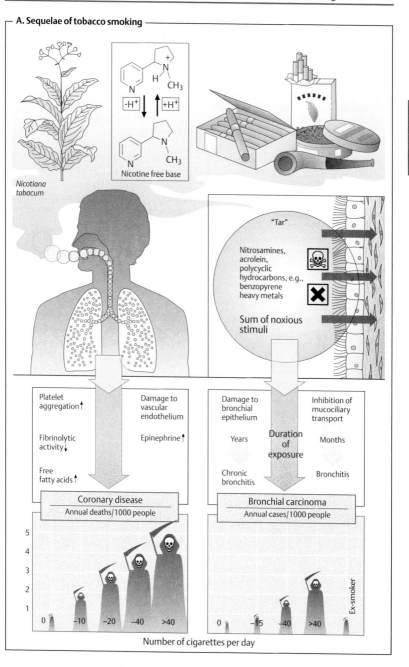

Nicotiana tabacum

Nicotine free base

"Tar"

Nitrosamines, acrolein, polycyclic hydrocarbons, e.g., benzopyrene heavy metals

Sum of noxious stimuli

Platelet aggregation↑

Damage to vascular endothelium

Fibrinolytic activity↓

Epinephrine↑

Free fatty acids↑

Damage to bronchial epithelium

Inhibition of mucociliary transport

Years

Duration of exposure

Months

Chronic bronchitis

Bronchitis

Coronary disease
Annual deaths/1000 people

Bronchial carcinoma
Annual cases/1000 people

5
4
3
2
1

0   −10   −20   −40   >40

0   −15   −40   >40   Ex-smoker

Number of cigarettes per day

□ Dopamine

As a *biogenic amine*, dopamine belongs to a group of substances produced in the organism by decarboxylation of amino acids. Besides dopamine and norepinephrine formed from it, this group includes many other messenger molecules such as histamine, serotonin, and γ-aminobutyric acid.

Dopamine actions and pharmacological implications (A). In the CNS, dopamine serves as a neuromediator. Dopamine receptors are also present in the periphery. Neuronally released dopamine can interact with various receptor subtypes, all of which are coupled to G-proteins. Two groupings can be distinguished: the family of D_1-like receptors (comprising subtypes D_1 and D_5) and the family of D_2-like receptors (comprising subtypes D_2, D_3, and D_4). The subtypes differ in their signal transduction pathways. Thus, synthesis of cAMP is stimulated by D_1-like receptors but inhibited by D_2-like receptors.

Released dopamine can be reutilized by neuronal reuptake and re-storage in vesicles or can be catabolized like other endogenous catecholamines by the enzymes MAO and COMT (p. 86).

Various drugs are employed therapeutically to influence dopaminergic signal transmission.

Antiparkinsonian agents. In Parkinson disease, nigrostriatal dopamine neurons degenerate. To compensate for the lack of dopamine, use is made of L-dopa as the dopamine precursor and of D_2 receptor agonists (cf. p. 188).

Prolactin inhibitors. Dopamine released from hypothalamic neurosecretory nerve cells inhibits the secretion of prolactin from the adenohypophysis (p. 238). Prolactin promotes production of breast milk during the lactation period; moreover it inhibits the secretion of gonadorelin. D_2 receptor agonists prevent prolactin secretion and can be used for weaning and the treatment of female infertility resulting from hyperprolactinemia.

The D_2 agonists differ in their duration of action and, hence, their dosing interval; e. g., bromocriptine 3 times daily, quinagolide once daily, and cabergoline once to twice weekly.

Antiemetics. Stimulation of dopamine receptors in the area postrema can elicit vomiting. D_2 receptor antagonists such as metoclopramide and domperidone are used as antiemetics (p. 342). In addition they promote gastric emptying.

Neuroleptics. Various CNS-permeant drugs that exert a therapeutic action in schizophrenia display antagonist properties at D_2 receptors; e. g., the phenothiazines and butyrophenone neuroleptics (p. 232).

Dopamine as a therapeutic agent (B). When given by infusion, dopamine causes a dilation of renal and splanchnic arteries that results from stimulation of D_1 receptors. This lowers cardiac afterload and augments renal blood flow, effects that are exploited in the treatment of cardiogenic shock. Because of the close structural relationship between dopamine and norepinephrine, it is easy to understand why, at progressively higher doses, dopamine is capable of activating β_1-adrenoceptors and finally α_1-receptors. In particular, α-mediated vasoconstriction would be therapeutically undesirable (symbolized by red warning sign).

Apomorphine is a dopamine agonist with a variegated pattern of usage. Given parenterally as an emetic agent to aid elimination of orally ingested poisons, it is not without hazards (hypotension, respiratory depression). In akinetic motor disturbances, it is a back-up drug. Taken orally, it supposedly is beneficial in erectile dysfunction.

A. Dopamine actions as influenced by drugs

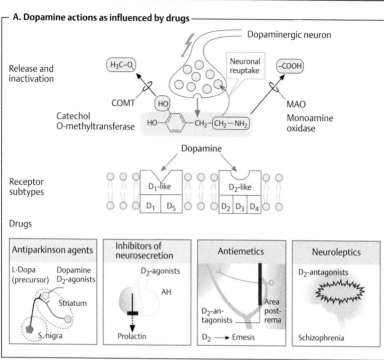

B. Dopamine as a therapeutic agent

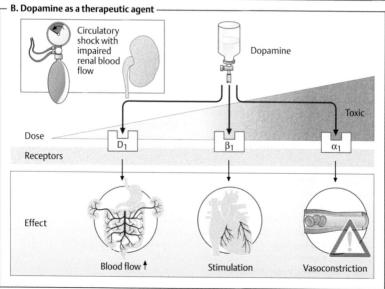

□ Histamine Effects and Their Pharmacological Properties

Functions. In the CNS histamine serves as a neurotransmitter/modulator, promoting *inter alia* wakefulness. In the gastric mucosa, it acts as a mediator substance that is released from enterochromaffin-like (ECL) cells to stimulate gastric acid secretion in neighboring parietal cells (p. 170). Histamine stored in blood basophils and tissue mast cells plays a mediator role in IgE-mediated allergic reactions (p. 72). By increasing the tone of bronchial smooth muscle, histamine may trigger an asthma attack. In the intestines, it promotes peristalsis, which is evidenced in food allergies by the occurrence of diarrhea. In blood vessels, histamine increases permeability by inducing the formation of gaps between endothelial cells of postcapillary venules, allowing passage of fluid into the surrounding, tissue (e.g., wheal formation). Blood vessels are dilated because histamine induces release of nitric oxide from the endothelium (p. 124) and because of a direct vasorelaxant action. By stimulating sensory nerve endings in the skin, histamine can evoke itching.

Receptors. Histamine receptors are coupled to G-proteins. The H_1 and H_2 receptors are targets for substances with antagonistic actions. The H_3 receptor is localized on nerve cells and may inhibit release of various transmitter substances, including histamine itself.

Metabolism. Histamine-storing cells form histamine by decarboxylation of the amino acid histidine. Released histamine is degraded; no reuptake system exists as for norepinephrine, dopamine, and serotonin.

Antagonists. The H_1 and H_2 receptors can be blocked by selective antagonists.

H_1-Antihistaminics. Older substances in this group (first generation) are rather non-specific and also block other receptors (e.g.,

muscarinic cholinoceptors). These agents are used for the symptomatic relief of allergies (e.g., bamipine, clemastine, dimetindene, mebhydroline, pheniramine); as antiemetics (meclizine, dimenhydrinate; p. 342); and as prescription-free sedatives/hypnotics (see p. 220). Promethazine represents the transition to psychopharmaceuticals of the type of neuroleptic phenothiazines (p. 232).

Unwanted effects of most H_1-antihistaminics are lassitude (impaired driving skills) and atropine-like reactions (e.g., dry mouth, constipation). Newer substances (second-generation H_1-antihistaminics) do not penetrate into the CNS and are therefore practically devoid of sedative effects. Presumably they are transported back into the blood by a P-glycoprotein located in the endothelium of the blood–brain barrier. Furthermore, they hardly have any anticholinergic activity. Members of this group are cetirizine (a racemate) and its active enantiomer levocetirizine, as well as loratadine and its active metabolite desloratadine. Fexofenadine is the active metabolite of terfenadine, which may reach excessive blood levels when biotransformation (via CYP3A4) is too slow; and which can then cause cardiac arrhythmias (prolongation of QT-interval). Ebastine and mizolastine are other new agents.

H_2-Blockers (cimetidine, ranitidine, famotidine, nizatidine) inhibit gastric acid secretion, and thus are useful in the treatment of peptic ulcers (p. 172). Cimetidine may lead to drug interactions because it inhibits hepatic cytochrome oxidases. The successor drugs (e.g., ranitidine) are of less concern in this respect.

Mast cell stabilizers. Cromoglycate (cromolyn) and nedocromil decrease, by an as yet unknown mechanism, the capacity of mast cells to release of histamine and other mediators during allergic reactions. Both agents are applied topically (p. 338).

A. Histamine actions as influenced by drugs

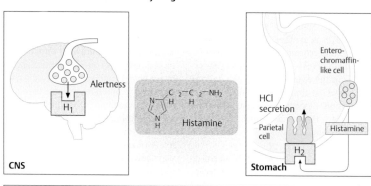

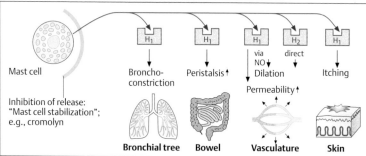

Receptor antagonists

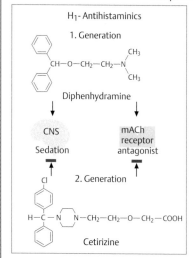

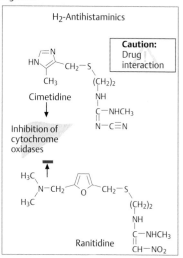

□ Serotonin

Occurrence. Serotonin (5-hydroxytrypta-mine, 5-HT) is synthesized from L-trypto-phan in enterochromaffin cells of the intestinal mucosa. 5-HT-synthesizing neurons occur also in the enteric nerve plexus and the CNS, where the amine fulfills a neuromediator function. Blood platelets are unable to synthesize 5-HT, but are capable of taking up, storing, and releasing it.

Serotonin receptors. Based on biochemical and pharmacological criteria, seven receptors classes can be distinguished. Of major pharmacotherapeutic importance are those designated: 5-HT_1, 5-HT_2, each with different subtypes, 5-HT_4, and 5-HT_7, all of which are G-protein-coupled, whereas the 5-HT_3 subtype represents a ligand-gated nonselective cation channel (p. 64).

Serotonin actions—cardiovascular system. The responses to 5-HT are complex, because multiple, in part opposing, effects are exerted via the different receptor subtypes. Thus, 5-HT_{2A} receptors on vascular smooth muscle cells mediate direct vasoconstriction. Vasodilation and lowering of blood pressure can occur by several indirect mechanisms: 5-HT_{1A} receptors mediate sympathoinhibition ($\rightarrow$ decrease in neurogenic vasoconstrictor tonus) both centrally and peripherally; 5-HT_1-like receptors on vascular endothelium promote release of vasorelaxant mediators (NO; prostacyclin). 5-HT released from platelets plays a role in thrombogenesis, hemostasis, and the pathogenesis of preeclamptic hypertension.

Sumatriptan is an antimigraine drug that possesses agonist activity at 5-HT receptors of the 1D and 1B subtypes (p. 334). It causes a constriction of cranial blood vessels, which may result from a direct vascular action or from inhibition of the release of neuropeptides that mediate "neurogenic inflammation." A sensation of chest tightness may occur and be indicative of coronary vaso-

spasm. Other "triptans" are naratriptan, zolmitriptan, and rizatriptan.

Gastrointestinal tract. Serotonin released from myenteric neurons or enterochromaffin (EC) cells acts on 5-HT_4 receptors to enhance bowel motility, enteral fluid secretion, and thus propulsive activity. To date, attempts at modifying the influence of serotonin on intestinal motility by agonistic or antagonistic drugs have not been very successful. Although the 5-HT_4 agonist cisapride was shown to be effective in increasing propulsive activity of the intestinal tract, its adverse effects were very pronounced. Since it is degraded via CYP3A4, it is liable to interact with numerous drugs. In particular, arrhythmias (in part severe) associated with QT prolongation were noted; the arrhythmogenic action is caused by blockade of K^+ channels. The drug is no longer available.

Central nervous system. Serotoninergic neurons play a part in various brain functions, as evidenced by the effects of drugs likely to interfere with serotonin.

Fluoxetine is an antidepressant which, by blocking reuptake, retards inactivation of released serotonin. Its activity spectrum includes significant psychomotor stimulation and depression of appetite.

Sibutramine, an inhibitor of the neuronal reuptake of 5-HT and norepinephrine, is marketed as an antiobesity drug (pp. 329).

Ondansetron, an antagonist at the 5-HT_3 receptor, possesses striking effectiveness against cytotoxic drug-induced emesis, evident both at the start of and during cytostatic therapy. Tropisetron and granisetron produce analogous effects.

LSD and other psychedelics (psychotomimetics) such as *mescaline* and *psilocybin* can induce states of altered awareness, or induce hallucinations and anxiety, probably mediated by 5-HT_{2A} receptors.

A. Serotonin actions as influenced by drugs

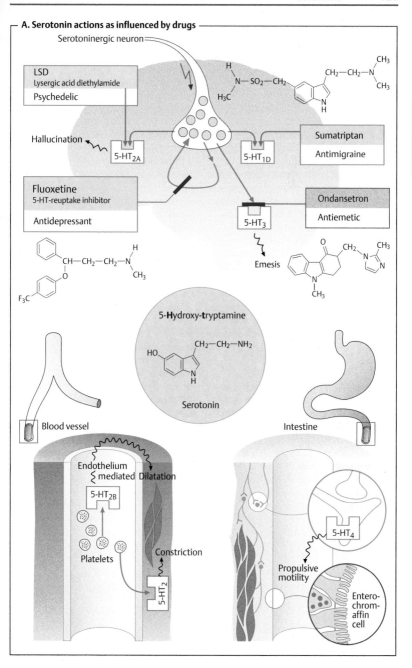

◻ Vasodilators—Overview

The distribution of blood within the circulation is a function of vascular caliber. Venous tone regulates the volume of blood returned to the heart and, hence, stroke volume and cardiac output. The luminal diameter of the arterial vasculature determines peripheral resistance. Cardiac output and peripheral resistance are prime determinants of arterial blood pressure (p. 324).

In (**A**), the clinically most important vasodilators are presented. Some of these agents possess different efficacy in affecting the venous and arterial limbs of the circulation.

Possible uses. *Arteriolar vasodilators* are given to lower blood pressure in hypertension (p. 314), to reduce cardiac work in angina pectoris (p. 318), and to reduce ventricular afterload (pressure load) in cardiac failure (p. 322). *Venous vasodilators* are used to reduce venous filling pressure (preload) in angina pectoris (p. 318) or congestive heart failure (p. 322). Practical uses are indicated for each drug group.

Counterregulation in acute hypotension due to vasodilators (B). Increased *sympathetic* drive raises heart rate (reflex tachycardia) and cardiac output and thus helps to elevate blood pressure. The patients experience palpitations. Activation of the *renin–angiotensin–aldosterone (RAA) system* serves to increase blood volume, hence cardiac output. Fluid retention leads to an increase in body weight and, possibly, edemas.

These counterregulatory processes are susceptible to pharmacological inhibition (β-blockers, ACE inhibitors, diuretics).

Mechanisms of action. The tonus of vascular smooth muscle can be decreased by various means.

Protection against vasoconstricting mediators. ACE inhibitors and angiotensin receptor antagonists protect against angiotensin II (p. 128); α-adrenoceptor antagonists interfere with (nor)epinephrine (p. 94); bosentan (see below) is an antagonist at receptors for endothelin, a powerful vasoconstrictor released by the endothelium.

Substitution of vasorelaxant mediators. Analogues of prostacyclin (from vascular endothelium), such as iloprost, or of prostaglandin E_1, such as alprostadil, stimulate the corresponding receptors; organic nitrates (p. 124) substitute for endothelial NO.

Direct action on vascular smooth muscle cells. Ca^{2+}-channel blockers (p. 126) and K^+ channel openers (diazoxide, minoxidil) act at the level of channel proteins to inhibit membrane depolarization and excitation of vascular smooth muscle cells. Phosphodiesterase (PDE) inhibitors retard the degradation of intracellular cGMP, which lowers contractile tonus. Several PDE isozymes with different localization and function are known.

The following sections deal with special aspects:

Erectile dysfunction. Sildenafil, vardenafil, and tardalafil are inhibitors of PDE-5 and are used to promote erection. During sexual arousal NO is released from nerve endings in the corpus cavernosum of the penis, which stimulates the formation of cGMP in vascular smooth muscle. PDE-5, which is important in this tissue, breaks down cGMP, thus counteracting erection. Blockers of PDE-5 "conserve" cGMP.

Pulmonary hypertension. This condition involves a narrowing of the pulmonary vascular bed resulting mostly from unknown causes. The disease often is progressive, associated with right ventricular overload, and all but resistant to treatment with conventional vasodilators. The endothelin antagonist, bosentan, offers a new therapeutic approach. Administration of NO by inhalation is under clinical trial.

A. Vasodilators

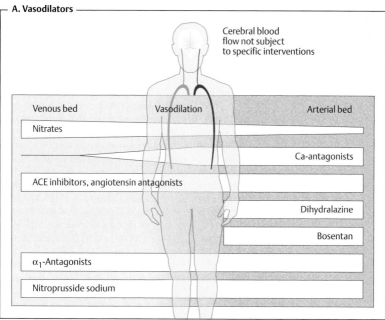

Cerebral blood flow not subject to specific interventions

Venous bed   Vasodilation   Arterial bed

Nitrates

Ca-antagonists

ACE inhibitors, angiotensin antagonists

Dihydralazine

Bosentan

α_1-Antagonists

Nitroprusside sodium

B. Counter-regulatory responses in hypotension due to vasodilators

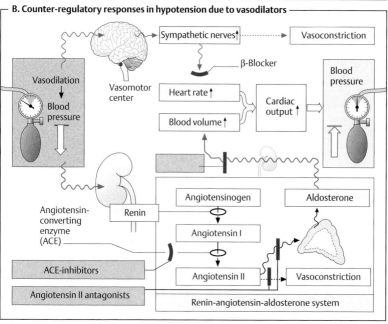

Sympathetic nerves↑ ┄┄► Vasoconstriction

β-Blocker

Vasodilation
↓
Blood pressure

Vasomotor center

Heart rate ↑

Blood volume ↑

Cardiac output ↑

Blood pressure

Angiotensin-converting enzyme (ACE)

Renin

Angiotensinogen

Aldosterone

Angiotensin I

Angiotensin II

Vasoconstriction

ACE-inhibitors

Angiotensin II antagonists

Renin-angiotensin-aldosterone system

□ Organic Nitrates

Various esters of nitric acid (HNO_3) and polyvalent alcohols relax vascular smooth muscle, e.g., nitroglycerin (glyceryl trinitrate) and isosorbide dinitrate. *The effect is more pronounced in venous than in arterial beds.*

These vasodilator effects produce hemodynamic consequences that can be put to therapeutic use. Owing to a decrease in both venous return (preload) and arterial afterload, cardiac work is decreased (p. 318). As a result, the cardiac oxygen balance improves. Spasmodic constriction of larger coronary vessels (coronary spasm) is prevented.

Uses. Organic nitrates are used chiefly in *angina pectoris* (p. 316), less frequently in severe forms of chronic and acute congestive heart failure. Continuous intake of higher doses with maintenance of steady plasma levels leads to loss of efficacy, inasmuch as the organism becomes refractory (tachyphylactic). This "nitrate tolerance" can be avoided if a daily "nitrate-free interval" is maintained, e. g., overnight.

At the start of therapy, **unwanted reactions** occur frequently in the form of a throbbing headache, probably caused by dilation of cephalic vessels. This effect also exhibits tolerance, even when daily "nitrate pauses" are observed. Excessive dosages give rise to hypotension, reflex tachycardia, and circulatory collapse.

Mechanism of action. The reduction in vascular smooth muscle tone is due to activation of guanylate cyclase and elevation of cyclic GMP levels. The causative agent is nitric oxide (NO) generated from the organic nitrate. NO is a physiological messenger molecule that endothelial cells release onto subjacent smooth muscle cells ("endothelium-derived relaxant factor," EDRF). Organic nitrates thus utilize a physiological pathway; hence their high efficacy. The enzymatically mediated generation of NO from organic nitrates (via a mitochondrial aldehyde dehydrogenase) within the smooth muscle cell depends on a supply of free sulfhydryl (–SH) groups; "nitrate-tolerance" is attributed to a cellular exhaustion of SH donors.

Nitroglycerin (NTG) is distinguished by a high membrane penetrability and very low stability. It is the drug of choice in the treatment of angina pectoris attacks. For this purpose, it is administered as a spray, or in sublingual or buccal tablets for transmucosal delivery. The onset of action is between 1 and 3 minutes. Due to a nearly complete presystemic elimination, it is poorly suited for oral administration. Transdermal delivery (nitroglycerin patch) also avoids presystemic elimination.

Isosorbide dinitrate (ISDN) penetrates well through membranes, is more stable than NTG, and is partly degraded into the weaker, but much longer acting, 5-isosorbide mononitrate (ISMN). ISDN can also be applied sublingually; however, it is mainly administered orally in order to achieve a prolonged effect. ISMN is not suitable for sublingual use because of its higher polarity and slower rate of absorption. Taken orally, it is absorbed and is not subject to first-pass elimination.

Molsidomine itself is inactive. After oral intake, it is slowly converted into an active metabolite, linsidomine. The differential effectiveness in arterial vs. venous beds is less evident compared to the drugs mentioned above. Moreover, development of "nitrate tolerance" is of less concern. These differences in activity profile appear to reflect a different mechanism of NO release. The same applies to the following sodium nitroprusside.

Sodium nitroprusside contains a nitroso (–NO) group, but is not an ester. It dilates venous and arterial beds equally. It is administered by infusion to achieve *controlled hypotension* under continuous close monitoring. Cyanide ions liberated from nitroprusside can be inactivated with sodium thiosulfate (p. 310).

A. Vasodilators: Nitrates

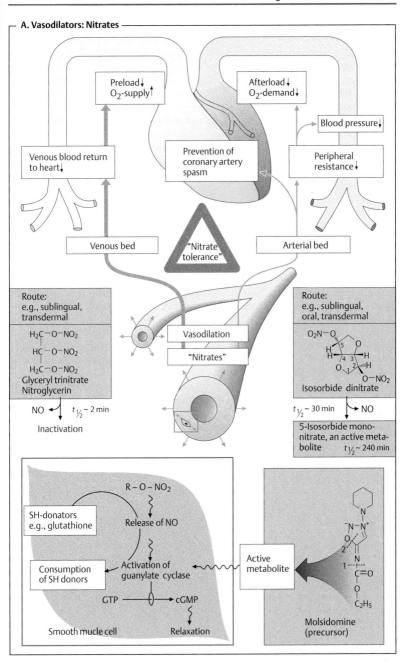

Preload↓
O₂-supply↑

Afterload↓
O₂-demand↓

Blood pressure↓

Venous blood return to heart↓

Prevention of coronary artery spasm

Peripheral resistance↓

Venous bed

"Nitrate tolerance"

Arterial bed

Route: e.g., sublingual, transdermal

$H_2C-O-NO_2$
$HC-O-NO_2$
$H_2C-O-NO_2$
Glyceryl trinitrate
Nitroglycerin

NO ← $t_{1/2}$ ~ 2 min

Inactivation

Vasodilation

"Nitrates"

Route: e.g., sublingual, oral, transdermal

O_2N-O
Isosorbide dinitrate

$t_{1/2}$ ~ 30 min   → NO

5-Isosorbide mono-nitrate, an active meta-bolite $t_{1/2}$ ~ 240 min

$R-O-NO_2$

SH-donators e.g., glutathione

Release of NO

Consumption of SH donors

Activation of guanylate cyclase

GTP → cGMP

Smooth mucle cell

Relaxation

Active metabolite

Molsidomine (precursor)

□ Calcium Antagonists

During electrical excitation of the cell membrane of heart or smooth muscle, different ionic currents are activated, including an inward Ca^{2+} current. The term Ca^{2+} antagonist is applied to drugs that inhibit the influx of Ca^{2+} ions without affecting inward Na^+ or outward K^+ currents to a significant degree. Other labels are *calcium entry blocker* or *Ca^{2+}-channel blocker*. Ca^{2+} antagonists used therapeutically can be divided into three groups according to their effects on heart and vasculature.

I. Dihydropyridine Derivatives

The dihydropyridines, e.g., **nifedipine**, are uncharged hydrophobic substances. They particularly induce a *relaxation* of vascular smooth muscle in *arterial beds*. An effect on cardiac function is practically absent at therapeutic dosage. (In pharmacological experiments on isolated cardiac muscle preparations, a clear negative inotropic effect is, however, demonstrable at high concentrations.) They are thus regarded as *vasoselective Ca^{2+} antagonists*. Because of the dilation of resistance vessels, blood pressure falls. Cardiac afterload is diminished (p. 318) and, therefore, also oxygen demand. Spasms of coronary arteries are prevented.

Indications. An indication for nifedipine is *angina pectoris* (p. 318). In angina pectoris, it is effective when given either prophylactically or during acute attacks. **Adverse effects** are palpitation (reflex tachycardia due to hypotension), headache, and pretibial edema.

The successor substances principally exert the same effects, but have different kinetic properties (slow elimination and, hence, steady plasma levels).

Nitrendipine, isradipine, and *felodipine* are used in the treatment of hypertension. *Nicardipine* and *nisoldipine* are also used in angina pectoris. *Nimodipine* is given prophylactically after subarachnoidal hemorrhage to prevent vasospasms. On its dihydropyridine ring, *amlodipine* possesses a side chain with a protonatable nitrogen and can therefore exist in a positively charged state. This influences its pharmacokinetics, as evidenced by the very long half-life of elimination (~40 hours).

II. Verapamil and Other Catamphiphilic Ca^{2+} Antagonists

Verapamil contains a nitrogen atom bearing a positive charge at physiological pH and thus represents a *cationic amphiphilic molecule*. It exerts inhibitory effects not only on *arterial smooth muscle*, but also on *heart muscle*. In the heart, Ca^{2+} inward currents are important in generating depolarization of sinoatrial node cells (impulse generation), in impulse propagation through the AV-junction (atrioventricular conduction), and in electromechanical coupling in the ventricular cardiomyocytes. Verapamil thus produces negative chronotropic, dromotropic, and inotropic effects.

Indications. Verapamil is used as an *antiarrhythmic drug* in supraventricular tachyarrhythmias. In atrial flutter or fibrillation, it is effective in reducing ventricular rate by virtue of inhibiting AV conduction. Verapamil is also employed in the prophylaxis of *angina pectoris attacks* (p. 318) and the treatment of *hypertension* (p. 314).

Adverse effects. Because of verapamil's effects on the sinus node, a drop in blood pressure fails to evoke a reflex tachycardia. Heart rate hardly changes; bradycardia may even develop. AV-block and myocardial insufficiency can occur. Patients frequently complain of constipation, because verapamil also inhibits intestinal musculature.

Gallopamil (= methoxyverapamil) is closely related to verapamil in terms of both structure and biological activity.

Diltiazem is a catamphiphilic benzothiazepine derivative with an activity profile resembling that of verapamil.

A. Vasodilators: calcium antagonists

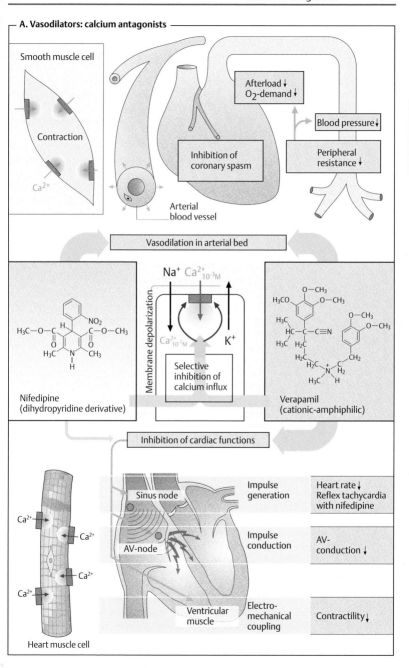

Smooth muscle cell

Contraction

Ca²⁺

Arterial
blood vessel

Inhibition of
coronary spasm

Afterload ↓
O₂-demand ↓

Blood pressure ↓

Peripheral
resistance ↓

Vasodilation in arterial bed

Membrane depolarization

Na⁺   Ca²⁺₁₀₋³ₘ

Ca²⁺₁₀₋⁷ₘ   K⁺

Selective
inhibition of
calcium influx

Nifedipine
(dihydropyridine derivative)

Verapamil
(cationic-amphiphilic)

Inhibition of cardiac functions

Sinus node

AV-node

Ventricular
muscle

Heart muscle cell

Ca²⁺

Impulse
generation

Heart rate ↓
Reflex tachycardia
with nifedipine

Impulse
conduction

AV-
conduction ↓

Electro-
mechanical
coupling

Contractility ↓

□ ACE Inhibitors

Angiotensin-converting enzyme (ACE) is a component of the antihypotensive renin–angiotensin–aldosterone (RAA) system. Renin is produced by specialized smooth muscle cells in the wall of the afferent arteriole of the renal glomerulus. These cells belong to the juxtaglomerular apparatus, the site of contact between afferent arteriole and distal tubule, which plays an important part in controlling nephron function. Stimuli eliciting *release of renin* are: drop in renal perfusion pressure, decreased rate of delivery of Na^+ or Cl^- to the distal tubules, as well as β-adrenoceptor-mediated sympathoactivation. The glycoprotein renin enzymatically cleaves the decapeptide angiotensin I from its circulating precursor substrate angiotensinogen. The enzyme ACE, in turn, produces biologically active angiotensin II from angiotensin I.

ACE is a rather nonspecific peptidase that can cleave C-terminal dipeptides from various peptides (dipeptidyl carboxypeptidase). As "kininase II," it contributes to the inactivation of kinins, such as bradykinin. ACE is also present in blood plasma; however, enzyme localized in the luminal side of vascular endothelium is primarily responsible for the formation of angiotensin II.

Angiotensin II can raise blood pressure in different ways, including (1) vasoconstriction in both the arterial and venous limb of the circulation; (2) stimulation of aldosterone secretion, leading to increased renal reabsorption of NaCl and water, hence an increased blood volume; (3) a central increase in sympathotonus and, peripherally, enhanced release and effects of norepinephrine. Chronically elevated levels of angiotensin II can increase muscle mass in heart and arteries (trophic effect).

ACE inhibitors, such as *captopril* and *enalaprilat*, the active metabolite of enalapril, occupy the enzyme as false substrates. Affinity significantly influences efficacy and rate of elimination. Enalaprilat has a stronger and longer-lasting effect than captopril.

Indications are *hypertension* and *cardiac failure.*

Lowering of elevated blood pressure is predominantly brought about by diminished production of angiotensin II. Impaired degradation of kinins that exert vasodilating actions may contribute to the effect.

In heart failure, cardiac output rises again after administration of an ACE inhibitor because ventricular afterload diminishes owing to a fall in peripheral resistance. Venous congestion abates as a result of (1) increased cardiac output and (2) reduction in venous return (decreased aldosterone secretion, decreased tonus of venous capacitance vessels).

Undesired effects. The magnitude of the antihypertensive effect of ACE inhibitors depends on the functional state of the RAA system. When the latter has been activated by loss of electrolytes and water (resulting from treatment with diuretic drugs), by cardiac failure, or by renal arterial stenosis, administration of ACE inhibitors may initially cause an excessive fall in blood pressure. Dry cough is a fairly frequent side effect, possibly caused by reduced inactivation of kinins in the bronchial mucosa. In most cases, ACE inhibitors are well tolerated and effective. Newer analogues include lisinopril, perindopril, ramipril, quinapril, fosinopril, benazepril, cilazapril, and trandolapril.

Antagonists at angiotensin II receptors. Two receptor subtypes can be distinguished: AT_1, which mediates the above actions of angiotensin II; and AT_2, whose physiological role is still unclear. *Losartan* is an AT_1 receptor antagonist whose main (antihypertensive) and side effects resemble those of ACE inhibitors. However, because it does not inhibit degradation of kinins, it does not cause dry cough. Losartan is used in the therapy of hypertension. Other analogues are valsartan, irbesartan, eprosartan, and candesartan.

A. Renin-angiotensin-aldosterone system and inhibitors

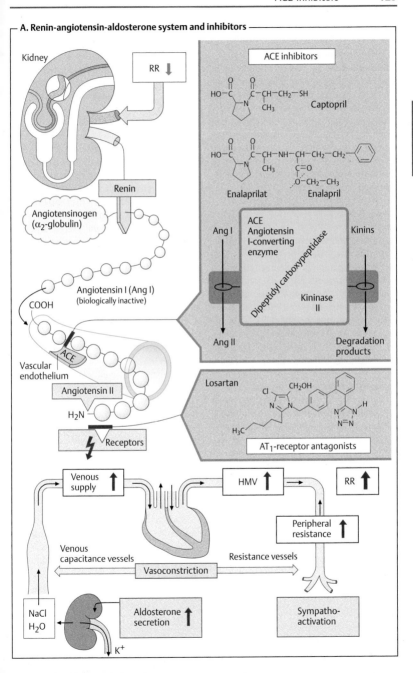

□ Drugs Used to Influence Smooth Muscle Organs

Bronchodilators. Narrowing of bronchioles raises airway resistance, e. g., in bronchial or bronchitic asthma. Several substances that are employed as *bronchodilators* are described elsewhere in more detail: β_2-sympathomimetics (p. 88; given by pulmonary, parenteral, or oral route), the methylxanthine *theophylline* (p. 338; given parenterally or orally), and the parasympatholytics *ipratropium* and *tiotropium* (p. 108).

Spasmolytics. *N-butylscopolamine* (p. 108) is used for the relief of painful spasms of the biliary or ureteral ducts. Its poor absorption (N.B. quaternary N; absorption rate < 10%) necessitates parenteral administration. Because the therapeutic effect is usually weak, a potent analgesic is given concurrently, e. g., the opioid meperidine. Note that some spasms of intestinal musculature can be effectively relieved by organic nitrates (in biliary colic) or by nifedipine (esophageal hypertension and achalasia).

Myometrial relaxants (tocolytics). β_2-Sympathomimetics such as fenoterol, given orally or parenterally, can prevent premature labor or interrupt labor in progress when dangerous complications necessitate caesarean section. Tachycardia is a side effect produced reflexly because of β_2-mediated vasodilation or a direct stimulation of cardiac β_1-receptors. Recently, *atosiban*, a structurally altered oxytocin derivative, has become available. It acts as an antagonist at oxytocin receptors, is given parenterally, and lacks the cardiovascular side effects of β_2-sympathomimetics, but often causes nausea and vomiting.

Myometrial stimulants. The neurohypophyseal hormone *oxytocin* (p. 238) is given parenterally (or by the nasal or buccal route) before, during, or after labor in order to prompt uterine contractions or to enhance them. Certain *prostaglandins* or analogues of them (p. 196; $F_2\alpha$, dinoprost; E_2, dinoprostone, sulprostone) are capable of inducing rhythmic uterine contractions and cervical relaxation at any time. They are mostly employed as abortifacients (local or parenteral application).

Ergot alkaloids are obtained from *Secale cornutum* (ergot), the sclerotium of a fungus (*Claviceps purpurea*) parasitizing rye. Consumption of flour from contaminated grain was once the cause of epidemic poisonings (*ergotism*) characterized by gangrene of the extremities (St. Anthony's fire) and CNS disturbances (hallucinations).

Ergot alkaloids contain lysergic acid (see ergotamine formula in **A**). They act on uterine and vascular muscle. *Ergometrine* particularly stimulates the uterus. It readily induces a tonic contraction of the myometrium (tetanus uteri). This jeopardizes placental blood flow and fetal oxygen supply. Ergometrine is not used therapeutically. The semisynthetic derivative *methylergometrine* is used only *after* delivery for uterine contractions that are too weak.

Ergotamine, as well as the ergotoxine alkaloids (ergocristine, ergocryptine, ergocornine), have a predominantly vascular action. Depending on the initial caliber, constriction or dilation may be elicited. The mechanism of action is unclear; a partial agonism at α-adrenoceptors may be important. Ergotamine is used in the treatment of migraine (p. 334). Its derivative, dihydroergotamine, is furthermore employed in orthostatic complaints (p. 324).

Other *lysergic acid derivatives* are the 5-HT antagonist methysergide, the dopamine agonist bromocriptine (p. 116), and the hallucinogen lysergic acid diethylamide (LSD, p. 236).

A. Drugs used to alter smooth-muscle function

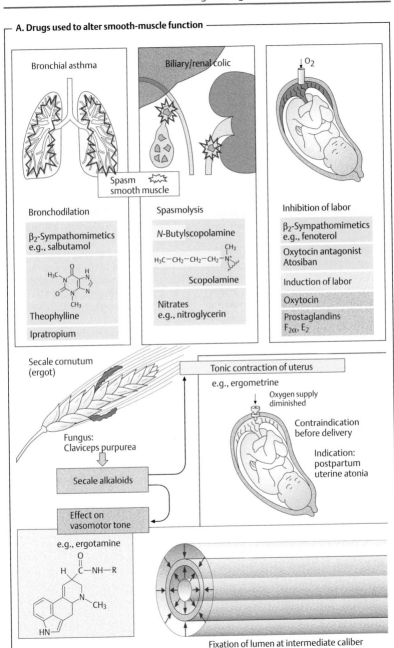

Bronchial asthma

Biliary/renal colic

↓ O₂

Spasm
smooth muscle

Bronchodilation

β₂-Sympathomimetics
e.g., salbutamol

H₃C ... CH₃

Theophylline

Ipratropium

Spasmolysis

N-Butylscopolamine

$H_3C-CH_2-CH_2-CH_2-N^+$ ... CH_3

Scopolamine

Nitrates
e.g., nitroglycerin

Inhibition of labor

β₂-Sympathomimetics
e.g., fenoterol

Oxytocin antagonist
Atosiban

Induction of labor

Oxytocin

Prostaglandins
$F_{2\alpha}$, E_2

Secale cornutum
(ergot)

Fungus:
Claviceps purpurea

Secale alkaloids

Effect on
vasomotor tone

e.g., ergotamine

Tonic contraction of uterus

e.g., ergometrine

Oxygen supply
diminished

Contraindication
before delivery

Indication:
postpartum
uterine atonia

Fixation of lumen at intermediate caliber

□ Cardiac Drugs

Possible ways of influencing heart function (A). The pumping capacity of the heart depends on different factors: with increasing heart rate, the force of contraction increases ("positive staircase"); the degree of diastolic filling regulates contraction amplitude (Starling's law of the heart). The sympathetic innervation with its transmitter norepinephrine and the hormone epinephrine promote contractile force generation (but also oxygen consumption), and raise beating rate and excitability (p. 88). The parasympathetic innervation lowers beat frequency because acetylcholine inhibits pacemaker cells (p. 104).

From the influence of the autonomic nervous system it follows that all sympatholytic or sympathomimetic and parasympatholytic or parasympathomimetic drugs can produce corresponding effects on cardiac performance. These possibilities are exploited therapeutically: for instance, β-blockers for suppressing excessive sympathetic drive (p. 96); ipratropium for treating sinus bradycardia (p. 108). An unwanted activation of the sympathetic system can result from anxiety, pain, and other emotional stress. In these cases, the heart can be protected from harmful stimulation by psychopharmaceuticals such as benzodiazepines (diazepam and others; important in myocardial infarction).

Cardiac work furthermore depends strongly on the state of the circulation system: physical rest or work demand appropriate cardiac performance; the level of mean blood pressure is an additional decisive factor. Chronic elevation of afterload leads to myocardial insufficiency. Therefore, all blood pressure-lowering drugs can have an important therapeutic influence on the myocardium. Vasodilator substances (e. g., nitrates) lower the venous return and/or peripheral resistance and, hence, exert a favorable effect in angina pectoris or heart failure.

The heart muscle cells can also be reached directly. Thus, cardiac glycosides bind to the Na$^+$/K$^+$-ATPases, (p. 134), the Ca-antagonists to Ca^{2+} channels (p. 126), and antiarrhythmics of the local anaesthetic type to Na$^+$ channels (p. 136) in the plasmalemma.

Events underlying contraction and relaxation (B). The signal triggering **contraction** is a propagated action potential (AP) generated in the sinoatrial node. *Depolarization* of the plasmalemma leads to a rapid *rise in cytosolic Ca^{2+} levels*, which causes contraction (**electromechanical coupling**). The level of Ca^{2+} concentration attained determines the degree of shortening, i. e., the force of contraction. Sources of calcium are: (a) extracellular calcium entering the cell through voltage-gated *Ca^{2+} channels*; (b) calcium stored in the *sarcoplasmic reticulum* (SR); (c) calcium bound to the inside of the *plasmalemma*. The plasmalemma of cardiomyocytes extends into the cell interior in the form of tubular invaginations (transverse tubuli).

The trigger signal for **relaxation** is the return of the membrane potential to its resting level. During repolarization Ca^{2+} levels fall below the threshold for activation of the myofilaments (3×10^{-7} M): the *plasmalemmal* Ca binding sites regain their Ca-binding capacity; calcium ions are pumped back into the SR lumen and the plasmalemmal *ATPases* move Ca^{2+} that entered during systole back out of the cell under expenditure of energy. Additionally, Ca^{2+} is extruded from the cell in exchange for Na$^+$ (Na/Ca *exchanger*).

A. Possible mechanisms for influencing heart function

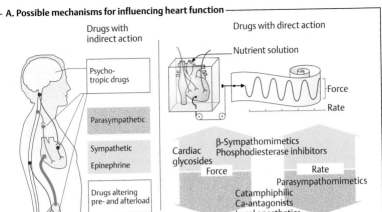

Drugs with indirect action

Psycho-tropic drugs

Parasympathetic

Sympathetic
Epinephrine

Drugs altering pre- and afterload

Drugs with direct action

Nutrient solution

Force
Rate

β-Sympathomimetics
Phosphodiesterase inhibitors
Cardiac glycosides
Force
Rate
Parasympathomimetics
Catamphiphilic
Ca-antagonists
Local anesthetics

B. Processes in myocardial contraction and relaxation

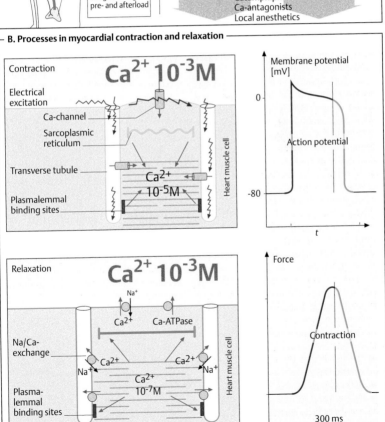

Contraction

Ca^{2+} 10^{-3}M

Electrical excitation

Ca-channel

Sarcoplasmic reticulum

Transverse tubule

Ca^{2+} 10^{-5}M

Plasmalemmal binding sites

Heart muscle cell

Membrane potential [mV]

0

Action potential

-80

t

Relaxation

Ca^{2+} 10^{-3}M

Na^+
Ca^{2+} Ca-ATPase

Na/Ca-exchange

Ca^{2+} Ca^{2+}
Na^+ Ca^{2+} 10^{-7}M Na^+

Plasma-lemmal binding sites

Heart muscle cell

Force

Contraction

300 ms

t

▫ Cardiac Glycosides

Diverse plants are sources of sugar-containing compounds (glycosides) that also contain a steroid ring system (structural formulas, **A**) and augment the contractile force of heart muscle: *cardiotonic glycosides, cardiosteroids, "digitalis."*

The cardiosteroids possess a small therapeutic margin, signs of intoxication are arrhythmia and contracture (**B**). This therapeutic drawback can be explained by the mechanism of action.

Cardiac glycosides (**CG**) bind to the extracellular domain of Na^+/K^+-ATPases and exclude this enzyme molecule for a time from further ion transport activity. The high-affinity binding of CG is restricted to a particular conformation that the enzyme adopts during its transport cycle. In the resting state, Na^+/K^+-ATPase molecules are not binding partners. Under normal conditions only a fraction of the Na^+/K^+-ATPase transport activity is required to maintain the high gradients of Na^+ and K^+ across the plasmalemma. Low therapeutic concentrations of CG occupy only a fraction of Na^+/K^+-ATPases; the decrease of the resulting pump activity can easily be compensated for by recruitment of resting ATPase molecules via a small increase of the intracellular Na^+ concentration.

Attached to the ATPases there are Na^+ channels which, upon binding of CG to the enzyme, lose their specificity for Na^+ and are converted to nonselective, promiscuous channels: during systole, Ca^{2+} will easily pass through this channel owing to its huge gradient (almost 4 orders of magnitude!). This results in an increased Ca^{2+}-influx and augmented contractile force. It should, however, be noted that the mode of action of cardiosteroids is still a matter of debate.

Mobilization of edema (weight loss) and lowering of heart rate are simple but decisive criteria for achieving optimal dosing. If ATPase activity is inhibited too much, K^+ and Na^+ homeostasis is disturbed: the membrane potential declines, arrhythmias occur. Intracellular flooding with Ca^{2+} prevents relaxation during diastole: *contracture.*

The **CNS effects** of CGs (**C**) are also due to binding to Na^+/K^+-ATPases. Enhanced vagal nerve activity causes a decrease in sinoatrial beating rate and velocity of atrioventricular conduction. In patients with heart failure improved circulation also contributes to the reduction in heart rate. Stimulation of the area postrema leads to nausea and vomiting.

Indications for CGs are:
1 *chronic congestive heart failure,*
2 *atrial fibrillation or flutter,* where inhibition of AV conduction protects the ventricles from excessive atrial impulse activity and thereby improves cardiac performance (**D**).

Signs of intoxication are:
1 *Cardiac arrhythmias,* which under certain circumstances are life-threatening, e.g., sinus bradycardia, AV-block, ventricular extrasystoles, ventricular fibrillation (ECG);
2 *CNS disturbances:* characteristically, altered color vision (xanthopsia), and also fatigue, disorientation, hallucinations;
3 anorexia, nausea, vomiting, diarrhea;
4 *renal:* loss of electrolytes and water; this must be differentiated from mobilization of edema fluid accumulated in front of the heart during congestive failure, an effect expected with therapeutic dosage.

Therapy of intoxication: *administration of* K^+, which *inter alia* reduces binding of CG, but may impair AV-conduction; administration of antiarrhythmics, such as *phenytoin or lidocaine* (p. 136); oral administration of *colestyramine* (p. 160) for binding and preventing absorption of digitoxin present in the intestines (enterohepatic cycle), and most importantly injection of *antibody (Fab) fragments* that bind and inactivate digitoxin and digoxin. Compared with full antibodies, fragments have superior tissue penetrability, more rapid renal elimination, and lower antigenicity.

A. Cardiac glycosides

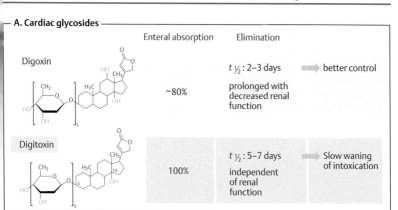

	Enteral absorption	Elimination	
Digoxin	~80%	$t\frac{1}{2}$: 2–3 days prolonged with decreased renal function	better control
Digitoxin	100%	$t\frac{1}{2}$: 5–7 days independent of renal function	Slow waning of intoxication

B. Therapeutic and toxic effects of cardiac glycosides (CG)

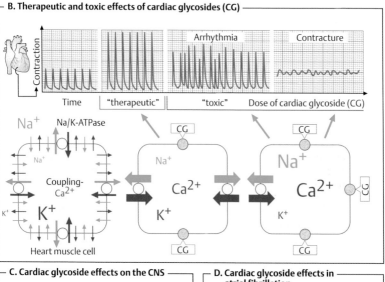

Contraction

Time   "therapeutic"   Arrhythmia   Contracture   "toxic"   Dose of cardiac glycoside (CG)

Na⁺   Na/K-ATPase

Na⁺

Coupling-Ca²⁺   Ca²⁺   CG   Na⁺   Ca²⁺   CG   CG

K⁺   K⁺   K⁺

Heart muscle cell   CG   CG

C. Cardiac glycoside effects on the CNS

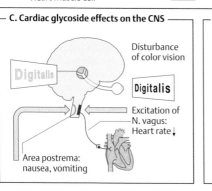

Digitalis

Disturbance of color vision

Digitalis

Excitation of N. vagus: Heart rate ↓

Area postrema: nausea, vomiting

D. Cardiac glycoside effects in atrial fibrillation

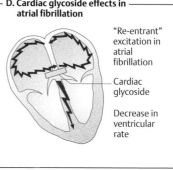

"Re-entrant" excitation in atrial fibrillation

Cardiac glycoside

Decrease in ventricular rate

□ Antiarrhythmic Drugs

The electrical impulse for contraction (propagated action potential; p.138) originates in pacemaker cells of the sinoatrial node and spreads through the atria, atrioventricular (AV) node, and adjoining parts of the His–Purkinje fiber system to the ventricles (**A**). Irregularities of heart rhythm can interfere dangerously with cardiac pumping function.

I. Drugs for Selective Control of Sinoatrial and AV Nodes

In some forms of arrhythmia, certain drugs can be used that are capable of selectively facilitating and inhibiting (green and red arrows, respectively) the pacemaker function of sinoatrial or atrioventricular cells.

Sinus bradycardia. An abnormally low sinoatrial impulse rate (< 60/min) can be raised by *parasympatholytics*. The quaternary *ipratropium* is preferable to atropine, because it lacks CNS penetrability (p.108). Sympathomimetics also exert a positive chronotropic action; they have the disadvantage of increasing myocardial excitability (and automaticity) and, thus, promoting ectopic impulse generation (tendency to extrasystolic beats). In **cardiac arrest**, *epinephrine*, given by intrabronchial instillation or intracardiac injection, can be used to reinitiate heart beat.

Sinus tachycardia (resting rate > 100 beats/min). β-Blockers eliminate sympatho-excitation and lower cardiac rate. Sotalol is noteworthy because of its good antiarrhythmic action (caution: QT-prolongation)

Atrial flutter or fibrillation. An excessive ventricular rate can be decreased by *verapamil* (p.126) or *cardiac glycosides* (p.134). These drugs inhibit impulse propagation through the AV node, so that fewer impulses reach the ventricles.

II. Nonspecific Drug Actions on Impulse Generation and Propagation

In some types of rhythm disorders, **antiarrhythmics of the local anesthetic, Na⁺-channel blocking type** are used for both prophylaxis and therapy. These substances block the Na^+ channel responsible for the fast depolarization of nerve and muscle tissues. Therefore, the elicitation of action potentials is impeded and impulse conduction is delayed. This effect may exert a favorable influence in some forms of arrhythmia, but can itself act arrhythmogenically. Unfortunately, antiarrhythmics of the local anesthetic, Na⁺-channel blocking type lack sufficient specificity in two respects: (1) other ion channels of cardiomyocytes, such as K^+ and Ca^+ channels, are also affected (abnormal QT prolongation); and (2) their action is not restricted to cardiac muscle tissue but also impacts on neural tissues and brain cells. Adverse effects on the heart include production of arrhythmias and lowering of heart rate, AV conduction, and systolic force. CNS side effects are manifested by vertigo, giddiness, disorientation, confusion, motor disturbances, etc.

Some antiarrhythmics are rapidly degraded in the body by cleavage (see arrows in **B**); these substances are not suitable for oral administration but must be given intravenously (e.g., lidocaine).

Irrespective of the cause underlying atrial fibrillation, formation of a thrombus may occur in the atria, because blood stagnates in the auricles. From such a thrombus an embolus may be dislodged and carried into the arterial supply of the brain, precipitating a *stroke*. It is therefore imperative to institute anticoagulant therapy in atrial fibrillation. For immediate effect, heparin preparations are indicated; subsequently, changeover to vitamin K antagonists (e.g., phenprocoumon) may be made. As long as episodes of arrhythmia occur, therapy must be continued.

A. Cardiac impulse generation and conduction

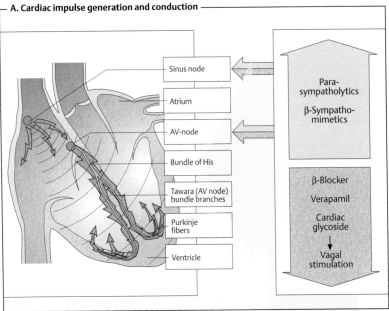

Sinus node

Atrium

AV-node

Bundle of His

Tawara (AV node) bundle branches

Purkinje fibers

Ventricle

Para-sympatholytics

β-Sympatho-mimetics

β-Blocker

Verapamil

Cardiac glycoside

↓

Vagal stimulation

B. Antiarrhythmics of the Na⁺-channel blocking type

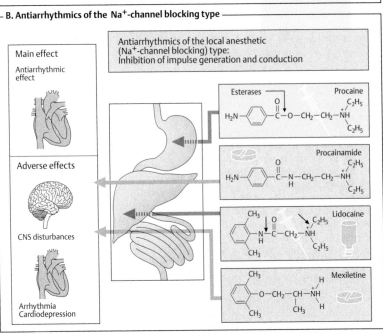

Antiarrhythmics of the local anesthetic (Na$^+$-channel blocking) type: Inhibition of impulse generation and conduction

Main effect

Antiarrhythmic effect

Adverse effects

CNS disturbances

Arrhythmia Cardiodepression

Procaine

Procainamide

Lidocaine

Mexiletine

☐ Electrophysiological Actions of Antiarrhythmics of the Na⁺-Channel Blocking Type

Action potential and ionic currents. The transmembrane electrical potential of cardiomyocytes can be recorded through an intracellular microelectrode. Upon electrical excitation, the resting potential shows a characteristic change—the action potential (AP). Its underlying cause is a sequence of transient ionic currents. During *rapid depolarization* (phase 0), there is a short-lived *influx of Na⁺* through the membrane. A subsequent *transient influx of Ca²⁺* (as well as of Na⁺) maintains the depolarization (phase 2, *plateau of AP*). A delayed *efflux of K⁺* returns the membrane potential (phase 3, *repolarization*) to its resting value (phase 4). The velocity of depolarization determines the speed at which the AP propagates through the myocardial syncytium.

The transmembrane ionic currents involve proteinaceous *membrane pores*: Na⁺, Ca²⁺, and K⁺ channels. In (**A**), the phasic change in the functional state of Na⁺ channels during an action potential is illustrated.

Na+-channel blocking antiarrhythmics *reduce the probability of Na⁺ channels* to open upon membrane depolarization ("**membrane stabilization**"). The potential consequences are (**A**, bottom): (1) A reduction in the velocity of depolarization and a decrease in the speed of impulse propagation; aberrant impulse propagation is impeded. (2) *Depolarization is entirely absent*; pathological impulse generation, e. g., in the marginal zone of an infarction, is suppressed. (3) The time required until a new depolarization can be elicited, i. e., the *refractory period, is increased*; prolongation of the AP (see below) contributes to the increase in refractory period. Consequently, premature excitation with risk of fibrillation is prevented.

Mechanism of action. Na⁺-channel blocking antiarrhythmics resemble most local anesthetics in being cationic amphiphilic molecules (p. 206; exception: phenytoin, p. 191). Possible molecular mechanisms of their inhibitory effects are outlined on p. 202 in more detail. Their low structural specificity is reflected by a low selectivity toward different cation channels. Besides the Na⁺ channel, *Ca²⁺and K⁺ channels* are also likely to be *blocked*. Accordingly, cationic amphiphilic antiarrhythmics affect both the depolarization and repolarization phases. Depending on the substance, AP duration can be increased (Class IA), decreased (Class IB), or remain the same (Class IC). *Antiarrhythmics representative of these categories* include: Class IA—quinidine, procainamide, ajmaline, disopyramide; Class IB—lidocaine, mexiletine, tocainide; Class IC—flecainide, propafenone.

K²⁺–channel blocking antiarrhythmics. The drug amiodarone and the β-blocker sotalol have been assigned to Class III, comprising agents that cause marked prolongation of AP with less effect on the velocity of depolarization. Note that Class II is represented by β-blockers and Class IV by the Ca²⁺-channel blockers verapamil and diltiazem (see p. 126).

Therapeutic uses. Because of their *narrow therapeutic margin*, antiarrhythmics are only employed when rhythm disturbances are of such severity as to impair the pumping action of the heart, or when there is a threat of other complications. Combinations of different antiarrhythmics are not recommended (e. g., quinidine plus verapamil). Some agents, such as amiodarone, are reserved for special cases. This iodine-containing substance has unusual properties: its elimination half-life is 50–70 days; depending on its electrical charge, it is bound to apolar and polar lipids, stored in tissues (corneal opacification, pulmonary fibrosis); and it interferes with thyroid function.

A. Effects of antiarrhythmics of the Na⁺-channel blocking type

Ionic currents during action potential

States of Na⁺-channels during an action potential

□ Drugs for the Treatment of Anemias

Anemia denotes a reduction in red blood cell count or hemoglobin content, or both.

Erythropoiesis (A)

Blood corpuscles develop from stem cells through several cell divisions ($n = 17!$). Hemoglobin is then synthesized and the cell nucleus is extruded. Erythropoiesis is stimulated by the hormone **erythropoietin** (a glycoprotein), which is released from the kidneys when renal oxygen tension declines. A nephrogenic anemia can be ameliorated by parenteral administration of recombinant erythropoietin (epoetin alfa) or hyperglycosylated erythropoietin (darbepoetin; longer half-life than epoetin).

Even in healthy humans, formation of red blood cells and, hence, the oxygen transport capacity of blood, is augmented by erythropoietin,. This effect is equivalent to high-altitude training and is employed as a doping method by high-performance athletes. Erythropoietin is inactivated by cleavage of sugar residues, with a biological half-life of ~ 5 hours after intravenous injection and a $t_{1/2}$ > 20 hours after subcutaneous injection.

Given adequate production of erythropoietin, a **disturbance of erythropoiesis** is due to two principal causes. (1) **Cell multiplication** is **inhibited** because DNA synthesis is insufficient. This occurs in deficiencies of *vitamin B_{12}* or *folic acid* (macrocytic hyperchromic anemia). (2) **Hemoglobin synthesis** is **impaired**. This situation arises in **iron deficiency**, since Fe^{2+} is a constituent of hemoglobin (microcytic hypochromic anemia).

Vitamin B_{12} (B)

Vitamin B_{12} (**cyanocobalamin**) is produced by bacteria; vitamin B_{12} generated in the colon, however, is unavailable for absorption. Liver, meat, fish, and milk products are rich sources of the vitamin. The **minimal requirement** is about 1 µg/day. Enteral absorption of vitamin B_{12} requires the so-called "**intrinsic factor**" from parietal cells of the stomach. The complex formed with this gly-coprotein undergoes endocytosis in the ileum. Bound to its transport protein, transcobalamin, vitamin B_{12} is destined for storage in the liver or uptake into tissues.

A frequent cause of **vitamin B_{12} deficiency** is atrophic gastritis leading to a *lack of intrinsic factor.* Besides megaloblastic anemia, damage to mucosal linings and degeneration of myelin sheaths with neurological sequelae will occur (**pernicious anemia**). The optimal **therapy** consists in **parenteral administration** of **cyanocobalamin** or **hydroxycobalamin** (vitamin B_{12a}; exchange of –CN for –OH group). Adverse effects, in the form of hypersensitivity reactions, are very rare.

Folic Acid (B)

Leafy vegetables and liver are rich in folic acid (FA). The **minimal requirement** is ~ 50 µg/day. Polyglutamine-FA in food is hydrolyzed to monoglutamine-FA prior to being absorbed. **Causes of deficiency** include insufficient intake, malabsorption, and increased requirements during pregnancy (hence the prophylactic administration during pregnancy). Antiepileptic drugs and oral contraceptives may decrease FA absorption, presumably by inhibiting the formation of monoglutamine-FA. Inhibition of dihydro-FA reductase (e. g., by methotrexate, p. 300) depresses the formation of the active species, tetrahydro-FA. *Symptoms* of deficiency are megaloblastic anemia and mucosal damage. **Therapy** consists in **oral administration** of FA.

Administration of FA can mask a vitamin B_{12} deficiency. Vitamin B_{12} is required for the conversion of methyltetrahydro-FA to tetrahydro-FA, which is important for DNA-synthesis (**B**). Inhibition of this reaction due to vitamin B_{12} deficiency can be compensated by increased FA intake. The anemia is readily corrected; however, nerve degeneration progresses unchecked and its cause is made more difficult to diagnose by the absence of hematological changes. Indiscriminate use of FA-containing multivitamin preparations can, therefore, be harmful.

A. Erythropoiesis in bone marrow

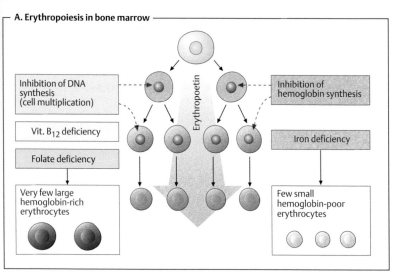

Inhibition of DNA synthesis (cell multiplication)

Inhibition of hemoglobin synthesis

Erythropoetin

Vit. B$_{12}$ deficiency

Folate deficiency

Iron deficiency

Very few large hemoglobin-rich erythrocytes

Few small hemoglobin-poor erythrocytes

B. Vitamin B$_{12}$ and folate metabolism

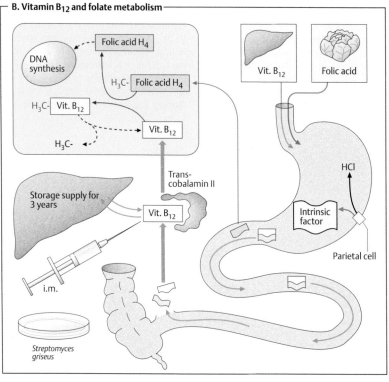

DNA synthesis

Folic acid H$_4$

H$_3$C- Folic acid H$_4$

H$_3$C- Vit. B$_{12}$

Vit. B$_{12}$

H$_3$C-

Vit. B$_{12}$

Folic acid

Trans-cobalamin II

Storage supply for 3 years

Vit. B$_{12}$

HCl

Intrinsic factor

Parietal cell

i.m.

Streptomyces griseus

☐ Iron Compounds

Not all iron ingested in food is equally absorbable. Trivalent Fe^{3+} is virtually not taken up from the neutral milieu of the small bowel, where the divalent Fe^{2+} is markedly better absorbed. Uptake is particularly efficient in the form of heme (present in hemoglobin and myoglobin). Within the mucosal cells of the gut, iron is oxidized and either deposited as ferritin (see below) or passed on to the transport protein, transferrin. The amount absorbed does not exceed that needed to balance losses due to epithelial shedding from skin and mucosae or hemorrhage (so-called "**mucosal block**"). In men this amount is ~ 1 mg/day, in women it is ~ 2 mg/day (because of menstrual blood loss); it corresponds to about 10% of the dietary intake. The transferrin–iron complex undergoes endocytotic uptake into erythrocyte precursors to be utilized for hemoglobin synthesis. About 70% of the total body store of iron (~ 5 g) is contained within erythrocytes. When these are degraded by macrophages of the mononuclear phagocyte system, iron is liberated from hemoglobin. Fe^{3+} can be stored as ferritin (= protein apoferritin + Fe^{3+}) or be returned to erythropoiesis sites via transferrin.

A frequent **cause of iron deficiency** is chronic blood loss due to gastric/intestinal ulcers or tumors. One liter of blood contains 500 mg of iron in healthy condition. Despite a significant increase in absorption rate, absorption is unable to keep up with losses and the body store of iron falls. Iron deficiency results in impaired synthesis of hemoglobin and **anemia**.

The **treatment** of choice (after the cause of bleeding has been found and eliminated) consists in the **oral administration of Fe^{2+}-compounds**, e.g., ferrous sulfate (daily dose 100 mg of iron, equivalent to 300 mg of $FeSO_4$, divided into multiple doses). Replenishing of iron stores may take several months. Oral administration, however, is advantageous in that it is impossible to overload the body with iron through an intact mucosa because of its demand-regulated absorption (mucosal block).

Adverse effects. The frequent gastrointestinal complaints (epigastric pain, diarrhea, constipation) necessitate intake of iron preparations with or after meals, although absorption is higher from the empty stomach.

Interactions. Antacids inhibit iron absorption. Combination with ascorbic acid (vitamin C) to protect Fe^{2+} from oxidation to Fe^{3+} is theoretically sound but practically is not needed.

Parenteral administration of Fe^{3+} salts is indicated only when adequate oral replacement is not possible. There is a risk of overdosage, with iron deposition in tissues (**hemosiderosis**). The binding capacity of transferrin is limited and free Fe^{3+} is toxic. Therefore, Fe^{3+} complexes are employed that can donate Fe^{3+} directly to transferrin or can be phagocytosed by macrophages, enabling iron to be incorporated into the ferritin store. Possible *adverse effects* are: with i.m. injection, persistent pain at the injection site and skin discoloration; with i.v. injection, flushing, hypotension, anaphylactic shock.

A. Iron: possible routes of administration and fate in the organism

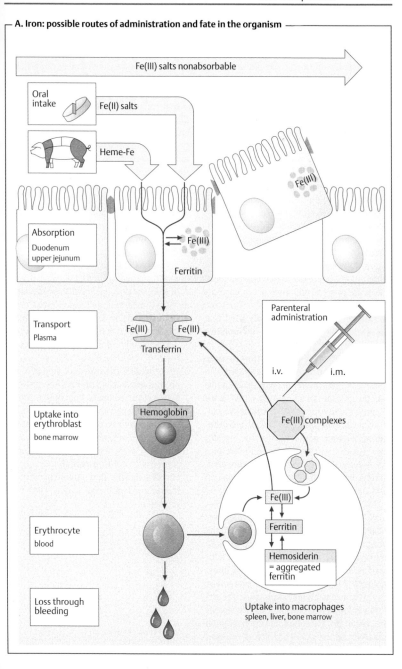

□ Prophylaxis and Therapy of Thromboses

Upon vascular injury, the coagulation system is activated: thrombocytes and fibrin molecules coalesce into a "plug" that seals the defect and halts bleeding (**hemostasis**). Unnecessary formation of an intravascular clot—a thrombosis—can be life-threatening. If the clot forms on an atheromatous plaque in a coronary artery, myocardial infarction is imminent; a thrombus in a deep leg vein can be dislodged and carried into a lung artery and can cause pulmonary embolism.

Drugs that *decrease the coagulability of blood*, such as **coumarins** and **heparin** (**A**) are employed for the **prophylaxis** of thromboses. In addition, attempts are directed, by means of acetylsalicylic acid, at inhibiting the aggregation of blood platelets, which are prominently involved in intra-arterial thrombogenesis (p. 152). For the **therapy** of thrombosis, drugs are used that dissolve the fibrin meshwork—**fibrinolytics** (p. 150).

An overview of the **coagulation cascade** and sites of action for coumarins and heparin is shown in (**A**). There are two ways to initiate the cascade (**B**): (1) conversion of factor XII into its active form (XII$_a$, intrinsic system) at intravascular sites denuded of endothelium; (2) conversion of factor VII into VII$_a$ (extrinsic system) under the influence of a tissue-derived lipoprotein (tissue thromboplastin). Both mechanisms converge via factor X into a common final pathway.

The **clotting factors** are protein molecules. "Activation" mostly means proteolysis (cleavage of protein fragments) and, with the exception of fibrin, conversion into protein-hydrolyzing enzymes (*proteases*). Some activated factors require the presence of phospholipids (PL) and Ca^{2+} for their proteolytic activity. Conceivably, Ca^{2+} ions cause the adhesion of factor to a phospholipid surface, as depicted in (**B**). Phospholipids are contained in platelet factor 3 (PF3), which is released from aggregated platelets, and in tissue thromboplastin (**A**). The sequential activation of several enzymes allows the aforementioned reactions to "snowball" (symbolized in **C** by increasing number of particles), culminating in massive production of fibrin.

Ca^{2+}-chelators (**B**) prevent the enzymatic activity of Ca^{2+}-dependent factors; they contain COO$^-$ groups that bind Ca^{2+} ions (**C**): **citrate** and **EDTA** (ethylenediaminetetraacetic acid) form soluble complexes with Ca^{2+}; **oxalate** precipitates Ca^{2+} as insoluble calcium oxalate. Chelation of Ca^{2+} cannot be used in vivo for therapeutic purposes because Ca^{2+} concentrations would have to be lowered to a level incompatible with life (hypocalcemic tetany). These compounds (sodium salts) are, therefore, used only for rendering blood incoagulable outside the body. This effect can be reversed at any time by addition of Ca^{2+} ions.

In vivo, the progression of the coagulation cascade can be inhibited as follows (**C**):

1. **Coumarin derivatives** decrease the blood concentrations of inactive factors II, VII, IX and X, by inhibiting their synthesis in the liver.

2. The complex consisting of **heparin** and antithrombin III neutralizes the protease activity of activated factors; unlike unfractionated heparin, *low-molecular-weight heparin fragments* or the "minimal molecular subunit of heparin," *fondaparinux*, inhibit only activated factor Xa when complexed with antithrombin III.

3. **Hirudin** and its derivatives (bivalirudin, lepirudin) block the active center of thrombin.

A. Activation of clotting

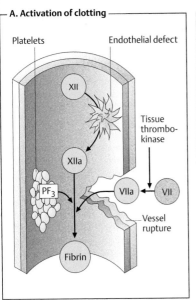

Platelets
Endothelial defect

XII

XIIa

PF₃

Tissue thrombo-kinase

VIIa   VII

Vessel rupture

Fibrin

B. Inhibition of clotting by removal of Ca²⁺

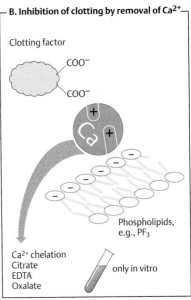

Clotting factor

COO^-

COO^-

Ca

Phospholipids, e.g., PF₃

Ca^{2+} chelation
Citrate
EDTA
Oxalate

only in vitro

C. Inhibition of clotting cascade in vivo

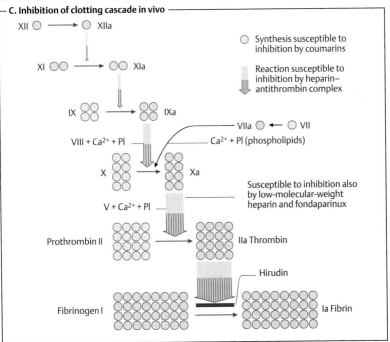

XII $\longrightarrow$ XIIa

○ Synthesis susceptible to inhibition by coumarins

XI $\longrightarrow$ XIa

Reaction susceptible to inhibition by heparin–antithrombin complex

IX $\longrightarrow$ IXa

VIIa ← VII

VIII + Ca²⁺ + Pl

Ca²⁺ + Pl (phospholipids)

X $\longrightarrow$ Xa

Susceptible to inhibition also by low-molecular-weight heparin and fondaparinux

V + Ca²⁺ + Pl

Prothrombin II $\longrightarrow$ IIa Thrombin

Hirudin

Fibrinogen I $\longrightarrow$ Ia Fibrin

□ Vitamin K Antagonists and Vitamin K

Vitamin K promotes the hepatic γ-carboxylation of glutamate residues on the precursors of factors II, VII, IX, and X. Carboxyl groups are required for Ca^{2+}-mediated binding to phospholipid surfaces (p.144). There are several vitamin K derivatives of different origins: K_1 (phytomenadione) from chlorophyllous plants; K_2 from gut bacteria; and K_3 (menadione) synthesized chemically. All are hydrophobic and require bile acids for absorption.

Oral anticoagulants. Structurally related to vitamin K, **4-hydroxycoumarins** act as "false" vitamin K and prevent regeneration of reduced (active) vitamin K from vitamin K epoxide, hence the synthesis of vitamin K-dependent clotting factors

Coumarins are well absorbed after oral administration. Their duration of action varies considerably. Synthesis of clotting factors depends on the intrahepatocytic concentration ratio between coumarins and vitamin K. The dose required for an adequate anticoagulant effect must be determined individually for each patient (monitoring of the International Normalized Ratio, INR).

Indications. Hydroxycoumarins are used for the prophylaxis of thromboembolism as, for instance, in atrial fibrillation or after heart valve replacement.

The **most important adverse effect is bleeding**. With coumarins, this can be counteracted by giving vitamin K_1. However, coagulability of blood returns to normal only after hours or days, when the liver has resumed synthesis and restored sufficient blood levels of carboxylated clotting factors. In urgent cases, deficient factors must be replenished directly (e.g., by transfusion of whole blood or of prothrombin concentrate).

Other notable adverse effects include: at the start of therapy, hemorrhagic skin necroses and alopecia; with exposure in utero, disturbances of fetal cartilage and bone formation and CNS injury (due to bleeding); enhanced risk of retroplacental bleeding.

□ Possibilities for Interference (B)

Adjusting the dosage of a hydroxycoumarin calls for a delicate balance between the opposing risks of bleeding (effect too strong) and of thrombosis (effect too weak). After the dosage has been titrated successfully, loss of control may occur if certain interfering factors are ignored. If the patient changes dietary habits and consumes more vegetables, vitamin K may predominate over the vitamin K antagonist. If vitamin K-producing gut flora is damaged in the course of antibiotic therapy, the antagonist may prevail. Drugs that increase hepatic biotransformation via enzyme induction (p. 38) may accelerate elimination of a hydroxycoumarin and thus lower its blood level. Inhibitors of hepatic biotransformation (e. g., the H_2 blocker cimetidine) augment the action of hydroxycoumarins. Apart from pharmacokinetic alterations, pharmacodynamic interactions must be taken into account. Thus, acetylsalicylic acid is contraindicated because (a) it retards hemostasis by inhibiting platelet aggregation and (b) it may cause damage to the gastric mucosa with erosion of blood vessels.

A. Vitamin K-antagonists of the coumarin type and vitamin K

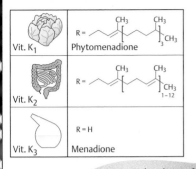

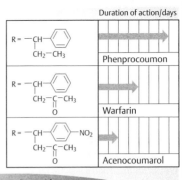

Duration of action/days

Vit. K₁ — Phytomenadione

Vit. K₂

Vit. K₃ — Menadione

R = H

Phenprocoumon

Warfarin

Acenocoumarol

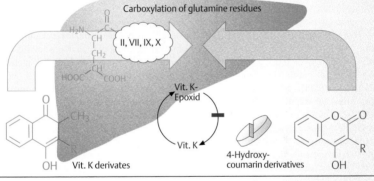

Carboxylation of glutamine residues

II, VII, IX, X

Vit. K-Epoxid

Vit. K

Vit. K derivates

4-Hydroxy-coumarin derivatives

B. Possible interactions

Risk of thrombosis	Optimal adjustment	Risk of bleeding
Increased intake of vitamin K-rich food		Damage to vitamin K-producing intestinal bacteria by antibiotics
Increase		Decrease

Vitamin K effect

Hydroxy-coumarin effect

Decrease		Increase
Inhibition of enteral coumarin absorption by adsorbents, e.g., antacids, medicinal charcoal

Acceleration of hepatic coumarin metabolism: enzyme induction, e.g., by carbamazepine, rifampicin | | Inhibition of hepatic coumarin metabolism, e.g., by cimetidine, metronidazole |

☐ Heparin (A)

Occurrence and structure. Heparin can be obtained from porcine gut, where it is present (together with histamine) in storage vesicles of mast cells. Heparin molecules are chains of amino sugars bearing $-COO^-$ and $-SO_3^-$ groups. Chain length is not constant and anticoagulant efficacy varies with chain length. The potency of a preparation is standardized in international units of activity (IU) by bioassay and comparison with a reference preparation. The molecular weight (MW) for *unfractionated heparin* ranges from 4000 to 40 000, with a peak around 15 000. *Low-molecular-weight fractionated heparin* can be produced by cleavage of native heparin; molecular size is less heterogeneous, with a mean MW of 5000 (e.g., certoparin, dalteparin, enoxaparin). The synthetic *fondaparinux* (MW 1728) resembles the basic pentasaccharide subunit of heparin, essential for activity. The numerous negative charges are significant in several respects: (1) they contribute to complex formation with antithrombin III that underlies the anticoagulant effect; (2) they permit binding of heparin to its antidote, **protamine** (a polycationic protein from salmon sperm); (3) they confer poor membrane penetrability, necessitating administration of heparin by injection.

Mechanism of action. *Antithrombin III (AT III)* is a circulating glycoprotein capable of inhibiting activated clotting factors by occupation and irreversible blockade of the active center. Heparin acts to inhibit clotting by accelerating formation of this complex more than 1000-fold. Activated clotting factors have differing requirements for optimal chain length of heparin. For instance, to inactivate thrombin, the heparin molecule must simultaneously contact the factor and AT III. With factor Xa, however, contact between heparin and AT III is sufficient for speeding up inactivation.

Indications. Heparin is used for the prophylaxis and therapy of thrombosis. For the former, low dosages, given subcutaneously, are sufficient. Unfractionated heparin must be injected about three time daily, fractionated heparins and fondaparinux can be administered once daily. For treatment of thrombosis, heparin must be infused intravenously in an increased daily dose.

Adverse effects. When bleeding is induced by heparin, the heparin action can be instantly reversed by protamine. Against fractionated heparins and fondaparinux, protamine is less or not effective. Heparin-induced thrombocytopenia type II (HIT II) is a dangerous complication. It results from formation of antibodies that precipitate with bound heparin on platelets. The platelets aggregate and give rise to vascular occlusions. Because of the thrombocytopenia, hemorrhages may occur. Fondaparinux is also contraindicated in HIT II.

The drug *danaparoid* consists mostly of the **heparinoid** heparan sulfate. Its chains are composed of a part of the heparin molecule (indicated by blue color underlay). Its effect is mediated by AT III.

☐ Hirudin and Derivatives (B)

The polypeptide **hirudin** from the saliva of the European medicinal leech inhibits clotting of the leech's blood meal by blockade of the active center of thrombin. This action is independent of AT III and thus also occurs in patients with AT III deficiency. *Lepirudin* and *desrudin* are yeast-derived recombinant analogues. They can be used in patients with HIT II.

Ximelagatran is a modified thrombin antagonist suitable for oral use.

A. Heparins: origin, structure, and mechanism of action

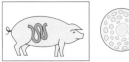

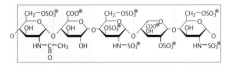

Mast cell

Pentasaccharide basic unit

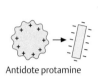

Antidote protamine

Standard heparin
unfractionated
mean
MW ~15 000

~3x daily s.c.

Low-MW heparin
fractionated
mean MW ~5000

~once daily s.c.

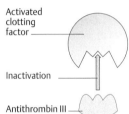

Activated
clotting
factor

Inactivation

Antithrombin III

Acceleration
of inactivation

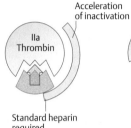

IIa
Thrombin

Standard heparin
required

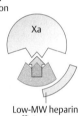

Xa

Low-MW heparin
sufficient

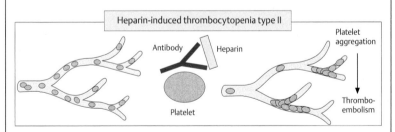

Heparin-induced thrombocytopenia type II

Antibody   Heparin

Platelet

Platelet
aggregation

Thrombo-
embolism

B. Hirudin and derivatives

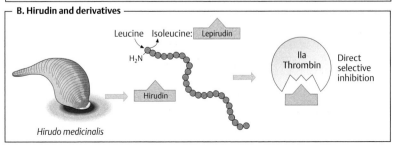

Leucine   Isoleucine: Lepirudin

H_2N

Hirudin

Hirudo medicinalis

IIa
Thrombin

Direct
selective
inhibition

□ Fibrinolytics

The fibrin meshwork of a blood clot can be cleaved by plasmin. As a protease, plasmin can break down not only fibrin but also fibrinogen and other proteins. Plasmin derives from an inactive precursor, plasminogen, present in blood. Under physiological conditions, specificity of action for fibrin is achieved because, among other things, activation takes place on the fibrin clot.

The **tissue plasminogen activator** (**t-PA**) is released into the blood from endothelial cells when blood flow stagnates. Next to its catalytic center, this protease possesses other functional domains, including docking sites for fibrin. During contact with fibrin, plasminogen–plasmin conversion rate is several-fold higher than in streaming blood. Plasminogen also contains a binding domain for fibrin.

Plasminogen activators available for therapeutic use are designated as fibrinolytics; they are infused intravenously in myocardial infarction, stroke, deep leg vein thrombosis, pulmonary embolism, and other thrombotic vascular occlusions. The earlier treatment is started after thrombus formation, the better is the chance of achieving patency of the occluded vessel.

The desired effect carries with it the risk of bleeding as the most important **adverse effect**, because, apart from the intravascular fibrin clot forming the thrombus, other fibrin coagula sealing defects in the vascular wall are dissolved as well. Moreover, use of fibrinolytics entails the risk that fibrinogen and other clotting factors circulating in blood will undergo cleavage ("systemic lytic state").

Streptokinase is the oldest available fibrinolytic. By itself it lacks enzymatic activity; only after binding to a plasminogen molecule is a complex formed that activates plasminogen. Streptokinase is produced by streptococcal bacteria. Streptokinase antibodies may be present as a result of previous streptococcal infections and may lead to incompatibility reactions.

Urokinase is an endogenous plasminogen activator that occurs in different organs. Urokinase used therapeutically is obtained from human cultured kidney cells. Circulating antibodies are not expected. The substance is more expensive than streptokinase and also does not depend on fibrin in its action.

Alteplase is a recombinant tissue plasminogen activator (rt-PA). As a result of its production in eukaryotic Chinese hamster ovary (CHO) cells, carbohydrate residues are present as in the native substance. At the therapeutically used dosage, alteplase loses its "fibrin dependence" and thus also activates circulating plasminogen. In fresh myocardial infarctions, alteplase appears to produce better results than does streptokinase.

Tenecteplase is a variant of alteplase that has been altered by six point mutations, resulting in a significant prolongation of its plasma half-life (tenecteplase $t_{1/2}$ = 20 minutes; alteplase $t_{1/2}$ = 3–4 minutes). Tenecteplase is dosed according to body weight and given by intravenous bolus injection.

Reteplase is a deletion variant of t-PA that lacks both fibrin-binding domains and oligosaccharide side chains (manufactured in prokaryotic *E. coli*). It is eliminated more slowly than alteplase. Whereas alteplase is given by infusion, reteplase can be administered in two bolus injections spaced 30 minutes apart

Plasmin inhibitors. *ε-Aminocaproic acid* as well as *tranexamic acid* and *p-aminomethylbenzoic acid* (PAMBA) are plasmin inhibitors that can be useful in bleeding complications. They exert an inhibitory effect by occupying the fibrin binding site of plasminogen or plasmin.

A. Fibrinolytics

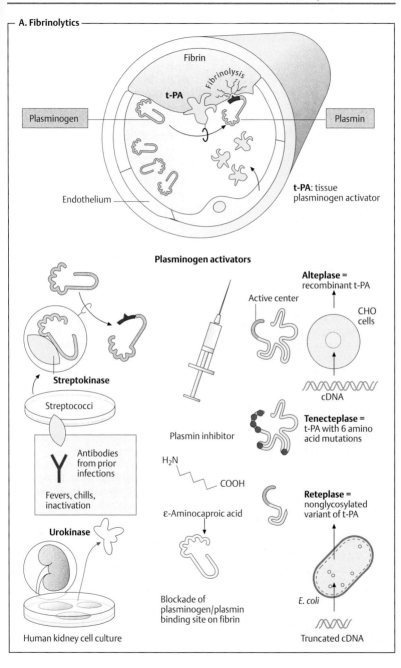

Fibrin

Fibrinolysis

t-PA

Plasminogen

Plasmin

t-PA: tissue plasminogen activator

Endothelium

Plasminogen activators

Streptokinase

Streptococci

Antibodies from prior infections

Fevers, chills, inactivation

Urokinase

Human kidney cell culture

Plasmin inhibitor

H_2N — COOH

ε-Aminocaproic acid

Blockade of plasminogen/plasmin binding site on fibrin

Active center

Alteplase = recombinant t-PA

CHO cells

cDNA

Tenecteplase = t-PA with 6 amino acid mutations

Reteplase = nonglycosylated variant of t-PA

E. coli

Truncated cDNA

□ Intra-arterial Thrombus Formation (A)

Activation of platelets, e.g., upon contact with collagen of the extracellular matrix after injury to the vascular wall, constitutes the immediate and decisive step in initiating the process of **primary hemostasis**, i.e., cessation of bleeding. However in the absence of vascular injury, platelets can be activated as a result of damage to the endothelial cell lining of blood vessels. Among the multiple functions of the endothelium, the production of prostacyclin and nitric oxide (NO) plays an important role because both substances inhibit the tendency of platelets to adhere to the endothelial surface. Impairment of endothelial function, e.g., due to chronic hypertension, chronic elevation of plasma LDL levels or of blood glucose, and cigarette smoking, increases the probability of adhesion between thrombocytes and endothelium. The deceleration of fast flowing platelets occurs through an interaction between the glycoprotein Ibα (GP I) in the platelet membrane and von Willebrand factor in the endothelium and basal membrane (denuded after endothelial injury). For the proper activation of the platelet, interaction with subendothelial collagen of an additional platelet glycoprotein (GP IV) is necessary. As soon as platelets are activated (see p. 154), they change their shape and gain affinity for fibrinogen. This results from a conformational change of glycoprotein IIb/IIIa in the platelet membrane. Platelets can now be linked to each other via fibrinogen bridges (**A**).

Platelet aggregation proceeds like an avalanche because, once activated, **one** platelet can activate **other** platelets. On the injured endothelial cell a thrombus is formed, which obstructs blood flow. Ultimately, the vascular lumen is occluded by the thrombus as the latter is solidified by vasoconstriction promoted by the release of serotonin and thromboxane A$_2$ from the aggregated platelets and by locally activated thrombin. Thrombin plays a twofold part in thrombus formation: as a protease, thrombin cleaves fibrinogen and thus initiates the formation of fibrin clot (blood coagulation, p. 144). The effects of thrombin on platelets and endothelial cells, however, involve a proteolytic activation of receptors coupled to G-proteins (so-called protease-activated receptors). When these events occur in a larger, functionally important artery, myocardial infarction or stroke may be the result.

Von Willebrand factor plays a key role in thrombogenesis. Lack of this factor is the cause of thrombasthenia, the inability to staunch bleeding by platelet aggregation. A relative deficiency of von Willebrand factor can be transiently relieved by injection of the vasopressin analogue desmopressin, because this substance makes factor available from stored supplies.

□ Formation, Activation, and Aggregation of Platelets (B)

Platelets are fragments of multicellular megakaryocytes. They constitute the smallest formed elements of blood (diameter 1–4 μm) and, devoid of a cell nucleus, are no longer capable of protein synthesis. Platelets can be activated by various stimuli, leading to:

- Change in shape
- Conversion of integrin GP IIb/IIIa into its active conformation
- Release of active substances such as serotonin, platelet-activating factor (PAF), ADP, and thromboxane A$_2$. All these substances activate other platelets.

A. Thrombogenesis

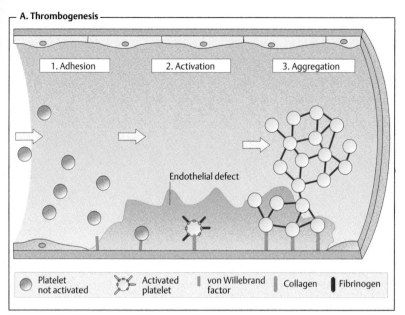

1. Adhesion   2. Activation   3. Aggregation

Endothelial defect

| Platelet not activated | Activated platelet | von Willebrand factor | Collagen | Fibrinogen |

B. Aggregation of platelets by the integrin GPIIb/IIIa

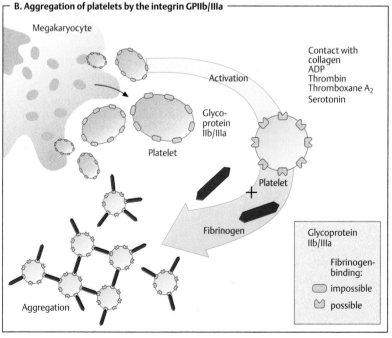

Megakaryocyte

Activation

Contact with collagen
ADP
Thrombin
Thromboxane A_2
Serotonin

Glyco-protein IIb/IIIa

Platelet

Platelet

Fibrinogen

Aggregation

Glycoprotein IIb/IIIa

Fibrinogen-binding:

impossible

possible

☐ Inhibitors of Platelet Aggregation (A)

Collagen, thrombin, ADP, and thromboxane A_2 are the most important mediators that induce maximal activation and aggregation of platelets. The first essential step in platelet activation is mediated by direct contact with collagen, which can bind to different proteins in the platelet membrane. The most important "collagen receptor" in the platelet membrane is glycoprotein VI (GP VI). Activation induces a change in platelet shape and triggers secretion of substances stored in intracellular platelet granula (e.g., ADP, serotonin). In addition, GP VI stimulates cyclooxygenase (COX-1), causing thromboxane A_2 to be produced and released from arachidonic acid (p. 196).

The propensity of platelets to aggregate can be inhibited by various pharmacological interventions.

Acetylsalicylic acid (**ASA**) prevents COX-1-mediated synthesis of thromboxane. Low daily doses (75–100 mg) may be sufficient. Indications include prophylaxis of re-infarction after myocardial infarction and of stroke. Despite the low dosage, adverse effects such as gastric mucosal damage or provocation of asthma attacks cannot be ruled out.

Available alternatives to ASA are the **ADP receptor antagonists** *ticlopidine* and *clopidrogel*, which can also be given orally. Similarly to ASA, ticlopidine and clopidrogel cause an irreversible inhibition of platelet function. Both substances are inactive precursors that are converted by hepatic cytochrome P450 to an active metabolite that binds covalently to a subtype ($P2Y_{12}$) of ADP receptors on platelets. Consequently, ADP-mediated platelet aggregation is inhibited for the duration of the platelet life cycle ($\sim$7–10 days). Ticlopidine may cause serious adverse effects, including neutropenia and thrombopenia. The successor substance, clopidrogel, is better tolerated.

Antagonists at the integrin glycoprotein IIb/IIIa. Available agents are suitable only for parenteral administration and, in clinical settings, are used in percutaneous coronary balloon distension or in unstable angina pectoris. They block the fibrinogen cross-linking protein and thus decrease fibrinogen-mediated meshing of platelets independently of the precipitating cause. *Abciximab* is a chimeric Fab-antibody fragment directed against GP IIb/IIIa protein. *Tirofiban* and *eptifibatide* act as competitive antagonists at the fibrinogen binding site. Because abciximab adheres to GPIIb/IIIa for a long time, 24–48 hours are required after injection of the drug before platelet aggregation again becomes possible. The effects of eptifibatide and tirofiban dissipate within a few hours. Because GP IIb/IIIa antagonists inhibit the common final pathway in platelet activation, they pose a risk of bleeding during treatment.

☐ Presystemic Effect of ASA

The inhibition of platelet aggregation by ASA results from acetylation and blockade of platelet COX-1 (**B**). The specificity of this reaction is achieved in the following manner: irreversible acetylation of the enzyme already occurs in the blood of the splanchnic region, that is, before the liver is reached. Since ASA is subject to extensive presystemic deacetylation, cyclooxygenases located posthepatically (e.g., in endothelial cells) are hardly affected. Confinement of COX-1 inhibition to platelets is further accentuated because enzyme can be re-synthesized in normal cells having a nucleus but not in the anuclear platelets.

A. Inhibitors of platelet aggregation

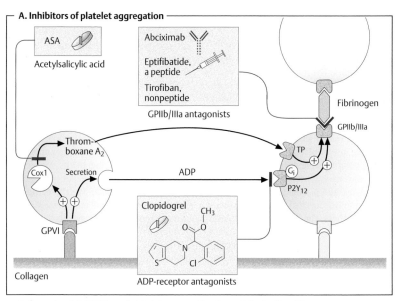

B. Presystemic inhibition of platelet aggregation by acetylsalicylic acid

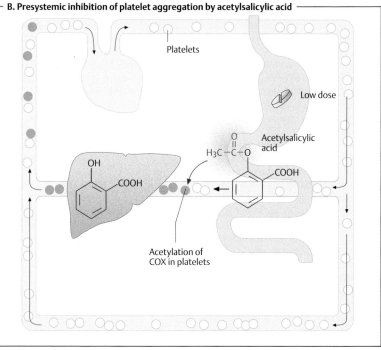

☐ Plasma Volume Expanders

Major blood loss entails the danger of life-threatening circulatory failure, i. e., hypovolemic shock. The immediate threat results not so much from the loss of erythrocytes, i. e., oxygen carriers, as from the reduction in volume of circulating blood.

To eliminate the threat of shock, replenishment of the circulation is essential. With moderate loss of blood, administration of a plasma volume expander may be sufficient. Blood plasma consists basically of water, electrolytes, and plasma proteins. However, a plasma substitute need not contain **plasma proteins**. These can be suitably **replaced** with **macromolecules** ("colloids") that, like plasma proteins, (1) *do not readily leave the circulation and are poorly filtrable in the renal glomerulus;* and (2) *bind water along with its solutes owing to their colloid osmotic properties.* In this manner, they will maintain circulatory filling pressure for many hours. On the other hand, complete elimination of these colloids from the body is clearly desirable.

Compared with whole blood or plasma, plasma substitutes offer several *advantages*: they can be produced more easily and at lower cost, have a longer shelf-life, and are free of pathogens such as hepatitis B and C or AIDS viruses.

Three colloids are currently employed as plasma volume expanders—the two polysaccharides dextran and hydroxyethyl starch, and the polypeptide gelatin.

Dextran is a polymer formed by bacteria and consisting of atypically linked (1→6 instead of 1→4 bond) glucose molecules. Commercially available plasma substitutes contain dextran of a *mean* molecular weight (MW) of 70 or 75 kDa (**dextran 70 or 75**) or 40 kDa (**dextran 40** or **low-molecular-weight dextran**). The chain length of single molecules varies widely, however. Smaller dextran molecules can be filtered at the glomerulus and slowly excreted in urine; the larger ones are eventually taken up and degraded by cells of the mononuclear phagocyte system. Apart from restoring blood volume, dextran solutions are used for hemodilution in the management of blood flow disorders.

As for microcirculatory improvement, it is occasionally emphasized that low -molecular-weight dextran, unlike dextran 70, may directly reduce the aggregability of erythrocytes by way of altering their surface properties. With prolonged use, larger molecules will accumulate owing to the more rapid renal excretion of the smaller ones. Consequently, the molecular weight of dextran circulating in blood will tend toward a higher mean molecular weight with the passage of time.

The most important adverse effect results from the antigenicity of dextrans, which may lead to an **anaphylactoid reaction**. Dextran antibodies can be intercepted without an immune response by injection of small dextran molecules (MW 1000), thus obviating any incompatibility reaction to subsequent infusion of the dextran plasma substitute solution.

Hydroxyethyl starch (hetastarch) is produced from starch. By virtue of its hydroxyethyl groups, it is metabolized more slowly and retained significantly longer in blood than would be the case with infused starch. Hydroxyethyl starch resembles dextrans in terms of its pharmacological properties and therapeutic applications. A particular adverse effect is pruritus of prolonged duration with deposition of the drug in peripheral nerves.

Gelatin colloids consist of cross-linked peptide chains obtained from collagen. They are employed for blood replacement but not for hemodilution in circulatory disturbances.

A. Plasma subtitutes

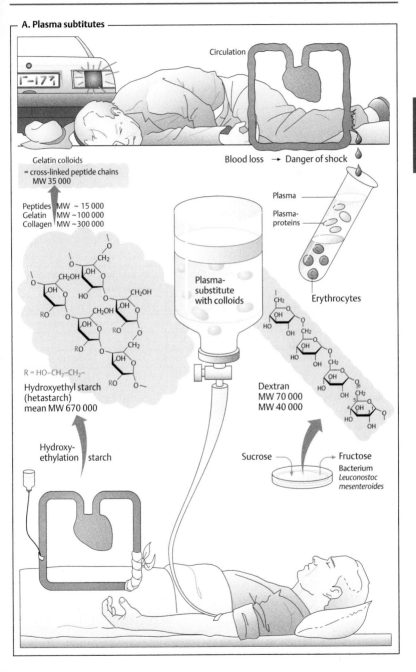

Circulation

Blood loss → Danger of shock

Gelatin colloids
= cross-linked peptide chains
MW 35 000

Peptides MW ~ 15 000
Gelatin MW ~100 000
Collagen MW ~300 000

Plasma

Plasma-
proteins

Plasma-
substitute
with colloids

Erythrocytes

R = HO–CH₂–CH₂–

Hydroxyethyl starch
(hetastarch)
mean MW 670 000

Dextran
MW 70 000
MW 40 000

Hydroxy-
ethylation starch

Sucrose → Fructose
Bacterium *Leuconostoc mesenteroides*

□ Lipid-lowering Agents

Triglycerides and cholesterol are essential constituents of the organism. Among other things, triglycerides represent a form of energy store and cholesterol is a basic building block of biological membranes. Both lipids are water insoluble and require appropriate "packaging" for transport in the aqueous media of lymph and blood. To this end, small amounts of lipid are coated with a layer of phospholipids, embedded in which are additional proteins—the apolipoproteins (**A**). According to the amount and the composition of stored lipids, as well as the type of apolipoprotein, one distinguishes four transport forms (see table).

other tissues with fatty acids. Left behind are LDL particles that either return into the liver or supply extrahepatic tissues with cholesterol.

LDL particles carry the apolipoprotein B-100, by which they are bound to receptors that mediate uptake of LDL into the cells, including the hepatocytes (receptor-mediated endocytosis, p. 26).

HDL particles are able to transfer cholesterol from tissue cells to LDL particles. In this way, cholesterol is transported from tissues to the liver.

Hyperlipoproteinemias can be caused genetically (primary hyperlipoproteinemia) or can occur in obesity and metabolic disorders (secondary hyperlipoproteinemia). Ele-

	Origin	Density (g/ml)	Mean time in blood plasma (h)	Diameter (nm)
Chylomicron	Gut epithelium	> 1.006	0.2	500 or more
VLDL particle	Liver	0.95–1.006	3	100–200
LDL particle	(Blood)	1.006–1.063	50	25
HDL particle	Liver	1.063–1.210	–	5–10

Lipoprotein metabolism. Enterocytes release absorbed lipids in the form of triglyceride-rich chylomicrons. Bypassing the liver, these enter the circulation mainly via the lymph and are hydrolyzed by extrahepatic endothelial lipoprotein lipases to liberate fatty acids. The remnant particles move on into liver cells and supply these with cholesterol of dietary origin.

The liver meets the larger part (60%) of its requirement for cholesterol by synthesis de novo from acetyl-coenzyme A. Synthesis rate is regulated at the step leading from hydroxymethylglutaryl-CoA (HMG-CoA) to mevalonic acid (p. 161**A**), with HMG-CoA reductase as the rate-limiting enzyme.

The liver requires cholesterol for synthesizing VLDL particles and bile acids. Triglyceride-rich VLDL particles are released into the blood and, like the chylomicrons, supply

vated LDL-cholesterol serum concentrations are associated with an increased risk of atherosclerosis, especially when there is a concomitant decline in HDL concentration (increase in LDL : HDL quotient).

Treatment. Various drugs are available that have different mechanisms of action and effects on LDL (cholesterol) and VLDL (triglycerides) (**A**). Their use is indicated in the therapy of primary hyperlipoproteinemias. In secondary hyperlipoproteinemias, the immediate goal should be to lower lipoprotein levels by dietary restriction, treatment of the primary disease, or both.

A. Lipoprotein metabolism

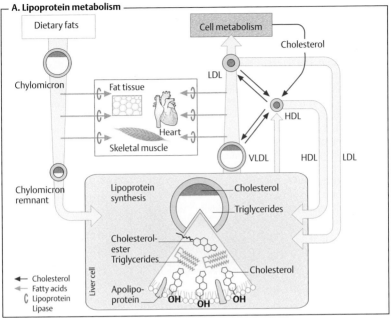

B. Cholesterol metabolism in liver cell and cholesterol-lowering drugs

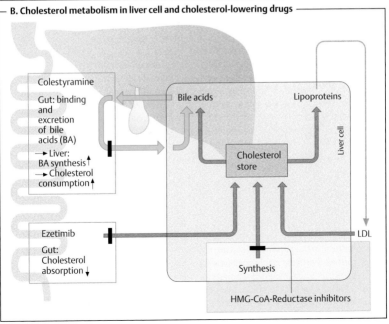

Drugs. As nonabsorbable anion-exchange resins, *colestyramine* and *colestipol* can bind bile acids in the gut lumen, which are thus removed from cholesterol metabolism. The required dosage is rather high (15–30 g/day) and liable to produce gastrointestinal disturbances. Consequently, patient compliance is low. Moreover, the resins trap needed drugs and vitamins. A more promising approach to lowering absorption of cholesterol derives from a novel mechanism of action probably based on the specific inhibition of intestinal cholesterol transporters that are required for absorption of cholesterol. An inhibitor of this type is *ezetimibe*.

β-Sitosterin is a plant steroid that is not absorbed after oral administration; in sufficiently high dosage it impedes enteral absorption of cholesterol. Treatment with sitosterin has become obsolete. The drug is no longer on the market.

The **statins** *lovastatin* and *fluvastatin* inhibit HMG-CoA reductase. They contain a molecular moiety that chemically resembles the physiological substrate of the enzyme (**A**). Lovastatin is a lactone that is rapidly absorbed by the enteral route, subjected to extensive first-pass extraction in the liver, and there hydrolyzed to active metabolites. Fluvastatin represents the active form and, as an acid, is actively transported by a specific anion carrier that moves bile acids from blood into liver and also mediates the selective uptake of the mycotoxin amanitin (**A**). Normally viewed as presystemic elimination, efficient hepatic extraction serves to confine the action of statins to the liver. Despite the inhibition of HMG-CoA reductase, hepatic cholesterol content does not fall because hepatocytes compensate any drop in cholesterol levels by increasing the synthesis of LDL receptor protein (along with the reductase). Since, in the presence of statins, the newly-formed reductase is inhibited as well, the hepatocyte must meet its cholesterol demand entirely by uptake of LDL from the blood (**B**). Accordingly, the concentration of circulating LDL falls. As LDL remains in blood

for a shorter time, the likelihood of LDL being oxidized to its proatherogenic degradation product decreases pari passu.

Other statins include *simvastatin* (also a lactone prodrug), *pravastatin*, *atorvastatin*, and *cerivastatin* (active form with open ring). The statins are the most important therapeutics for lowering cholesterol levels. Their notable cardiovascular protective effect, however, appears to involve additional actions.

The combination of a statin with an inhibitor of cholesterol absorption (e.g., *ezetimibe*) can lower LDL levels even further.

A rare but dangerous adverse effect of statins is damage to skeletal muscle (rhabdomyolysis). This risk is increased by combined use of fibric acid agents (see below). Cerivastatin has proved particularly toxic. Besides muscle damage associated with myoglobinuria and renal failure, severe hepatotoxicity has also been noted, prompting withdrawal of the drug.

Nicotinic acid and its derivatives (*pyridylcarbinol, xanthinol nicotinate,* and *acipimox*) activate endothelial lipoprotein lipase and thereby mainly lower triglyceride levels. At the start of therapy, a prostaglandin-mediated vasodilation occurs (flushing, hypotension) that can be prevented by low doses of acetylsalicylic acid.

Clofibrate and derivatives (*bezafibrate, fenofibrate, and gemfibrozil*) lower concentrations of VLDL (triglycerides) along with LDL (cholesterol). They may cause damage to liver and skeletal muscle (myalgia, myopathy, rhabdomyolysis with myoglobinemia and renal failure). The mechanism of action of fibrates is not completely understood. They bind to a peroxisome proliferator-activated receptor (PPARα) and thereby influence genes regulating lipid metabolism.

A. Accumulation and effect of HMG-CoA reductase inhibitors in liver

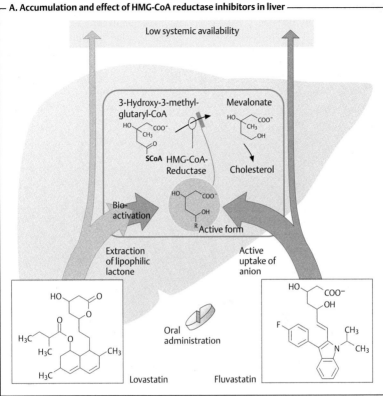

B. Regulation by cellular cholesterol concentration of HMG-CoA reductase and LDL-receptors

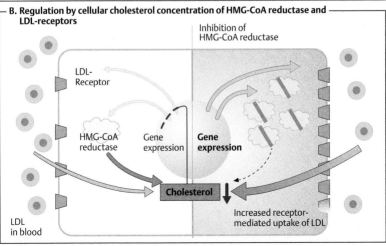

□ Diuretics—An Overview

Diuretics (saluretics) elicit increased production of urine (diuresis). In the strict sense, the term is applied to drugs with a direct renal action. The predominant action of such agents is to augment urine excretion by inhibiting the reabsorption of NaCl and water.

The most important **indications** for diuretics are the following.

Mobilization of edemas (A). In edema there is swelling of tissues owing to accumulation of fluid, chiefly in the extracellular (interstitial) space. When a diuretic is given, increased renal excretion of Na^+ and H_2O causes a reduction in plasma volume with hemoconcentration. As a result, plasma protein concentration rises along with oncotic pressure. As the latter operates to attract water, fluid will shift from interstitium into the capillary bed. The fluid content of tissues thus falls and the edemas recede. The decrease in plasma volume and interstitial volume means a diminution of the extracellular fluid volume (EFV). Depending on the condition, use is made of thiazides, loop diuretics, aldosterone antagonists, and osmotic diuretics.

Antihypertensive therapy. Diuretics have been used as drugs of first choice for lowering elevated blood pressure (p. 314). Even at low dosage, they decrease peripheral resistance (without significantly reducing EFV) and thereby normalize blood pressure.

Therapy of congestive heart failure. By lowering peripheral resistance, diuretics aid the heart in ejecting blood (reduction in afterload, p. 322); cardiac output and exercise tolerance are increased. Owing to the increased excretion of fluid, EFV and venous return decrease (reduction in preload). Symptoms of venous congestion, such as ankle edema and hepatic enlargement, subside. The drugs principally used are thiazides (possibly combined with K^+-sparing diuretics) and loop diuretics.

Prophylaxis of renal failure. In circulatory failure (shock), e. g., secondary to massive hemorrhage, renal production of urine may cease (anuria). By means of diuretics, an attempt is made to maintain urinary flow. Use of either osmotic or loop diuretics is indicated.

Massive use of diuretics entails a hazard of **adverse effects (A)**:

1. The decrease in blood volume can lead to hypotension and *collapse*.
2. Blood viscosity rises owing to the increase in erythrocyte and thrombocyte concentrations, bringing an increased risk of intravascular coagulation or *thrombosis*.

When depletion of NaCl and water (EFV reduction) occurs as a result of diuretic therapy, the body can initiate **counterregulatory responses (B)**, namely, activation of the renin–angiotensin–aldosterone system (p. 128). Because of the diminished blood volume, renal blood flow is jeopardized. This leads to release from the kidneys of the hormone renin, which enzymatically catalyzes the formation of angiotensin I. Angiotensin I is converted to angiotensin II by the action of "angiotensin-converting enzyme" (ACE). Angiotensin II stimulates release of aldosterone. The mineralocorticoid promotes renal reabsorption of NaCl and water and thus counteracts the effect of diuretics. ACE inhibitors (p. 128) and angiotensin II antagonists augment the effectiveness of diuretics by preventing this counterregulatory response.

A. Mechanism of edema fluid mobilization by diuretics

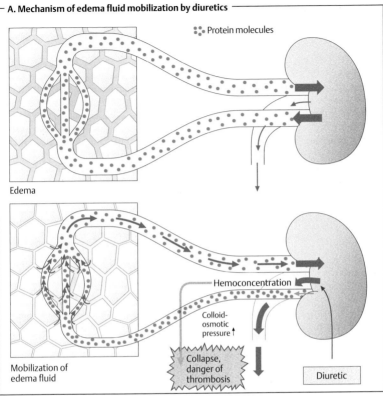

Edema

Mobilization of
edema fluid

Protein molecules

Hemoconcentration

Colloid-
osmotic
pressure ↑

Collapse,
danger of
thrombosis

Diuretic

B. Possible counter-regulatory responses during long-term diuretic therapy

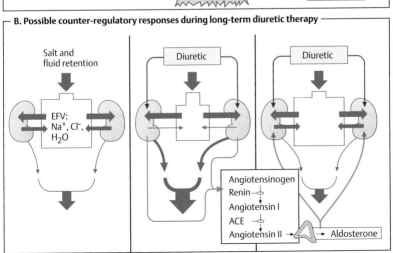

Salt and
fluid retention

EFV:
Na$^+$, Cl$^-$,
H$_2$O

Diuretic

Diuretic

Angiotensinogen
Renin
Angiotensin I
ACE
Angiotensin II → Aldosterone

◻ NaCl Reabsorption in the Kidney (A)

The smallest functional unit of the kidney is the **nephron**. In the glomerular capillary loops, ultrafiltration of plasma fluid into Bowman's capsule yields primary urine. In the proximal tubules (pT), ~70% of the ultrafiltrate is retrieved by iso-osmotic reabsorption of NaCl and water. Downstream, in the thick portion of the ascending limb of Henle's loop, NaCl is absorbed unaccompanied by water. The differing properties of the limbs of Henle's loop, together with the parallel arrangement of vasa recta, are the prerequisites for the **hairpin countercurrent mechanism** that allows build-up of a very high NaCl concentration in the renal medulla. NaCl is again reabsorbed in the distal convoluted tubules, the connecting segment, and the collecting ducts, accompanied by a compensatory secretion of K^+ in the (cortical) collecting tubules. In the connecting tubules and collecting ducts, vasopressin (antidiuretic hormone, ADH) increases the epithelial permeability for water by insertion of aquaporin molecules into the luminal plasmalemma. The driving force for the passage of water comes from the hyperosmolar milieu of the renal medulla. In this manner, water is retained in the body, and concentrated urine can leave the kidney. The efficient mechanisms of reabsorption permit the production of ~1 l/day of final urine from 150–180 l/day of primary urine.

Na^+ transport through the tubular cells basically occurs in similar fashion in all segments of the nephron. The intracellular concentration of Na^+ is significantly below that in primary urine because the Na^+/K^+-ATPase of the basolateral membrane continuously pumps Na^+ from the cell into the interstitium. Along the resulting luminal–intracellular concentration gradient, movement of sodium ions across the membrane proceeds by a carrier mechanism. All diuretics inhibit Na^+ reabsorption. This effect is based on two mechanisms: either the inward movement is diminished or the outward transport impaired.

◻ Aquaporins (AQP)

By virtue of their structure, cell membranes are water-impermeable. Therefore, special pores are built into the membrane to allow permeation of water. These consist of proteins called **aquaporins** that, of necessity, occur widely and with many variations in both the plant and animal kingdoms. In the human kidney, the following types exist:

- AQP-1 localized in the proximal tubulus and the descending limb of Henle's loop.
- AQP-2 localized in the connecting tubuli and collecting ducts; its density in the luminal plasmalemma is regulated by vasopressin.
- AQP-3 and AQP-4 present in the basolateral membrane region to allow passage of water into the interstitium.

◻ Osmotic Diuretics (B)

These include *mannitol* and *sorbitol* which act mainly in the proximal tubules to prevent reabsorption of water. These polyhydric alcohols cannot be absorbed and therefore bind a corresponding volume of water. Since body cells lack transport mechanisms for these substances (structure on p. 175), they also cannot be absorbed through the intestinal epithelium and thus need to be given by intravenous infusion. The result of osmotic diuresis is a large volume of dilute urine, as in decompensated diabetes mellitus. Osmotic diuretics are indicated in the prophylaxis of renal hypovolemic failure, the mobilization of brain edema, and the treatment of acute glaucoma attacks (p. 346).

A. Renal actions of diuretics

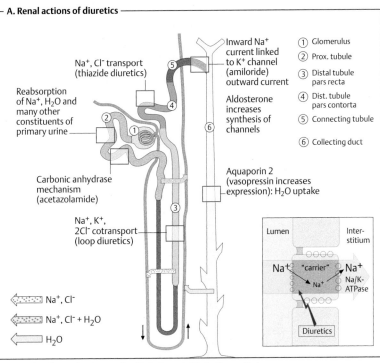

Na+, Cl− transport
(thiazide diuretics)

Reabsorption
of Na+, H2O and
many other
constituents of
primary urine

Carbonic anhydrase
mechanism
(acetazolamide)

Na+, K+,
2Cl− cotransport
(loop diuretics)

Inward Na+
current linked
to K+ channel
(amiloride)
outward current

Aldosterone
increases
synthesis of
channels

Aquaporin 2
(vasopressin increases
expression): H2O uptake

① Glomerulus
② Prox. tubule
③ Distal tubule
   pars recta
④ Dist. tubule
   pars contorta
⑤ Connecting tubule
⑥ Collecting duct

Na+, Cl−

Na+, Cl− + H2O

H2O

Lumen — Inter-stitium

Na+ — "carrier" — Na+
   → Na+ → Na/K-ATPase

Diuretics

B. NaCl reabsorption in proximal tubule and effect of mannitol

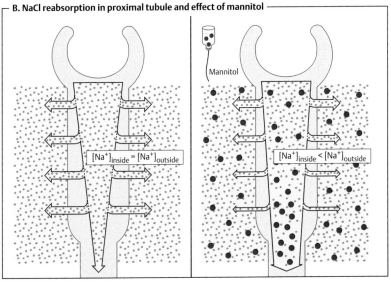

$[Na^+]_{inside} = [Na^+]_{outside}$

Mannitol

$[Na^+]_{inside} < [Na^+]_{outside}$

☐ Diuretics of the Sulfonamide Type

These drugs contain the sulfonamide group $-SO_2NH_2$ and are suitable for oral administration. In addition to being filtered at the glomerulus, they are subject to tubular secretion. Their concentration in urine is higher than in blood. They act on the tubule cells from the luminal side. Loop diuretics have the highest efficacy. Thiazides are most frequently used. The carbonic anhydrase inhibitors no longer serve as diuretics but have important other therapeutic uses; accordingly, their mode of action is considered here.

Acetazolamide is a **carbonic anhydrase (CAH) inhibitor** that acts predominantly in the proximal convoluted tubules. Its mechanism of action can be summarized as follows. Reabsorption of Na^+ is decreased because fewer H^+ ions are available for the Na^+/H^+ antiporter. As a result, excretion of Na^+ and H_2O increases. CAH accelerates attainment of equilibrium of CO_2 hydration/dehydration reactions:

$$\overset{(1)}{} \qquad \overset{(2)}{}$$
$$H^+ + HCO_3- \rightleftharpoons H_2CO_3 \rightleftharpoons H_2O + CO_2$$

Cytoplasmic enzyme is used in tubulus cells to generate H^+ (reaction 1), which is secreted into the tubular fluid in exchange for Na^+. There, H^+ captures HCO_3^-. CAH localized in the luminal membrane catalyzes reaction 2 (dehydration) to yield again H_2O and CO_2, which can easily permeate through the cell membrane. In the tubulus cell, H^+ and HCO_3^- are regenerated. When the enzyme is inhibited, these reactions occur too slowly, so that less Na^+, HCO_3^- and water are reabsorbed from the fast-flowing tubular fluid. Loss of HCO_3^- leads to acidosis. The diuretic effectiveness of CAH inhibitors decreases with prolonged use. CAH is also involved in the production of ocular aqueous humor. Present indications for drugs in this class include: acute glaucoma, acute mountain sickness, and epilepsy.

Dorzolamide can be applied topically to the eye to lower intraocular pressure in glaucoma (p. 346).

Loop diuretics include *furosemide* (frusemide), *piretanide*, and others. After oral administration of furosemide, a strong diuresis occurs within 1 hour but persists for only about 4 hours. The site of action of these agents is the thick ascending limb of Henle's loop, where they inhibit $Na^+/K^+/2Cl^-$ cotransport. As a result, these electrolytes, together with water, are excreted in larger amounts. Excretion of Ca^{2+} and Mg^{2+} also increases. Special *adverse effects* include (reversible) hearing loss and enhanced sensitivity to nephrotoxic agents. *Indications*: pulmonary edema (added advantage of i.v. injection in left ventricular failure: immediate dilation of venous capacitance vessels, → preload reduction); refractoriness to thiazide diuretics; e. g., in renal failure with creatinine clearance reduction (< 30 ml/min); prophylaxis of acute renal hypovolemic failure. Ethacrynic acid is classed in this group although it is not a sulfonamide.

Thiazide diuretics (benzothiadiazines) include *hydrochlorothiazide, trichlormethiazide* and *butizide*. *Chlorthalidone* is a long-acting analogue. These drugs affect the distal convoluted tubules, where they inhibit Na^+/Cl^- cotransport in the luminal membrane of tubulus cells. Thus, reabsorption of NaCl and water is inhibited. Renal excretion of Ca^{2+} decreases, that of Mg^{2+} increases. *Indications* are hypertension, congestive heart failure, and mobilization of edema. Frequently, they are combined with the K^+ sparing diuretics triamterene or amiloride (p. 168).

Unwanted effects of sulfonamide-type diuretics: (a) *hypokalemia* is a consequence of an increased secretion of K^+ in the connecting tubule and the collecting duct because more Na^+ becomes available for exchange against K^+; (b) *hyperglycemia*; (c) increase in serum urate levels (*hyperuricemia*), which may precipitate gout in predisposed patients. Sulfonamide diuretics compete with urate for the tubular organic anion secretory system.

A. Diuretics of the sulfonamide type

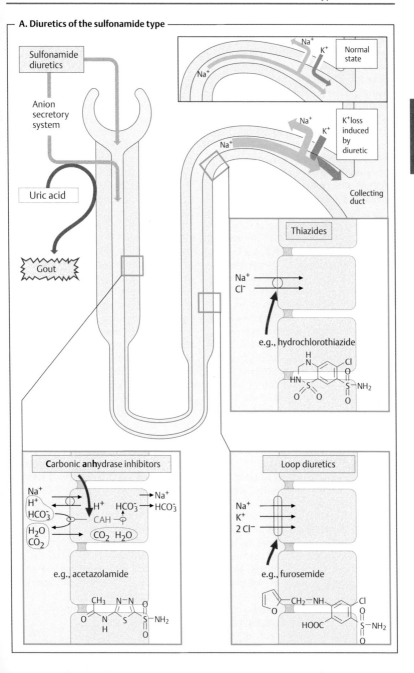

□ Potassium-sparing Diuretics (A)

These agents act in the connecting tubules and the proximal part of the collecting ducts where Na$^+$ is reabsorbed and K$^+$ is secreted. Their diuretic effectiveness is relatively minor. In contrast to sulfonamide diuretics (p. 166), there is no increase in K$^+$ secretion; rather, there is a risk of hyperkalemia. These drugs are suitable for oral administration.

a *Triamterene* and *amiloride*, in addition to glomerular filtration, undergo secretion in the proximal tubule. They act on cortical collecting tubule cells from the luminal side. Both inhibit the entry of Na$^+$ into the cell, whereby K$^+$ secretion is diminished. They are mostly used in combination with thiazide diuretics, e. g., hydrochlorothiazide, because the opposing effects on K$^+$ excretion cancel each other, while the effects on secretion of NaCl and water complement each other.

b *Aldosterone antagonists.* The mineralocorticoid aldosterone increases synthesis of Na-channel proteins and Na$^+$/K$^+$-ATPases in principal cells of the connecting tubules and the cortical collecting ducts, thereby promoting the reabsorption of Na$^+$ (Cl$^-$ and H$_2$O follow), and simultaneously enhancing secretion of K$^+$. *Spironolactone*, as well as its *metabolite canrenone*, are antagonists at the aldosterone receptor and attenuate the effect of the hormone. The diuretic effect of spironolactone develops fully only with continuous administration for several days. Two possible explanations are: (1) the conversion of spironolactone into and accumulation of the more slowly eliminated metabolite canrenone; (2) an inhibition of aldosterone-stimulated protein synthesis would become noticeable only if existing proteins had become nonfunctional and needed to be replaced by de-novo synthesis.

A particular *adverse effect* results from interference with gonadal hormones, as evidenced by the development of gynecomastia. *Clinical uses* include conditions of increased aldosterone secretion (e. g., liver cirrhosis with ascites) and congestive heart failure.

□ Vasopressin and Derivatives (B)

Vasopressin (ADH), a nonapeptide, is released from the posterior pituitary gland and promotes reabsorption of water in the kidney. This response is mediated by vasopressin receptors of the V$_2$ subtype. AVP enhances the permeability of connecting tubules and medullary collecting duct epithelium for H$_2$O (but not electrolytes) in the following manner: H$_2$O-channel proteins (type 2 aquaporins) are stored in tubulus cells within vesicles. When AVP binds to V$_2$ receptors, these vesicles fuse with the luminal cell membrane, allowing influx of H$_2$O along its osmotic gradient (the medullary zone is hyperosmolar). AVP thus causes urine volume to shrink from 15 l/day at this point of the nephron to the final 1.5 l/day. This aquaporin type can be reutilized after internalization into the cell. Nicotine augments (p. 112) and ethanol decreases release of AVP. At concentrations above those required for antidiuresis, AVP stimulates smooth musculature, including that of blood vessels ("**vasopressin**"). The latter response is mediated by V$_1$ receptors. Blood pressure rises; coronary vasoconstriction can precipitate angina pectoris.

Lypressin (8-L-lysine-vasopressin) acts like AVP. Other derivatives may display only one of the two actions.

Desmopressin is used for the therapy of diabetes insipidus (AVP deficiency), primary nocturnal enuresis and von Willebrand disease (p. 152); it is given by injection or via the nasal mucosa (as "snuff").

Felypressin and *ornipressin* serve as adjunctive vasoconstrictors in infiltration local anesthesia (p. 204).

A. Potassium-sparing diuretics

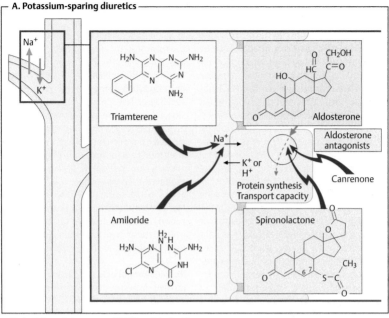

Triamterene

Aldosterone

Na⁺

K⁺

Na⁺

K⁺ or H⁺

Protein synthesis
Transport capacity

Aldosterone antagonists

Canrenone

Amiloride

Spironolactone

B. Antidiuretic hormone (ADH) and derivatives

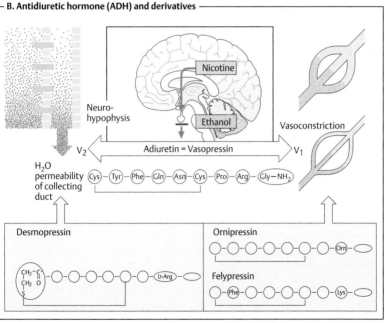

Neuro-hypophysis

Nicotine

Ethanol

Vasoconstriction

Adiuretin = Vasopressin

V_2

V_1

H₂O permeability of collecting duct

(Cys)—(Tyr)—(Phe)—(Gln)—(Asn)—(Cys)—(Pro)—(Arg)—(Gly—NH₂)

Desmopressin

Ornipressin

Felypressin

□ Drugs for Gastric and Duodenal Ulcers

In the area of a gastric or duodenal peptic ulcer, the mucosa has been attacked by digestive juices to such an extent as to expose the subjacent connective tissue layer (submucosa). This "self-digestion" occurs when the equilibrium between the corrosive hydrochloric acid and acid-neutralizing mucus, which forms a protective cover on the mucosal surface, is disturbed. Mucosal damage can be promoted by *Helicobacter pylori* bacteria that colonize the gastric mucus.

Drugs are employed with the following **therapeutic aims**: (a) to relieve pain; (b) to accelerate healing; and (c) to prevent ulcer recurrence. Therapeutic approaches are threefold : (I) to reduce aggressive forces by lowering H$^+$ output, (II) to increase protective forces by means of mucoprotectants; and (III) to eradicate *Helicobacter pylori.*

I. Lowering of Acid Concentration

Ia. Agents for acid neutralization (A). H$^+$-binding groups such as CO_3^{2-}, HCO_3^- or OH^-, together with their counter ions, are contained in **antacid drugs**. Neutralization reactions occurring after intake of $CaCO_3$ and $NaHCO_3$, respectively, are shown in (**A**). With nonabsorbable antacids, the counter ion is dissolved in the acidic gastric juice in the process of neutralization. Upon mixture with the alkaline pancreatic secretion in the duodenum, it is largely precipitated again by basic groups, e.g., as $CaCO_3$ or $AlPO_4$, and excreted in feces. Therefore, systemic absorption of counter ions or basic residues is minor. In the presence of renal insufficiency, however, absorption of even small amounts may cause an increase in plasma levels of counter ions (e.g., magnesium intoxication with paralysis and cardiac disturbances). Precipitation in the gut lumen is responsible for other side effects, such as reduced absorption of other drugs due to their adsorption to the surface of precipitated antacid; or

phosphate depletion of the body with excessive intake of $Al(OH)_3$.

Na$^+$ ions remain in solution even in the presence of HCO_3^--rich pancreatic secretions and are subject to absorption, like HCO_3^-. Because of the uptake of Na$^+$, use of $NaHCO_3$ must be avoided in conditions requiring restriction of NaCl intake, such as hypertension, cardiac failure, and edema.

Since food has a buffering effect, antacids are taken between meals (e. g., 1 and 3 hours after meals and at bedtime). Nonabsorbable antacids are preferred. Because $Mg(OH)_2$ produces a laxative effect (cause: osmotic action, p. 174, release of cholecystokinin by Mg^{2+}, or both) and $Al(OH)_3$ produces constipation (cause: astringent action of Al^{3+}, p. 180), these two antacids are frequently used in combination (e. g., magaldrate).

Ib. Inhibitors of acid production (B). Acting on their respective receptors, the transmitter acetylcholine, the hormone gastrin, and histamine released intramucosally stimulate the parietal cells of the gastric mucosa to increase output of HCl. Histamine comes from enterochromaffin-like (ECL) cells; its release is stimulated by the vagus nerve (via M$_1$ receptors) and hormonally by gastrin. The effects of acetylcholine and histamine can be abolished by orally applied antagonists that reach parietal cells via the blood. Proton pump inhibitors are drugs of first choice for promoting healing of ulcers. Infection with *H. pylori* should be treated resolutely (p. 172) to lower the risk of ulcer recurrence, chronic gastritis, gastric carcinomas, and gastric lymphomas.

The cholinoceptor antagonist **pirenzepine** preferentially blocks cholinoceptors of the M$_1$ type; its use in peptic ulcer therapy is now obsolete.

A. Drugs used to neutralize gastric acid

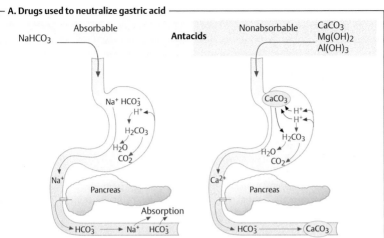

B. Drugs used to lower gastric acid production

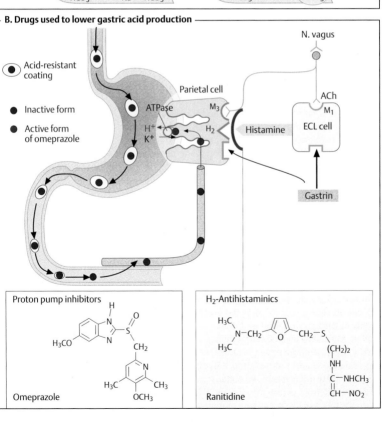

Histamine receptors on the parietal cells belong to the H_2 type and are blocked by **H_2 antihistaminics** (p. 118). Because histamine plays a pivotal role in the activation of parietal cells, H_2 antihistaminics also diminish responsivity to other stimulants, e. g., gastrin (in gastrin-producing pancreatic tumors, Zollinger–Ellison syndrome). The first H_2-blocker used clinically, *cimetidine*, only rarely produces adverse effects (CNS disturbances such as confusion; endocrine effects in the male such as gynecomastia, decreased libido, impotence); however, it inhibits the hepatic biotransformation of many other drugs. The more recently introduced substances *ranitidine*, *nizatidine*, and *famotidine* are effective at lower dosages. Evidently, inhibition of microsomal enzymes decreases with reduced drug load; thus, these substances are less likely to interfere with the therapeutic use of other pharmaceuticals.

Omeprazole (p. 171) can cause maximal inhibition of HCl secretion. Given orally in gastric juice-resistant capsules, it reaches parietal cells via the blood. In the acidic milieu of the mucosa, an active metabolite is formed and binds covalently to the ATP-driven proton pump (H^+/K^+-ATPase) that transports H^+ in exchange for K^+ into the gastric juice. *Lansoprazole, pantoprazole*, and *rabeprazole* produce analogous effects. Omeprazole is a racemate. With respect to dosage, the now available (*S*)-omeprazole (*esomeprazole*) represents the more potent enantiomer, but this offers no therapeutic advantage.

II. Protective Drugs

Sucralfate (**A**) contains numerous aluminum hydroxide residues. However, it is not an antacid because it fails to lower the overall acidity of gastric juice. After oral intake, sucralfate molecules undergo cross-linking in gastric juice, forming a paste that adheres to mucosal defects and exposed deeper layers. Here sucralfate intercepts H^+. Protected from acid, and also from pepsin, trypsin, and bile acids, the mucosal defect can heal more rap-

idly. Sucralfate is taken on an empty stomach (1 hour before meals and at bedtime). It is well tolerated, but released Al^{3+} ions can cause constipation.

Misoprostol (**B**) is a semisynthetic prostaglandin derivative with greater stability than natural prostaglandin, permitting absorption after oral administration. Locally released prostaglandins ($PGF_{2\alpha}$, PGE_2) promote mucus production in superficial cells and inhibit acid secretion of parietal cells (**B**). Inhibition of physiological PG synthesis by drugs (e. g., NSAIDS, p. 200) explains the mucosal injury from these pharmaceuticals: protection by the mucus layer is diminished and acid production is enhanced. Misoprostol mimics the action of the prostaglandins on the mucosal tunic and thus can attenuate the adverse effects produced by inhibitors of PG synthesis, at least as regards the gastric mucosa. Additional systemic effects (frequent diarrhea; risk of precipitating contractions of the gravid uterus) significantly restrict its therapeutic utility.

III. Eradication of Helicobacter pylori (**C**)

This organism plays an important role in the pathogenesis of chronic gastritis and peptic ulcer disease. The combination of antibacterial drugs and omeprazole has proved effective. If amoxicillin (p. 272) or clarithromycin (p. 278) cannot be tolerated, metronidazole (p. 276) may serve as a substitute. Colloidal bismuth compounds are also effective; however, as they entail the problem of heavy-metal exposure, this treatment can no longer be recommended.

A. Chemical structure and protective effect of sucralfate

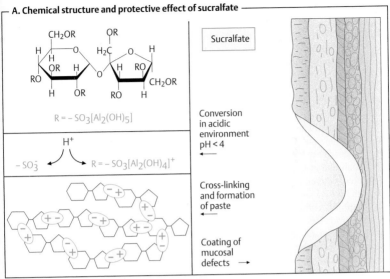

Sucralfate

$R = - SO_3[Al_2(OH)_5]$

H^+

$- SO_3^-$ $R = - SO_3[Al_2(OH)_4]^+$

Conversion in acidic environment pH < 4

Cross-linking and formation of paste

Coating of mucosal defects

B. Structure and protective effect of misoprostol

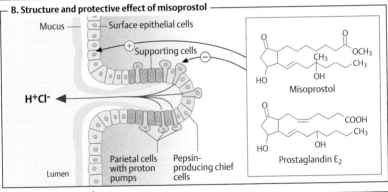

Mucus — Surface epithelial cells

Supporting cells

H^+Cl^-

Lumen

Parietal cells with proton pumps

Pepsin-producing chief cells

OCH_3

CH_3

CH_3

HO   OH

Misoprostol

COOH

CH_3

HO   OH

Prostaglandin E_2

C. Helicobacter eradication

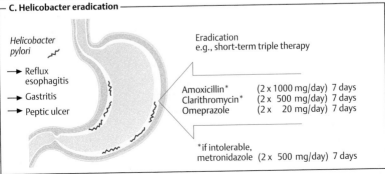

Helicobacter pylori

→ Reflux esophagitis

→ Gastritis

→ Peptic ulcer

Eradication
e.g., short-term triple therapy

Amoxicillin*   (2 x 1000 mg/day) 7 days
Clarithromycin*   (2 x 500 mg/day) 7 days
Omeprazole   (2 x   20 mg/day) 7 days

*if intolerable,
metronidazole (2 x 500 mg/day) 7 days

☐ Laxatives

Laxatives promote and facilitate bowel evacuation by acting locally to stimulate intestinal peristalsis, to soften bowel contents, or both.

1. Bulk Laxatives

Distension of the intestinal wall by bowel contents stimulates propulsive movements of the gut musculature (peristalsis). Activation of intramural mechanoreceptors induces a neurally mediated ascending reflex contraction (red in **A**) and descending relaxation (blue) whereby the intraluminal bolus is moved in the anal direction.

Hydrophilic colloids or **bulk gels** (**B**) comprise insoluble and nonabsorbable substances that expand on taking up water in the bowel. *Vegetable fibers* in the diet act in this manner. They consist of the indigestible plant cell walls containing homoglycans that are resistant to digestive enzymes, e. g., *cellulose* ($1 \rightarrow 4\beta$-linked glucose molecules vs. $1 \rightarrow 4\alpha$-glucoside bond in starch; p.157). *Bran*, a grain milling waste product, and *linseed* (flaxseed) are both rich in cellulose. Other hydrophilic colloids derive from the seeds of *Plantago* species or *karaya gum*. Ingestion of hydrophilic gels for the prophylaxis of constipation usually entails a low risk of side effects. However, when fluid intake is very low and a pathological stenosis exists in the bowel, mucilaginous viscous materials could cause an ileus.

Osmotically active laxatives (**C**) are soluble but nonabsorbable particles that retain water in the bowel by virtue of their osmotic action. The osmotic pressure of bowel contents always corresponds to that of the extracellular space because the intestinal mucosa is unable to maintain a higher or lower osmotic pressure of the luminal contents. Therefore, absorption of molecules (e. g., glucose, NaCl) occurs iso-osmotically, i. e., solute molecules are followed by a corresponding amount of water. Conversely, water remains in the bowel when molecules cannot be absorbed.

With *Epsom salt* ($MgSO_4$) and *Glauber's salt* (Na_2SO_4), the SO_4^{2-} anion is hardly absorbable and retains cations to maintain electroneutrality. Mg^{2+} ions are also believed to promote release of cholecystokinin/pancreozymin, a polypeptide that also stimulates peristalsis, from the duodenal mucosa. These so-called saline cathartics elicit a watery bowel discharge 1–3 hours after administration (preferably in isotonic solution). They are used to purge the bowel (e. g., before bowel surgery) or to hasten the elimination of ingested poisons. Contraindications arise because a small part of cations is absorbed. Thus, Glauber's salt is contraindicated in hypertension, congestive heart failure, and edema because of its high Na^+ content. Epsom salt is contraindicated in renal failure (risk of Mg^{2+} intoxication).

Osmotic laxative effects are also produced by the polyhydric alcohols *mannitol* and *sorbitol*, which unlike glucose cannot be transported through the intestinal mucosa.

Since the disaccharide *lactulose* cannot be hydrolyzed by digestive enzymes, it also acts as an osmotic laxative. Fermentation of lactulose by colon bacteria leads to acidification of bowel contents and a reduced number of bacteria. Lactulose is used in liver failure to forestall hepatic coma by preventing bacterial production of ammonia and its subsequent absorption (absorbable $NH_3 \rightarrow$ nonabsorbable NH_4^+). Another disaccharide, *lactitol*, produces a similar effect.

A. Stimulation of persistalsis by an intraluminal bolus

Stretch receptors

Contraction

Relaxation

B. Bulk laxatives

H_2O H_2O

Cellulose, agar-agar, bran, linseed

C. Osmotically active laxatives

H_2O
Na^+, Cl^-
H_2O H_2O H_2O
Na^+, Cl^- Na^+, Cl^-
H_2O H_2O H_2O
Na^+, Cl^-
H_2O H_2O H_2O
Na^+, Cl^- Na^+, Cl^-
H_2O H_2O H_2O
Na^+, Cl^-
H_2O

Iso-osmotic absorption

G H_2O H_2O G
G
H_2O

G = Glucose

H_2O H_2O H_2O
Na^+, Cl^- Na^+, Cl^- Na^+, Cl^-
H_2O H_2O H_2O
H_2O
Na^+, Cl^-
H_2O
H_2O H_2O H_2O
Na^+, Cl^- Na^+, Cl^- Na^+, Cl^-
H_2O H_2O H_2O

G H_2O

G   G
H_2O H_2O

H_2O
$2 Na^+ SO_4^{2-}$ H_2O H_2O
H_2O

Mannitol
H_2O

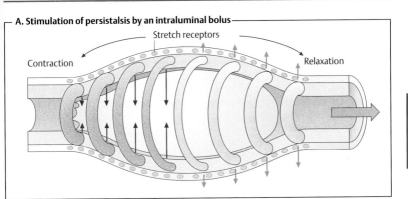

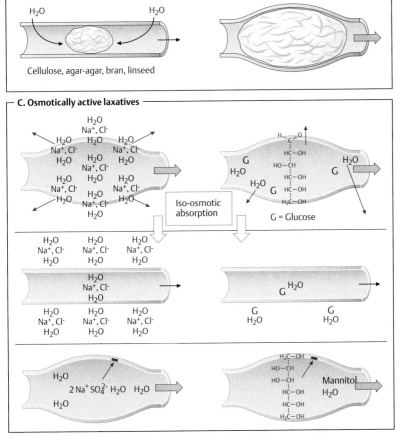

2. Irritant Laxatives

Laxatives in this group exert an irritant action on the enteric mucosa (**A**). Consequently, less fluid is absorbed than is secreted. The increased filling of the bowel promotes peristalsis; excitation of sensory nerve endings elicits enteral hypermotility. According to the site of irritation, one distinguishes the small-bowel irritant castor oil from the large-bowel irritants anthraquinone and diphenylmethane derivatives (for details see p. 178).

Misuse of laxatives. It is a widely held belief that at least one bowel movement per day is essential for health; yet three bowel evacuations per week is quite normal. The desire for frequent bowel emptying probably stems from the time-honored, albeit mistaken, notion that absorption of colon contents is harmful. Thus, purging has long been part of standard therapeutic practice. Nowadays it is known that intoxication from intestinal substances is impossible as long as the liver functions normally. Nonetheless, purgatives continue to be sold as remedies to "cleanse the blood" or to rid the body of "corrupt humors."

There can be no objection to the ingestion of bulk substances for the purpose of supplementing low-residue "modern diets." However, use of irritant purgatives or cathartics is not without hazards. Specifically, there is a risk of laxative dependence, i. e., the inability to do without them. Chronic intake of irritant purgatives disrupts the water and electrolyte balance of the body and can thus cause symptoms of illness (e. g., cardiac arrhythmias secondary to hypokalemia).

Causes of purgative dependence (B). The defecation reflex is triggered when the sigmoid colon and rectum are filled. A natural defecation empties the descending colon. The interval between natural stool evacuations depends on the speed with which this colon segment is refilled. A large-bowel irritant purgative clears out the entire colon.

Accordingly, a longer period is needed until the next natural defecation can occur. Fearing constipation, the user becomes impatient and again resorts to the laxative, which then produces the desired effect as a result of emptying out the upper colonic segments. Thus, a "compensatory pause" following cessation of laxative use must not give cause for concern (**B**).

In the colon, semifluid material entering from the small bowel is thickened by absorption of water and salts (from about 1000 ml to 150 ml per day). If, owing to the action of an irritant purgative, the colon empties prematurely, an enteral loss of NaCl, KCl and water will be incurred. In order to forestall depletion of NaCl and water, the body responds with an increased release of aldosterone (p. 168), which stimulates their reabsorption in the kidney. However, the action of aldosterone is associated with increased renal excretion of KCl. The enteral and renal K^+ losses add up to K^+ depletion of the body, evidenced by a fall in serum K^+ concentration (hypokalemia). This condition is accompanied by a reduction in intestinal peristalsis (bowel atonia). The affected individual infers "constipation" and again partakes of the purgative, and the vicious circle is closed.

A. Stimulation of peristalsis by mucosal irritation

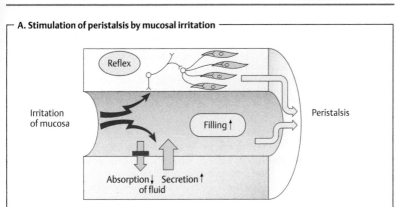

Reflex

Irritation of mucosa

Filling ↑

Peristalsis

Absorption ↓ Secretion ↑
of fluid

B. Causes of laxative habituation

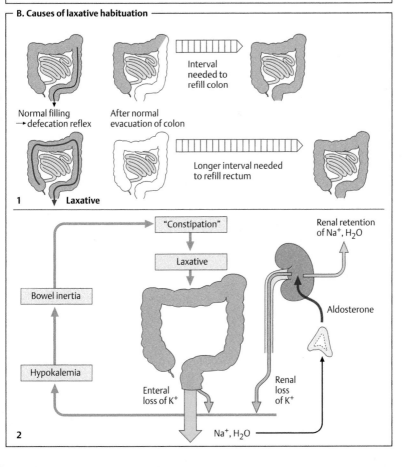

Interval needed to refill colon

Normal filling → defecation reflex

After normal evacuation of colon

Longer interval needed to refill rectum

1   **Laxative**

"Constipation"

Laxative

Renal retention of Na⁺, H₂O

Bowel inertia

Aldosterone

Hypokalemia

Enteral loss of K⁺

Renal loss of K⁺

Na⁺, H₂O

2

2a. Small-Bowel Irritant Purgative

Ricinoleic acid. Castor oil comes from *Ricinus communis* (castor bean; panel **A**: sprig, panicle, seed). The oil is obtained from the first cold-pressing of the seed (shown in natural size). Oral administration of 10–30 ml of castor oil is followed within 0.5–3 hours by discharge of a watery stool. Ricinoleic acid, but not the oil itself, is active. The acid arises as a result of the regular processes involved in fat digestion: the duodenal mucosa releases the enterohormone cholecystokinin/pancreozymin into the blood. The hormone elicits contraction of the gallbladder and discharge of bile acids via the bile duct, as well as release of lipase from the pancreas (intestinal peristalsis is also stimulated). Lipase liberates ricinoleic acids from castor oil; these irritate the small bowel and thus stimulate peristalsis. Because of its massive effect, castor oil is hardly suitable for the treatment of ordinary constipation. It can be employed after oral ingestion of a toxin in order to hasten elimination and to reduce absorption of toxin from the gut. Castor oil is not indicated after the ingestion of lipophilic toxins likely to depend on bile acids for their absorption.

2b. Large-Bowel Irritant Purgatives

Anthraquinone derivatives are of plant origin. They occur in the leaves (*Folia sennae*) or fruits (*Fructus sennae*) of the *senna* plant, the bark of *Rhamnus frangulae* and *Rh. purshiana* (*Cortex frangulae, Cascara sagrada*), the roots of rhubarb (*Rhizoma rhei*), or the leaf extract from *Aloë* species. The structural features of anthraquinone derivatives are illustrated by the prototype structure depicted in panel (**B**). Among other substituents, the anthraquinone nucleus contains hydroxyl groups, one of which is bound to a sugar (glucose, rhamnose). Following ingestion of galenical preparations or of the anthraquinone glycosides, discharge of soft stool occurs after a latency of 6–8 hours. The anthraquinone glycosides themselves are inactive but are converted by colon bacteria to the active free aglycones.

Diphenolmethane derivatives were developed from *phenolphthalein*, an accidentally discovered laxative, use of which had been noted to result in rare but severe allergic reactions. *Bisacodyl* and *sodium picosulfate* are converted by gut bacteria into the active colon-irritant principle. Given by the enteral route, bisacodyl is subject to hydrolysis of acetyl residues, absorption, conjugation in liver to glucuronic acid (or also to sulfate), and biliary secretion into the duodenum. Oral administration is followed after ~6–8 hours by discharge of soft formed stool. When given by suppository, bisacodyl produces its effect within one hour.

Indications for colon-irritant purgatives are the prevention of straining at stool following surgery, myocardial infarction, or stroke; and provision of relief in painful diseases of the anus, e. g., fissure, hemorrhoids.

Purgatives must not be given in abdominal complaints of unclear origin.

3. Lubricant laxatives

Liquid paraffin (*paraffinum subliquidum*) is almost nonabsorbable and makes feces softer and passed easier. It interferes with the absorption of fat-soluble vitamins by trapping them. The few absorbed paraffin particles may induce formation of foreign-body granulomas in enteric lymph nodes (paraffinomas). Aspiration into the bronchial tract can result in lipoid pneumonia. Because of these adverse effects, its use is not advisable.

Antiflatulents (carminatives) serve to alleviate *meteorism* (excessive accumulation of gas in the gastrointestinal tract). Aboral propulsion of intestinal contents is impeded when these are mixed with gas bubbles. Defoaming agents, such as *dimeticone* (dimethylpolysiloxane) and *simethicone*, in combination with charcoal, are given orally to promote separation of gaseous and semisolid contents.

A. Plants containing laxative substances

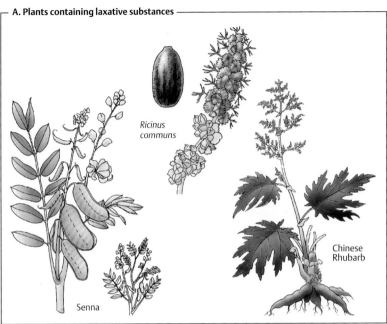

Ricinus communs

Senna

Chinese Rhubarb

B. Large-bowel irritant laxatives: anthraquinone derivatives

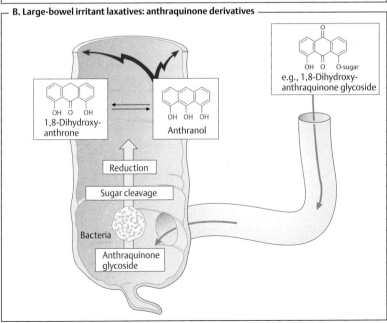

OH O   O-sugar
e.g., 1,8-Dihydroxy-anthraquinone glycoside

OH O   OH
1,8-Dihydroxy-anthrone

OH OH OH
Anthranol

Reduction

Sugar cleavage

Bacteria

Anthraquinone glycoside

□ Antidiarrheal Agents

Causes of diarrhea. Many bacteria (e.g., *Vibrio cholerae*) secrete toxins that inhibit the ability of mucosal enterocytes to absorb NaCl and water and, at the same time, stimulate mucosal secretory activity. **Bacteria** or **viruses** that invade the gut wall cause inflammation characterized by increased fluid secretion into the lumen. The enteric musculature reacts with increased peristalsis.

The aims of antidiarrheal therapy are (1) to prevent dehydration and electrolyte depletion (exsiccosis) of the body, and (2) to prevent the distressing, though nonthreatening, frequent bowel movements. The different therapeutic approaches listed are variously suited for these purposes.

Adsorbent powders are nonabsorbable materials with a large surface area. These bind diverse substances including toxins, permitting them to be inactivated and eliminated. *Medicinal charcoal* has a particularly large surface because of the preserved cell structures. The recommended effective antidiarrheal dose is in the range of 4–8 g. *Kaolin* (hydrated aluminum silicate) is another adsorbent.

Oral rehydration solution (in g/l of boiled water: NaCl 3.5, glucose 20, NaHCO₃ 2.5, KCl 1.5). Oral administration of glucose-containing salt solutions enables fluids to be absorbed because toxins do not impair the co-transport of Na^+ and glucose (as well as of H_2O) through the mucosal epithelium. In this manner, although frequent discharge of stool is not prevented, dehydration is successfully corrected (important in therapy of cholera).

Opioids. Activation of opioid receptors in the enteric nerve plexus results in inhibition of propulsive motor activity and enhancement of segmentation activity. This antidiarrheal effect was formerly induced by application of *opium tincture* (*paregoric*) containing *morphine*. Because of the CNS effects (sedation, respiratory depression, physical dependence), derivatives with mainly peripheral actions have been developed. Whereas *diphenoxylate* can still produce clear CNS effects, *loperamide* does not affect brain functions at normal dosage because it is pumped back into the blood by a P-glycoprotein located in capillary endothelial cells of the blood–brain barrier.

Loperamide is, therefore, the opioid antidiarrheal of first choice. The prolonged contact time for intestinal contents and mucosa may also improve absorption of fluid. With overdosage, there is a hazard of ileus. The drug is contraindicated in infants below age 2 years.

Antibacterial drugs. Use of these agents (e.g., co-trimoxazole, p. 274) is only rational when bacteria are the cause of diarrhea. This is rarely the case. Note that antibiotics also damage the intestinal flora, which in turn can give rise to diarrhea.

Astringents such as tannic acid (home remedy: black tea) or metal salts precipitate surface proteins and are thought to help "seal" the mucosal epithelium. Protein denaturation must not include cellular proteins, for this would mean cell death. Although astringents induce constipation (cf. Al^{3+} salts, p. 170), a therapeutic effect in diarrhea is doubtful.

Demulcents, e.g., pectin (home remedy: grated apples) are carbohydrates that expand on absorbing water. They improve the consistency of bowel contents; beyond that they are devoid of any favorable effect.

A. Antidiarrheals and their sites of action

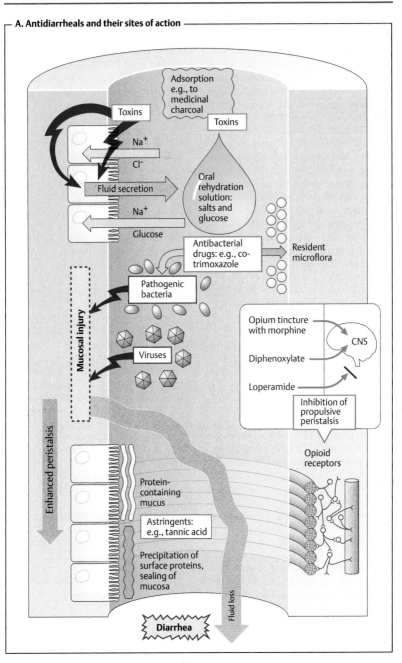

□ Drugs Affecting Motor Function

The smallest structural unit of skeletal musculature is the striated muscle fiber. It contracts in response to an impulse of "its" motor nerve. In executing motor programs, the brain sends impulses to the spinal cord. These converge on α-motoneurons in the anterior horn of the spinal medulla. Bundled in motor nerves, efferent axons course to skeletal muscles. Simple reflex contractions to sensory stimuli, conveyed via the dorsal roots to the motoneurons, occur without participation of the brain. Neural circuits that propagate afferent impulses into the spinal cord contain inhibitory interneurons. These serve to prevent a possible overexcitation of motoneurons (or excessive muscle contractions) due to the constant barrage of sensory stimuli.

Neuromuscular transmission (**B**) of motor nerve impulses to the striated muscle fiber takes place at the motor end plate. The nerve impulse liberates acetylcholine (ACh) from the axon terminal. ACh binds to *nicotinic cholinoceptors* at the motor end plate. This causes depolarization of the postsynaptic membrane, which in turn elicits a propagated action potential (AP) in the surrounding sarcolemma. The AP triggers a release of Ca^{2+} from its storage organelles, the sarcoplasmic reticulum (SR), within the muscle fiber; the rise in Ca^{2+} concentration induces a contraction (electromechanical coupling). Meanwhile, ACh is hydrolyzed by acetylcholinesterase (p. 104); excitation of the end plate subsides. If no AP follows, Ca^{2+} is taken up again by the SR and the myofilaments relax.

Centrally-acting muscle relaxants (**A**) lower muscle tone by augmenting the activity of intraspinal inhibitory interneurons. They are used in the treatment of painful muscle spasms, e. g., in spinal disorders. *Benzodiazepines* enhance the effectiveness of the inhibitory transmitter GABA (p. 222) at GABA$_A$ receptors, which are ligand-gated ion channels. *Baclofen* stimulates GABA$_B$ receptors, which are G-protein coupled.

The **convulsants toxins** *tetanus toxin* (cause of wound tetanus) and *strychnine*, diminish the efficacy of interneuronal synaptic inhibition mediated by the amino acid glycine (**A**). As a consequence of an unrestrained spread of impulses in the spinal cord, motor convulsions develop. Spasms of respiratory muscle groups endanger life.

Botulinus toxin from *Clostridium botulinum* is the most potent poison known. The estimated lethal dose for 50% of an exposed human population is $\sim 1 \times 10^{-9}$ g/kg (i. e., about 75 *nano*grams for an adult individual). The toxin, a zinc endopeptidase, blocks exocytosis of ACh in motor (and also parasympathetic) nerve endings. Death is caused by paralysis of respiratory muscles.

Targeted intramuscular injection of the toxin can produce a long-lasting localized paralysis. This procedure is used to treat pathological or painful muscle spasms (e. g., blepharospasm, esophageal achalasia, cervical dystonia). The same method is increasingly practiced in cosmetic surgery for removal of facial wrinkles ("face lift"). In focal hyperhidrosis (palmar, axillary, plantar), local injection of the toxin disrupts cholinergic sympathetic innervation, the effect of a single treatment lasting for several weeks.

A pathological rise in *serum Mg^{2+}* levels also causes inhibition of neuromuscular transmission.

Dantrolene interferes with electromechanical coupling in the muscle cell by inhibiting Ca^{2+} release from the SR. It is used to treat painful muscle spasms attending spinal diseases and skeletal muscle disorders involving excessive release of Ca^{2+} (malignant hyperthermia).

A. Mechanisms for influencing skeletal muscle tone

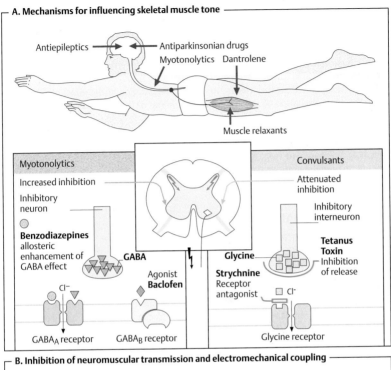

Antiepileptics

Antiparkinsonian drugs

Myotonolytics

Dantrolene

Muscle relaxants

Myotonolytics

Increased inhibition

Inhibitory neuron

Benzodiazepines allosteric enhancement of GABA effect

GABA

Cl^-

Agonist **Baclofen**

$GABA_A$ receptor

$GABA_B$ receptor

Convulsants

Attenuated inhibition

Inhibitory interneuron

Tetanus Toxin Inhibition of release

Glycine

Strychnine Receptor antagonist

Cl^-

Glycine receptor

B. Inhibition of neuromuscular transmission and electromechanical coupling

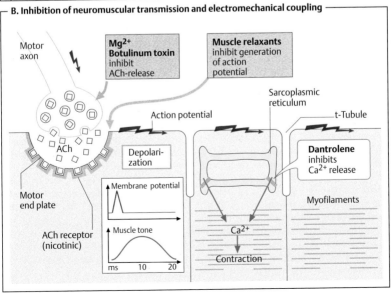

Motor axon

Mg^{2+} Botulinum toxin inhibit ACh-release

Muscle relaxants inhibit generation of action potential

Sarcoplasmic reticulum

Action potential

t-Tubule

ACh

Depolarization

Dantrolene inhibits Ca^{2+} release

Motor end plate

ACh receptor (nicotinic)

Membrane potential

Muscle tone

ms   10   20

Myofilaments

Ca^{2+}

Contraction

□ Muscle Relaxants

Muscle relaxants cause a *flaccid paralysis of skeletal musculature* by binding to motor end plate cholinoceptors, thus blocking *neuromuscular transmission* (p. 182). According to whether receptor occupancy leads to a blockade or an excitation of the end plate, one distinguishes **nondepolarizing** from **depolarizing** muscle relaxants (p. 186). As adjuncts to general anesthetics, muscle relaxants help to ensure that surgical procedures are not disturbed by muscle contractions of the patient (p. 214).

□ Nondepolarizing Muscle Relaxants

Curare is the term for plant-derived arrow poisons of South American natives. When struck by a curare-tipped arrow, an animal suffers paralysis of skeletal musculature within a short time after the poison spreads through the body; death follows because respiratory muscles fail ("peripheral respiratory paralysis"). Killed game can be eaten without risk because absorption of the poison from the gastrointestinal tract is virtually nil. The curare ingredient of greatest medicinal importance is **d-tubocurarine**. This compound contains a quaternary nitrogen atom (N) and, at the opposite end of the molecule, a tertiary N that is protonated at physiological pH. These two positively charged N atoms are common to all other muscle relaxants. The fixed positive charge of the quaternary N accounts for the poor enteral absorbability. *d*-Tubocurarine is given by i.v. injection (average dose ~ 10 mg). It binds to the end-plate nicotinic cholinoceptors without exciting them, acting as a competitive antagonist toward ACh. By preventing the binding of released ACh, it blocks neuromuscular transmission. Muscular paralysis develops within about 4 minutes. *d*-Tubocurarine does not penetrate into the CNS. The patient would thus experience motor paralysis and inability to breathe, while remaining fully conscious but incapable of expressing anything. For this reason, care must be taken to eliminate consciousness by administration of an appropriate drug (general anesthesia) before using a muscle relaxant. The effect of a single dose lasts about 30 minutes.

The duration of the effect of *d*-tubocurarine can be shortened by administering an acetylcholinesterase inhibitor, such as neostigmine (p. 106). Inhibition of ACh breakdown causes the concentration of ACh released at the end plate to rise. Competitive "displacement" by ACh of *d*-tubocurarine from the receptor allows transmission to be restored.

Unwanted effects produced by *d*-tubocurarine result from a non-immune-mediated release of histamine from mast cells leading to bronchospasm, urticaria, and hypotension. More commonly, a fall in blood pressure can be attributed to ganglionic blockade by *d*-tubocurarine.

Pancuronium is a synthetic compound now frequently used and not likely to cause histamine release or ganglionic blockade. Increased heart rate and blood pressure are attributed to blockade of cardiac M_2-cholinoceptors.

Other nondepolarizing muscle relaxants include the pancuronium congeners **vecuronium** and **rocuronium**, in addition to **alcuronium** derived from the alkaloid toxiferin. **Atracurium** is remarkable because it undergoes spontaneous nonenzymatic cleavage; termination of its effect therefore does not depend on hepatic or renal elimination. **Mivacurium** is structurally related to alcuronium; it is rapidly cleaved by cholinesterases and, hence, is short-acting like the depolarizing blocker succinylcholine (p. 186). Rocuronium possesses the fastest onset of action (90 seconds) in this group of substances. The onset of action of nondepolarizing muscle relaxants can be shortened by giving a small nonrelaxant dose minutes before the intubation dose ("priming principle").

A. Nondepolarizing muscle relaxants

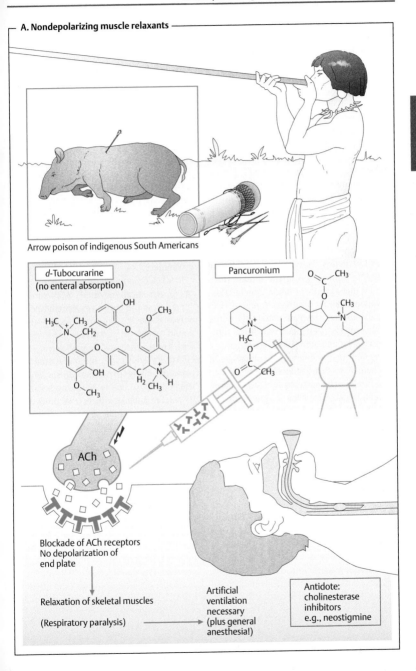

Arrow poison of indigenous South Americans

d-Tubocurarine
(no enteral absorption)

Pancuronium

ACh

Blockade of ACh receptors
No depolarization of
end plate

Relaxation of skeletal muscles

(Respiratory paralysis)

Artificial
ventilation
necessary
(plus general
anesthesia!)

Antidote:
cholinesterase
inhibitors
e.g., neostigmine

□ Depolarizing Muscle Relaxants

In this drug class, only **succinylcholine** (succinyldicholine, suxamethonium, **A**) is of clinical importance. Structurally, it can be described as a double ACh molecule. Like ACh, succinylcholine acts as agonist at end-plate nicotinic cholinoceptors, yet it produces muscle relaxation. Unlike ACh, it is not hydrolyzed by acetylcholinesterase. However, it is a substrate of nonspecific plasma cholinesterase (serum cholinesterase, p. 104). Succinylcholine is degraded more slowly than is ACh and therefore remains in the synaptic cleft for several minutes, causing an end plate depolarization of corresponding duration. This depolarization initially triggers a propagated action potential (AP) in the surrounding muscle cell membrane leading to contraction of the muscle fiber. After i.v. injection, fine muscle twitches (fasciculations) can be observed. A new AP can be elicited near the end plate only if the membrane has been unexcited for a sufficient interval and allowed to repolarize.

The AP is due to opening of voltage-gated Na-channel proteins, allowing Na^+ ions to flow through the sarcolemma and to cause depolarization. After a few milliseconds, the Na^+ channels close automatically ("inactivation"), the membrane potential returns to resting levels, and the AP is terminated. As long as the membrane potential remains incompletely repolarized, renewed opening of Na^+ channels, hence a new AP, is impossible. In the case of released ACh, rapid breakdown by ACh esterase allows repolarization of the end plate and thus a return of Na^+ channel excitability in the adjacent sarcolemma. With succinylcholine, however, there is a persistent depolarization of the end plate and adjoining membrane regions. Because the Na^+ channels remain inactivated, an AP cannot be triggered in the adjacent membrane.

The effect of a standard dose of succinylcholine lasts only about 10 minutes. It is often given at the start of anesthesia to facilitate intubation of the patient. As expected, cholinesterase inhibitors are unable to counteract the effect of succinylcholine. In the few patients with a genetic deficiency in pseudocholinesterase (= nonspecific cholinesterase), the succinylcholine effect is significantly prolonged.

Since the persistent depolarization of end plates is associated with an efflux of K^+ ions, hyperkalemia can result (risk of cardiac arrhythmias). Only in a few muscle types (e.g., extraocular muscle) are muscle fibers supplied with multiple end plates and therefore capable of a graded response. Here succinylcholine causes depolarization distributed over the entire fiber, which responds with a contracture. Intraocular pressure rises, which must be taken into account during eye surgery.

In skeletal muscle fibers whose motor nerve has been severed, ACh receptors spread over the entire cell membrane after a few days. In this case, succinylcholine would evoke a persistent depolarization with contracture and hyperkalemia. These effects are likely to occur in polytraumatized patients undergoing follow-up surgery. The use of succinylcholine is waning because of its marked adverse effects (rhabdomyolysis; hyperkalemia; cardiac arrest)

Clinical use of muscle relaxants. Among the available neuromuscular blockers, succinylcholine displays the fastest onset of action. The patient can be intubated as early as 30–60 seconds after intravenous injection ("rapid sequence intubation"), which is important in emergency situations with an increased risk of aspiration (e.g., ileus, full stomach, head trauma). Postoperative muscle pain due to succinylcholine can be prevented by preinjection of a small dose of a nondepolarizing blocker ("precurarization"). In combination with propofol p. 218), rocuronium (p. 184) creates intubation conditions comparable to those obtained with succinylcholine.

A. Action of the depolarizing relaxant succinylcholine

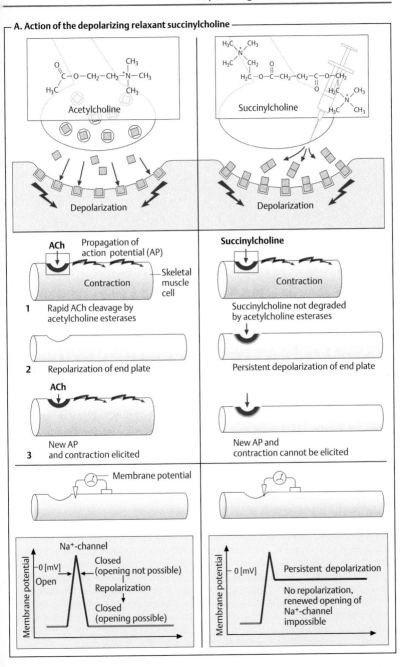

Acetylcholine

Succinylcholine

Depolarization

Depolarization

ACh — Propagation of action potential (AP)

Contraction — Skeletal muscle cell

1 Rapid ACh cleavage by acetylcholine esterases

2 Repolarization of end plate

ACh

New AP
3 and contraction elicited

Membrane potential

Na⁺-channel
Closed (opening not possible)

Open

Repolarization

Closed (opening possible)

Succinylcholine

Contraction

Succinylcholine not degraded by acetylcholine esterases

Persistent depolarization of end plate

New AP and contraction cannot be elicited

Membrane potential

Persistent depolarization

No repolarization, renewed opening of Na⁺-channel impossible

□ Antiparkinsonian Drugs

The central nervous programming of purposive movements depends on neuronal circuits interconnecting cortical regions, the thalamus, the cerebellum, and the basal ganglia (corpus striatum; subthalamic nucleus). The basal ganglia, in particular, play an important part in the initiation and scaling of movement as well as the programming of target acquisition. A disorder primarily involving basal ganglionic motor function is known as idiopathic **Parkinson disease** (shaking palsy). The disease typically manifests at an advanced age and is characterized by poverty of movement (akinesia), muscle stiffness (rigidity), tremor at rest, postural instability, gait disturbance, and a progressive impairment in the quality of life. The primary cause of this disease and its syndromal forms is a degeneration of dopamine neurons in the substantia nigra that project to the corpus striatum (specifically, the caudate nucleus and putamen) and exert an inhibitory influence. Cholinergic interneurons in the striatum promote neuronal excitation.

Pharmacotherapeutic measures are aimed at compensating striatal dopamine deficiency or suppressing unopposed cholinergic activity.

L-Dopa. Dopamine itself cannot penetrate the blood–brain barrier; however, its natural precursor, L-**d**ihydr**o**xy**p**henyl**a**lanine (levo-dopa), is effective in replenishing striatal dopamine levels, because it is transported across the blood–brain barrier via an amino acid carrier and is subsequently decarboxylated by dopa decarboxylase, present in striatal tissue. Decarboxylation also takes place in peripheral organs where dopamine is not needed and is likely to cause undesirable effects (vomiting; hypotension; p.116). Extracerebral production of dopamine can be prevented by inhibitors of dopa decarboxylase (carbidopa, benserazide) that do not penetrate the blood–brain barrier, leaving intracerebral decarboxylation unaffected.

Excessive elevation of brain dopamine levels may lead to undesirable reactions such as involuntary movements (dyskinesias) and mental disturbances.

Dopamine receptor agonists. Striatal dopamine deficiency can be compensated by lysergic acid derivatives such as *bromocriptine* (p.116), *lisuride*, *cabergoline*, and *pergolide* and by the non-ergot compounds *ropinirole* and *pramipexole*.

Inhibitors of monoamine oxidase-B (MAO_B). Monoamine oxidase occurs in the form of two isozymes: MAO_A and MAO_B. The corpus striatum is rich in MAO_B. This isozyme can be inhibited by *selegiline*. Degradation of biogenic amines in peripheral organs is not affected because MAO_A remains functional.

Inhibitor of catecholamine O-methyltransferase (COMT). The CNS-impermeant entacapone inhibits peripheral degradation of L-dopa and thus enhances availability of L-dopa for the brain. Accordingly, it is suitably only for combination therapy with L-dopa.

Anticholinergics. Antagonists at muscarinic cholinoceptors such as *benztropine* and *biperiden* (p.110) can be used to suppress the sequelae of the relative predominance of cholinergic activity in the striatum (in particular, tremor). Atropine-like peripheral side effects and impairment of cognitive function limit the tolerable dosage. Complete disappearance of symptoms cannot be achieved.

Amantadine. Early or mild parkinsonian manifestations may be relieved temporarily by amantadine. The underlying mechanisms of action may involve, inter alia, blockade of ligand-gated ion channels of the glutamate/NMDA subtype, ultimately leading to diminished release of acetylcholine.

Treatment of advanced Parkinson disease requires combined administration of the above drugs for ameliorating the symptoms of this grave condition. Commonly, additional signs of central degeneration develop as the disease progresses.

A. Antiparkinsonian drugs

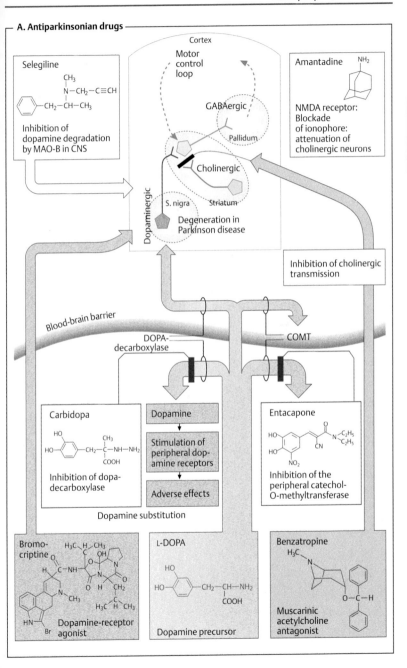

Cortex

Motor control loop

GABAergic

Pallidum

Cholinergic

Striatum

S. nigra

Degeneration in Parkinson disease

Dopaminergic

Blood-brain barrier

Selegiline

CH₃
|
N—CH₂—C≡CH
|
CH₂—CH—CH₃

Inhibition of dopamine degradation by MAO-B in CNS

Amantadine

NH₂

NMDA receptor: Blockade of ionophore: attenuation of cholinergic neurons

Inhibition of cholinergic transmission

DOPA-decarboxylase

COMT

Carbidopa

HO
HO—CH₂—C—NH—NH₂
|
CH₃
|
COOH

Inhibition of dopa-decarboxylase

Dopamine

Stimulation of peripheral dopamine receptors

Adverse effects

Dopamine substitution

Entacapone

HO
HO—
O₂N—C—CN
||
C—N(C₂H₅)₂

Inhibition of the peripheral catechol-O-methyltransferase

Bromocriptine

H₃C   CH₃

Dopamine-receptor agonist

L-DOPA

HO
HO—CH₂—CH—NH₂
|
COOH

Dopamine precursor

Benzatropine

H₃C
N

O—C—H

Muscarinic acetylcholine antagonist

□ Antiepileptics

Epilepsy is a *chronic* brain disease of diverse etiology; it is characterized by *recurrent paroxysmal* episodes of uncontrolled excitation of brain neurons. Involving larger or smaller parts of the brain, the electrical discharge is evident in the electroencephalogram (EEG) as synchronized rhythmic activity and manifests itself in motor, sensory, psychic, and vegetative (visceral) phenomena. As both the affected brain region and the cause of abnormal excitability may differ, epileptic seizures can take on many forms. From a pharmacotherapeutic viewpoint, these may be classified as:

- Generalized vs. partial (focal) seizures
- Seizures with or without loss of consciousness
- Seizures with or without specific modes of precipitation

The brief duration of a single epileptic fit makes acute drug treatment unfeasible. Instead, antiepileptics are used to *prevent* seizures and therefore need to be given chronically. Only in the case of *status epilepticus* (succession of several tonic-clonic seizures), is acute anticonvulsant therapy indicated—usually with benzodiazepines given i.v. or, if needed, rectally.

The initiation of an epileptic attack involves "pacemaker" cells; these differ from other nerve cells by their unstable resting membrane potential; i.e., a depolarizing membrane current persists after the action potential terminates.

Therapeutic interventions aim to stabilize neuronal resting potential and, hence, to lower excitability. In specific forms of epilepsy, initially a single drug is tried to achieve control of seizures, *valproate* usually being the drug of first choice in generalized seizures, and *carbamazepine* being preferred for partial (focal), especially partial complex, seizures. Dosage is increased until seizures are no longer present or adverse effects become unacceptable. Only when monotherapy with different agents proves inadequate

can change-over to a second-line drug or combined use ("add on") be recommended (**B**), provided that the possible risk of pharmacokinetic interactions is taken into account (see below). The precise mode of action of antiepileptic drugs remains unknown. Some agents appear to lower neuronal excitability by several mechanisms of action. In principle, responsivity can be decreased by inhibiting excitatory or activating inhibitory neurons. The transmitters utilized by most excitatory and inhibitory neurons are glutamate and γ-aminobutyric acid (GABA), respectively (p. 193**A**).

Glutamate receptors comprise three subtypes, of which the *NMDA subtype* has the greatest therapeutic importance. (*N*-methyl-D-aspartate is a synthetic selective agonist.) This receptor is a ligand-gated ion channel that, upon stimulation with glutamate, permits entry of both Na^+ and Ca^{2+} into the cell. Valproic acid inhibits both Na^+ and Ca^{2+} channels. The antiepileptics *lamotrigine*, *phenytoin*, and *phenobarbital* inhibit, among other things, the release of glutamate. *Felbamate* is a glutamate antagonist.

Benzodiazepines and *phenobarbital* augment the activation of the GABA$_A$ receptor by physiologically released amounts of GABA (**B**) (see pp. 193, 222). Chloride influx is increased, counteracting depolarization. *Progabide* is a direct GABA-mimetic but not an approved drug. *Tiagabine* blocks removal of GABA from the synaptic cleft by decreasing its reuptake. *Vigabatrin* inhibits GABA catabolism. *Gabapentin* augments the availability of glutamate as a precursor in GABA synthesis (**B**).

A. Epileptic attack, EEG, and antiepileptics

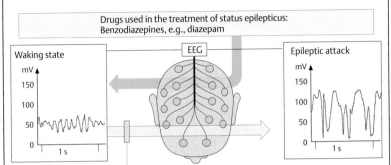

Drugs used in the treatment of status epilepticus:
Benzodiazepines, e.g., diazepam

Waking state

mV

150

100

50

0

1 s

EEG

Epileptic attack

mV

150

100

50

0

1 s

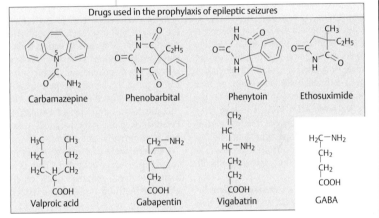

Drugs used in the prophylaxis of epileptic seizures

Carbamazepine

Phenobarbital

Phenytoin

Ethosuximide

Valproic acid

Gabapentin

Vigabatrin

GABA

B. Indications for antiepileptics

		I.	II.	III. Choice
Focal seizures	Simple seizures	Carbamazepine	Valproic acid, Phenytoin	Primidone, Phenobarbital
	Complex or secondarily generalized	+ Lamotrigine or Vigabatrin or Gabapentin		
Generalized attacks	Tonic-clonic attack (grand mal) Tonic attack Clonic attack Myoclonic attack	Valproic acid	Carbamazepine, Phenytoin	Lamotrigine, Primidone, Phenobarbital
		+ Lamotrigine or Vigabatrin or Gabapentin		
	Absence seizure		Ethosuximide	
			+ Lamotrigine or Clonazepam	

The tricyclic *carbamazepine*, its analogue *oxycarbazepine*, and *phenytoin* enhance inactivation of voltage-gated sodium and calcium channels and limit the spread of electrical excitation by inhibiting sustained high-frequency firing of neurons.

Ethosuximide blocks a neuronal T-type Ca^{2+} channel (**A**); and represents a special class because it is effective only in absence seizures.

All antiepileptics are likely, albeit in different degrees, to produce **adverse effects**. *Sedation, difficulty concentrating*, and *slowing of psychomotor drive* encumber practically all antiepileptic therapy. Moreover, cutaneous, hematological, and hepatic changes may necessitate a change in medication. Phenobarbital, primidone, and phenytoin may lead to *osteomalacia* (vitamin D prophylaxis) or *megaloblastic anemia* (folate prophylaxis). During treatment with phenytoin, *gingival hyperplasia* may develop in ~20% of patients. **Valproic acid** (**VPA**) is less sedating than other anticonvulsants. Tremor, gastrointestinal upset, and weight gain are frequently observed; reversible hair loss is a rarer occurrence. Its hepatotoxicity should be kept in mind.

Adverse reactions to **carbamazepine** include nystagmus, ataxia, and diplopia, particularly if the dosage is raised too fast. Gastrointestinal problems and skin rashes are frequent. It exerts an antidiuretic effect (sensitization of collecting ducts to vasopressin).

Valproate, carbamazepine, and other anticonvulsants pose teratogenic risks. Despite this, treatment should continue during *pregnancy*, as the potential threat to the fetus by a seizure is greater. However, it is mandatory to apply the lowest dose affording safe and effective prophylaxis. Concurrent high-dose administration of folate may prevent neural tube defects.

Carbamazepine, phenytoin, phenobarbital, and other anticonvulsants induce hepatic enzymes responsible for drug biotransformation; valproate is a potent inhibitor. *Combinations between anticonvulsants* or with other drugs may result in **clinically important interactions** (plasma level monitoring!).

Carbamazepine is also used to treat trigeminal neuralgia and neuropathic pain.

For the often intractable **childhood epilepsies**, various other agents are used including ACTH and the glucocorticoid dexamethasone. Multiple (mixed) seizures associated with the slow spike-wave (Lennox–Gastaut) syndrome may respond to valproate, lamotrigine, and felbamate, the last being restricted to drug resistant seizures owing to its potentially fatal liver and bone marrow toxicity.

Benzodiazepines are the drugs of choice for status epilepticus (see above); however, development of tolerance renders them less suitable for long-term therapy. *Clonazepam* is used for myoclonic and atonic seizures. *Clobazam*, a 1,5-benzodiazepine exhibiting an increased anticonvulsant/sedative activity ratio, has a similar range of clinical uses. Personality changes and paradoxical excitement are potential side effects.

Clomethiazole can also be effective for controlling status epilepticus but is used mainly to treat agitated states, especially alcoholic delirium tremens and associated seizures.

Topiramate, derived from D-fructose, has complex, long-lasting anticonvulsant actions that cooperate to limit the spread of seizure activity; it is effective in partial and generalized seizures and as add-on in Lennox–Gastaut syndrome.

It should be noted that certain drugs (e.g., neuroleptics, isoniazid, and high-dose β-lactam antibiotics) lower seizure threshold and are therefore contraindicated in epileptic patients.

Outlook: Among the newer antiepileptics, gabapentin, oxycarbazepine, lamotrigine, and topiramate are now endorsed as *primary monotherapeutics* for both partial and generalized seizures. Their pharmacokinetic characteristics are generally more desirable than those of the older drugs.

A. Neuronal sites of action of antiepileptics

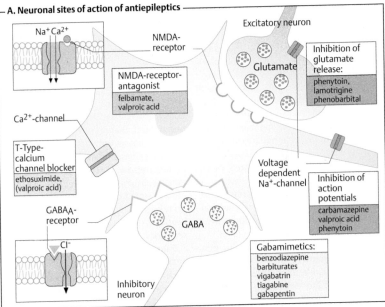

Excitatory neuron

Na^+ Ca^{2+}

NMDA-receptor

Glutamate

Inhibition of glutamate release:
phenytoin, lamotrigine phenobarbital

NMDA-receptor-antagonist
felbamate, valproic acid

Ca^{2+}-channel

T-Type-calcium channel blocker
ethosuximide, (valproic acid)

Voltage dependent Na^+-channel

Inhibition of action potentials
carbamazepine valproic acid phenytoin

$GABA_A$-receptor

Cl^-

GABA

Inhibitory neuron

Gabamimetics:
benzodiazepine
barbiturates
vigabatrin
tiagabine
gabapentin

B. Sites of action of antiepileptics in GABAergic synapse

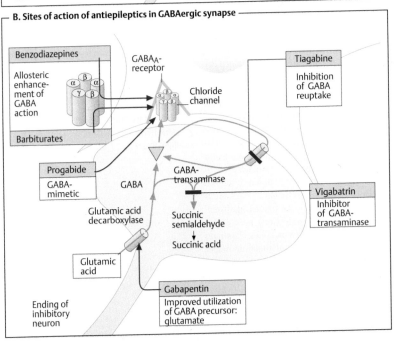

Benzodiazepines

Allosteric enhancement of GABA action

α β α
γ β

$GABA_A$-receptor

Chloride channel

Tiagabine

Inhibition of GABA reuptake

Barbiturates

Progabide

GABA-mimetic

GABA

GABA-transaminase

Succinic semialdehyde

Succinic acid

Vigabatrin

Inhibitor of GABA-transaminase

Glutamic acid decarboxylase

Glutamic acid

Gabapentin

Improved utilization of GABA precursor: glutamate

Ending of inhibitory neuron

□ Pain Mechanisms and Pathways

Pain is a designation for a spectrum of sensations of highly divergent character and intensity ranging from unpleasant to intolerable. Pain stimuli are detected by physiological receptors (sensors, nociceptors) least differentiated morphologically, viz., free nerve endings. The body of the bipolar afferent first-order neuron lies in the dorsal root ganglia. Nociceptive impulses are conducted via unmyelinated (C-fibers, conduction velocity 0.2–2 m/s) and myelinated axons (Aδ-fibers, 10–30 m/s). The free endings of Aδ-fibers respond to intense pressure or heat, those of C-fibers respond to chemical stimuli (H^+, K^+, histamine, bradykinin, etc.) arising from tissue trauma.

Irrespective of whether chemical, mechanical, or thermal stimuli are involved, they become significantly more effective in the presence of prostaglandins (p. 196).

Chemical stimuli also underlie pain secondary to inflammation or ischemia (angina pectoris, myocardial infarction). The intense pain that occurs during overdistension or spasmodic contraction of smooth muscle abdominal organs may be maintained by local anoxemia developing in the area of spasm (visceral pain).

Aδ- and C-fibers enter the spinal cord via the dorsal root, ascend in the dorsolateral funiculus, and then synapse on second-order neurons in the dorsal horn. The axons of the second-order neurons cross the midline and ascend to the brain as the anterolateral pathway or spinothalamic tract. Based on phylogenetic age, a neospinothalamic tract and a palaeospinothalamic tract are distinguished. The second-order (projection) neurons of both tracts lie in different zones (laminae) of the dorsal horn. Lateral thalamic nuclei receiving neospinothalamic input project to circumscribed areas of the postcentral gyrus. Stimuli conveyed via this path are experienced as sharp, clearly localizable pain. The medial thalamic regions receiving palaeospinothalamic input project to the postcentral gyrus as well as the frontal, limbic cortex and most likely represent the pathway subserving pain of a dull, aching, or burning character, i.e., pain that can be localized only poorly.

Impulse traffic in the neospinothalamic and palaeospinothalamic pathways is subject to modulation by descending projections that originate from the reticular formation and terminate at second-order neurons, at their synapses with first-order neurons or spinal segmental interneurons (**descending antinociceptive system**). This system can inhibit substance P-mediated impulse transmission from first- to second-order neurons via release of endogenous opiopeptides (enkephalins) or monoamines (norepinephrine, serotonin).

Pain sensation can be influenced or modified as follows:

- Elimination of the cause of pain
- Lowering of the **sensitivity of nociceptors** (antipyretic analgesics, local anesthetics)
- Interrupting **nociceptive conduction** in sensory nerves (local anesthetics)
- Suppression of **transmission of nociceptive impulses** in the spinal medulla (opioids)
- Inhibition of **pain perception** (opioids, general anesthetics)
- Altering emotional responses to pain, i.e., pain behavior (antidepressants as co-analgesics)

A. Pain mechanisms and pathways

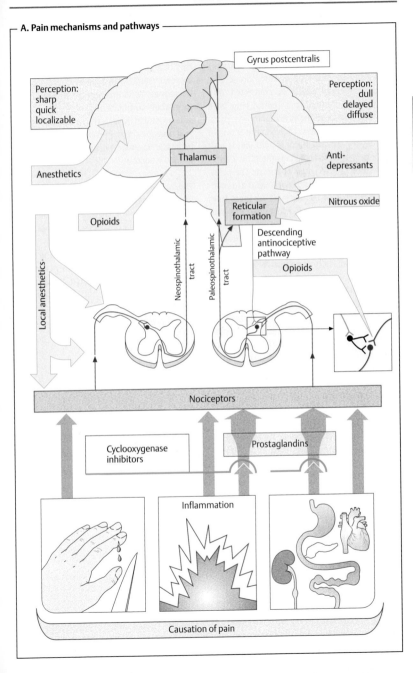

□ Eicosanoids

Under the influence of cyclooxygenases (COX-1, COX-2, and their splice variants), the extended molecule of arachidonic acid (eicosatetraenoic acid[1]) is converted into compounds containing a central ring with two long substituents: prostaglandins, prostacyclin, and thromboxanes. Via the action of a lipoxygenase, arachidonic acid yields leukotrienes, in which ring closure in the center of the molecule (**A**) does not occur. The products formed from arachidonic acid are inactivated very rapidly; they act as **local hormones**. The groups of prostaglandins and leukotrienes each comprise a large number of closely related compounds. In the present context, only the most important prostaglandins and their constitutive actions are considered.

Prostaglandin (PG)E$_2$ inhibits gastric acid secretion, increases production of mucus (mucosa-protective action), and elicits bronchoconstriction. **PGF$_{2\alpha}$** stimulates uterine motility. **PGI$_2$** (prostacyclin) produces vasodilatation and promotes renal excretion of Na$^+$. In addition, prostaglandins synthesized by COX-2 participate in inflammatory processes by sensitizing nociceptors, thus lowering pain threshold; by promoting inflammatory responses by release of mediators such as interleukin-1 and tumor-necrosis factor α; and by evoking fever.

Prostacyclin is produced in vascular endothelium and plays a role in the regulation of blood flow. It elicits vasodilation and prevents aggregation of platelets (functional antagonist of thromboxane).

Thromboxane A$_2$ is a local hormone of platelets; it promotes their aggregation. Small defects in the vascular or capillary wall elicit the formation of thromboxane.

Leukotrienes[2] are produced mainly in leukocytes and mast cells. Newly formed leukotrienes can bind to glutathione. From this complex, glutamine and glycine can be cleaved, resulting in a larger number of local hormones. Leukotrienes are pro-inflammatory; they stimulate invasion of leukocytes and enhance their activity. In anaphylactic reactions, they produce vasodilation, increase vascular permeability, and cause vasoconstriction.

Therapeutic uses of synthetic eicosanoids. Efforts to synthesize stable derivatives of prostaglandins for therapeutic applications have not been very successful to date. Dinoprostone (PGE$_2$), carboprost (15-methyl-PGF$_{2\alpha}$) and mifeprostone are uterine stimulants (p. 130, 254). Misoprostol is meant to afford protection of the gastric mucosa but has pronounced systemic side effects. All these substances lack organ specificity.

---

[1] Name derived from Greek *eikosi* = twenty for the number of carbon atoms and *tetra* = 4 for the number of double bonds

[2] Note the change in chemical nomenclature: -*triene* (tri=three), although leukotrienes possess four double bonds; however, of these only the conjugated ones are counted

A. Origin and actions of prostaglandins

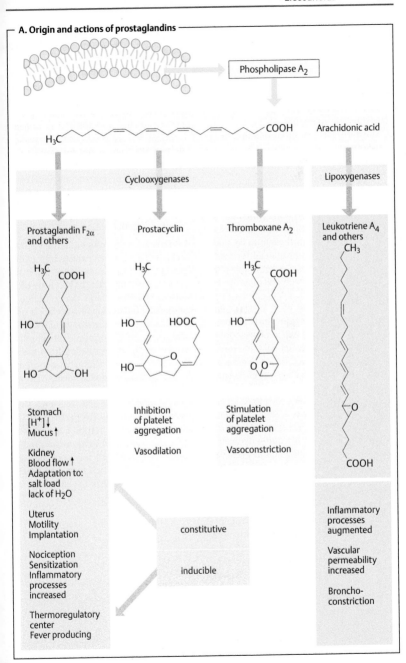

☐ Antipyretic Analgesics

The large and important family of drugs for the treatment of pain, inflammation, and fever has to be subdivided into two groups that differ in their mechanism of action and spectrum of activity, namely,

1. **Antipyretic analgesics**
2. **Nonsteroidal anti-inflammatory drugs (NSAIDs)**

all of which have the chemical character of acids.

Antipyretic analgesics represent *p*-aminophenol or pyrazolone derivatives with clinically useful analgesic and antipyretic efficacy. Their mechanism of action is not completely understood but thought to be mediated via inhibition of prostanoid formation by variants of COX enzymes. Acetaminophen (paracetamol), phenazone, and dipyrone belong in this group.

Acetaminophen has good analgesic efficacy in commonplace pain, such as toothache and headaches, but is of less use in inflammatory and visceral pain. It exerts a strong antipyretic effect. The adult dosage is 0.5–1.0 g up to 4 times daily; the elimination half-life is about 2 hours. Acetaminophen is eliminated renally after conjugation to sulfuric or glucuronic acid. A small portion of the dose is converted by hepatic CYP450 to a reactive metabolite that requires detoxification by coupling to glutathione. In suicidal or accidental poisoning with acetaminophen (10 g), the depleted store of thiol groups must be replaced by administration of acetylcysteine. This measure can be life-saving. Long-term therapy with pure acetaminophen preparations does not cause renal damage, reported earlier after use of stimulant combination preparations. Fixed combinations with codeine may be used with hardly any reservation.

Dipyrone (metamizole) is a pyrazolone derivative. It produces strong analgesia, even in pain of colic, and has an additional spasmolytic effect. The antipyretic effect is marked. The usual dosage is about 500 mg orally. Higher doses (up to 2.5 g) are needed for biliary colic. The effect of a standard dose lasts ~6 hours.

Use of dipyrone is compromised by a very rare but serious adverse reaction, viz., bone marrow depression. The incidence of agranulocytosis remains controversial; probably, one case occurs in >100 000 treatments. Hypotension may occur after intravenous injection. **Dipyrone is not for routine use**; however, short-term administration is recommended for appropriate individual cases.

☐ Nonsteroidal Anti-inflammatory Drugs (NSAIDs)

This term subsumes drugs other than COX-2 inhibitors that (a) are characterized chemically by an acidic moiety linked to an aromatic residue; and that (b) by virtue of inhibiting cyclooxygenases, are effective in suppressing inflammation, alleviating pain, and lowering fever. Cyclooxygenases (COX) localized to the endoplasmic reticulum are responsible for the formation from arachidonic acid of a group of local hormones comprising the prostaglandins, prostacyclin, and thromboxanes. NSAIDs (except ASA) are reversible inhibitors of COX enzymes. These enzymes possess an elongated pore into which the substrate arachidonic acid is inserted and converted to an active product. NSAIDs penetrate into this pore and thus prevent access for arachidonic acid, leading to reversible blockade of the enzyme.

A. Comparison of antipyretic analgesics with a nonsteroidal anti-inflammatory drug

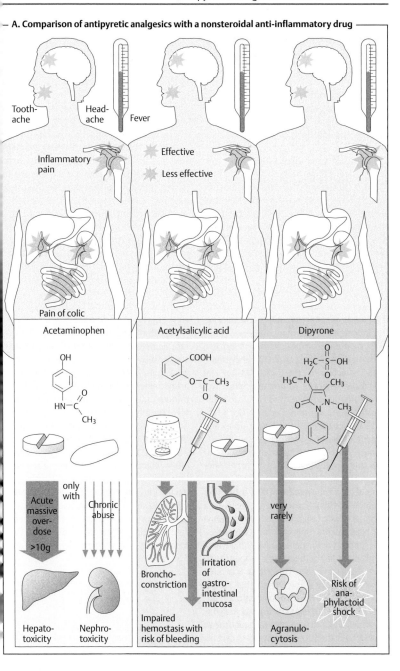

□ Cyclooxygenase (COX) Inhibitors

Two principal types of COX can be distinguished:

COX-1 is constitutive, that is, always present and active; it contributes to the physiological function of organs. Inhibition inevitably produces unwanted effects, such as mucosal injury, renal damage, hemodynamic changes, and disturbances of uterine function.

COX-2 is induced by inflammatory processes and produces prostaglandins that sensitize nociceptors, evoke fever, and promote inflammation by causing vasodilation and an increase in vascular permeability. However, in some organs, COX-2 is also expressed constitutively (kidney, vascular endothelium, uterus, and CNS).

Nonselective COX inhibitors derive from salicylic acid. The majority are carbonic acids, such as *ibuprofen*, *naproxene*, *diclofenac*, *indometacin*, and many more; or enolic acids, such as *azapropazone* and *meloxicam*. All these drugs inhibit both COX enzymes.

The molecules of COX-1 and COX-2 reveal a pharmacologically important difference: the enzymatic pore width of COX-2 exceeds that of COX-1. The nonselective COX inhibitors can also enter the narrower pores and thus inhibit both cyclooxygenases.

Efforts have succeeded to develop inhibitors that readily enter the slightly wider pores of COX-2 but not the COX-1 pores, giving rise to the **specific COX-2 inhibitors** (denoted **coxibs**). These drugs consist of a hetero-aromatic ring bearing two phenyl ring substituents, one of which contains a $-SO_2$ group (see formulas in **A**). The advantage of coxibs lies in their lesser propensity to cause mucosal injury. This effect has been reported in large clinical trials (but subsequently queried). However, a number of adverse reactions are now known that are consistent with COX-2 also serving constitutive functions. Furthermore, one needs to consider that COX-1 functions may be more or less affected at sufficiently large dosages. Selectivity factors (COX-1/COX-2 ratio) determined biochemically in vitro range from 30 to 400.

Coxibs available at present include: *celecoxib* (daily dosage 200–400 mg), *valdecoxib* (10–20 mg) (no longer available in the US) and its prodrug *parecoxib* (40 mg i.v.!).

Coxibs are not drugs for routine use and should only be employed in a targeted manner, in particular when antiarthritis treatment with nonselective NSAIDs has led to gastrointestinal mucosal damage (bleeding, gastritis, ulcerations). Contraindications must be heeded, in particular, advanced congestive heart failure, hepatic and renal diseases, inflammatory bowel diseases, and asthma. Concern over an increased risk of stroke and myocardial infarction in vulnerable patient populations has led to withdrawal of rofecoxib (Sept. 2004), raising strong suspicion that this represents a coxib class effect.

Acetylsalicylic acid (**ASA**) merits a separate comment. Acetylation of salicylic acid significantly reduces its ability to induce mucosal injury. After absorption of ASA, the acetyl moiety is cleaved with a $t_{1/2}$ of 15–20 minutes, salicylic acid then being present in vivo. For anti-inflammatory therapy, the required dosage of ASA lies above 3 g daily. For treatment of ordinary pain, a dose of ~500 mg is needed. At low dosage (100–200 mg daily), following absorption into the portal circulation, ASA causes a long-lasting blockade of COX-1-mediated thromboxane synthesis in platelets because of an irreversible acetylation of the enzyme. Since platelets represent anuclear cell fragments, they are unable to synthesize new COX molecules.

A. Nonsteroidal anti-inflammatory drugs (NSAIDs)

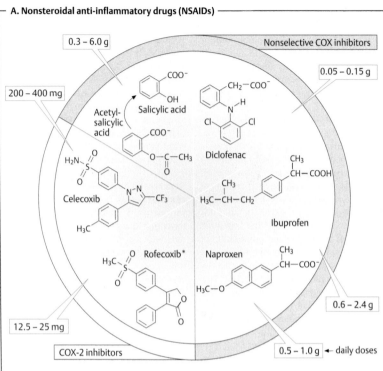

Nonselective COX inhibitors

0.3 – 6.0 g

0.05 – 0.15 g

200 – 400 mg

Salicylic acid

Acetyl-salicylic acid

Diclofenac

Celecoxib

Ibuprofen

Rofecoxib*

Naproxen

12.5 – 25 mg

COX-2 inhibitors

0.6 – 2.4 g

0.5 – 1.0 g ← daily doses

B. Adverse effects of nonsteroidal anti-inflammatory drugs

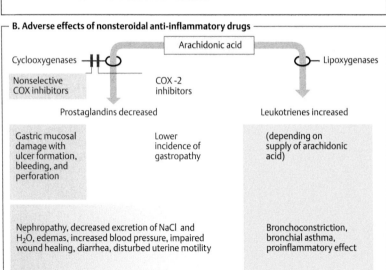

Arachidonic acid

Cyclooxygenases

Nonselective COX inhibitors

COX -2 inhibitors

Lipoxygenases

Prostaglandins decreased

Leukotrienes increased

Gastric mucosal damage with ulcer formation, bleeding, and perforation

Lower incidence of gastropathy

(depending on supply of arachidonic acid)

Nephropathy, decreased excretion of NaCl and H_2O, edemas, increased blood pressure, impaired wound healing, diarrhea, disturbed uterine motility

Bronchoconstriction, bronchial asthma, proinflammatory effect

◻ Local Anesthetics

Local anesthetics reversibly inhibit impulse generation and propagation in nerves. In sensory nerves, such an effect is desired when painful procedures must be performed, e. g., surgical or dental operations.

Mechanism of action. Axonal impulse conduction occurs in the form of an action potential. The change in potential involves a rapid influx of Na^+ (**A**) through a membrane channel protein that, upon being opened (activated), permits rapid inward movement of Na^+ down a chemical gradient ($[Na^+]_{outside}$ ~150 mM, $[Na^+]_{inside}$ ~7 mM). Local anesthetics are capable of inhibiting this rapid influx of Na^+; initiation and propagation of excitation are therefore blocked (**A**).

Most local anesthetics exist in part in the cationic amphiphilic form (cf. p. 206). This physicochemical property favors incorporation into membrane interphases between polar and apolar domains. These are found in phospholipid membranes and also in ion channel proteins. Some evidence suggests that Na^+-channel blockade results from binding of local anesthetics to the channel protein. It appears certain that the site of action is reached from the cytosol, implying that the drug must first penetrate the cell membrane (p. 204).

Local anesthetic activity is also shown by uncharged substances, suggesting a binding site in apolar regions of the channel protein or the surrounding lipid membrane.

Mechanism-specific adverse effects. Since local anesthetics block Na^+ influx not only in sensory nerves but also in other excitable tissues (**A** and p. 206), they are applied locally. Depression of excitatory processes in the heart, while undesired during local anesthesia, can be put to therapeutic use in cardiac arrhythmias (p. 138).

Forms of local anesthesia. Local anesthetics are applied via different routes, including infiltration of the tissue (**infiltration anesthesia**) or injection next to the nerve branch carrying fibers from the region to be anesthetized (**conduction anesthesia** of the nerve, **spinal anesthesia** of segmental dorsal roots), or by application to the surface of the skin or mucosa (**surface anesthesia**). In each case, the local anesthetic drug is required to diffuse to the nerves concerned from a depot placed in the tissue or on the skin.

High sensitivity of sensory, low sensitivity of motor nerves. Impulse conduction in sensory nerves is inhibited at a concentration lower than that needed for motor fibers. This difference may be due to the higher impulse frequency and longer action potential duration in nociceptive as opposed to motor fibers. Alternatively, it may relate to the thickness of sensory and motor nerves, as well as the distance between nodes of Ranvier. In saltatory impulse conduction, only the nodal membrane is depolarized. Because depolarization can still occur after blockade of three or four nodal rings, the area exposed to a drug concentration sufficient to cause blockade must be larger for motor fibers (p. 203**B**).

This relationship explains why sensory stimuli that are conducted via myelinated Aδ-fibers are affected later and to a lesser degree than are stimuli conducted via unmyelinated C-fibers. Since autonomic postganglionic fibers lack a myelin sheath, they are susceptible to blockade by local anesthetics. As a result, vasodilation ensues in the anesthetized region, because sympathetically driven vasomotor tone decreases. This local vasodilation is undesirable (see opposite).

A. Effects of local anesthetics

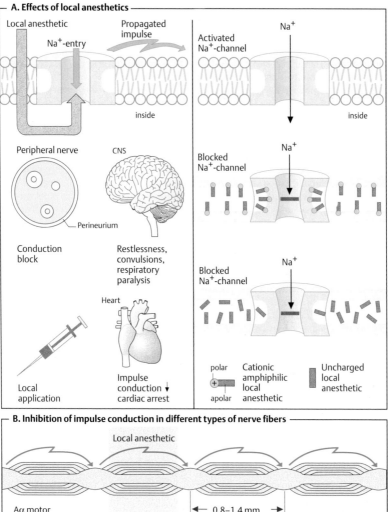

Local anesthetic
Propagated impulse
Na⁺-entry
inside

Activated Na⁺-channel
Na⁺
inside

Peripheral nerve
CNS
Perineurium

Blocked Na⁺-channel
Na⁺

Conduction block

Restlessness, convulsions, respiratory paralysis

Heart

Local application

Impulse conduction ↓ cardiac arrest

Blocked Na⁺-channel
Na⁺

polar
apolar
Cationic amphiphilic local anesthetic

Uncharged local anesthetic

B. Inhibition of impulse conduction in different types of nerve fibers

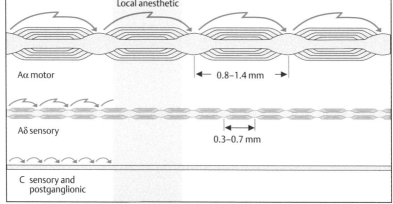

Local anesthetic

Aα motor
0.8–1.4 mm

Aδ sensory
0.3–0.7 mm

C sensory and postganglionic

Diffusion and effect. During diffusion from the injection site (i. e., the interstitial space of connective tissue) to the axon of a sensory nerve, the local anesthetic must traverse the **perineurium**. The multilayered perineurium is formed by connective tissue cells linked by *zonulae occludentes* (p. 22) and therefore constitutes a closed lipophilic barrier.

Local anesthetics in clinical use are usually tertiary amines; at the pH of interstitial fluid these exist partly as the neutral lipophilic base (symbolized by particles marked with two red dots) and partly as the protonated form, i. e., amphiphilic cation (symbolized by particles marked with one blue and one red dot). The uncharged form can penetrate the perineurium and enters the **endoneural space**, where a fraction of the drug molecules regains a positive charge in keeping with the local pH. The same process repeats itself when the drug penetrates through the axonal membrane (axolemma) into the **axoplasm** from which it exerts its action on the sodium channel; and again when it diffuses out of the endoneural space through the unfenestrated endothelium of capillaries into the blood.

The concentration of local anesthetic at the site of action is, therefore, determined by the speed of penetration into the endoneurium and axoplasm and the speed of diffusion into the capillary blood. To enable a sufficiently fast build-up of drug concentration at the site of action, there must be a correspondingly large concentration gradient between drug depot in the connective tissue and the endoneural space. Injection of solutions of low concentration will fail to produce an effect; however, too high concentrations must also be avoided because of the danger of intoxication resulting from too rapid systemic absorption into the blood.

To ensure a reasonably long-lasting local effect with minimal systemic action, a **vasoconstrictor** (epinephrine, less frequently norepinephrine or vasopressin derivatives) is often co-administered in an attempt to confine the drug to its site of action. As blood flow is diminished, diffusion from the endoneural space into the capillary blood decreases. Addition of a vasoconstrictor, moreover, helps to create a relative ischemia in the surgical field. Potential disadvantages of catecholamine-type vasoconstrictors include the reactive hyperemia following washout of the constrictor agent (p. 94) and cardiostimulation when epinephrine enters the systemic circulation. In lieu of epinephrine, the vasopressin analogue felypressin can be used as adjunctive vasoconstrictor (less pronounced reactive hyperemia, no arrhythmogenic action, but danger of coronary constriction). Vasoconstrictors must not be applied in local anesthesia involving the appendages (e. g., fingers, toes).

A. Disposition of local anesthetics in peripheral nerve tissue

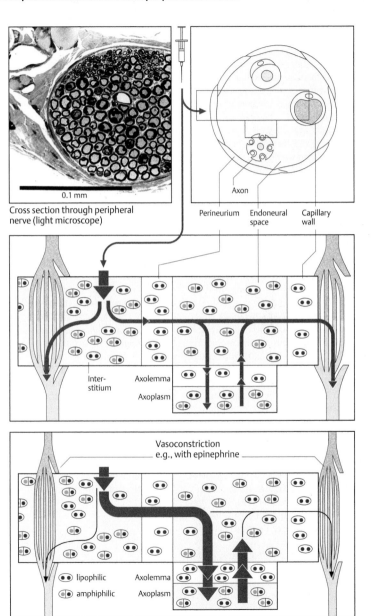

Cross section through peripheral nerve (light microscope)

0.1 mm

Axon

Perineurium Endoneural space Capillary wall

Inter-stitium

Axolemma

Axoplasm

Vasoconstriction e.g., with epinephrine

Axolemma

Axoplasm

lipophilic

amphiphilic

Characteristics of chemical structure. Local anesthetics possess a uniform structure. Generally they are secondary or tertiary amines. The nitrogen is linked through an intermediary chain to a lipophilic moiety—most often an aromatic ring system.

The amine function means that local anesthetics exist either as the neutral amine or as the positively charged ammonium cation, depending upon their dissociation constant (pK_a value) and the actual pH value. The pK_a of typical local anesthetics lies between 7.5 and 9. In its protonated form, the molecule possesses both a polar hydrophilic moiety (protonated nitrogen) and an apolar lipophilic moiety (ring system)—it is *amphiphilic*.

Depending on the pK_a, from 50% to 5% of the drug may be present at physiological pH in the uncharged lipophilic form. This fraction is important because it represents the lipid membrane-permeable form of the local anesthetic (p. 26), which must take on its cationic amphiphilic form in order to exert its action (p. 202).

Clinically used local anesthetics are either esters or amides. Even drugs containing a methylene bridge, such as chlorpromazine (p. 233) or imipramine (p. 229) would exert a local anesthetic effect with appropriate application. Ester-type local anesthetics are subject to inactivation by tissue esterases. This is advantageous because of the diminished danger of systemic intoxication. On the other hand, the high rate of bioinactivation and, therefore, shortened duration of action is a disadvantage.

Procaine cannot be used as surface anesthetic because it is inactivated faster than it can penetrate the dermis or mucosa. In *mepivacaine*, the nitrogen atom usually located at the end of the side chain forms part of a cyclohexane ring.

Lidocaine is broken down primarily in the liver by oxidative N-dealkylation. This step can occur only to a restricted extent in *prilocaine* and *carticaine* because both carry a substituent on the C-atom adjacent to the nitrogen group. Carticaine possesses a carboxymethyl group on its thiophene ring. At this position, ester cleavage can occur, resulting in the formation of a polar COO^- group, loss of the amphiphilic character, and conversion to an inactive metabolite.

Benzocaine is a member of the group of local anesthetics lacking a nitrogen atom that can be protonated at physiological pH. It is used exclusively as a surface anesthetic.

Other agents employed for surface anesthesia include the uncharged *polidocanol* and the catamphiphilic *tetracaine* and *lidocaine* (e.g. as a 5% gel).

Adverse effects of local anesthetics (LAs). The cellular point of attack of LAs is a "fast" Na^+ channel, opening of which initiates the action potential. LAs block this channel. Fast sodium channels also operate in other excitable tissues including nerve cells of the brain and muscle or specialized conducting tissues of the heart. The action of LAs is thus not confined to nerve tissue; it is not organ-specific. Accordingly, serious adverse effects occur when LAs enter the circulation too rapidly or in too high concentrations. In the heart, impulse conduction is disrupted, as evidenced by atrioventricular block or, at worst, ventricular arrest. In the CNS, different regions are perturbed with a resultant loss of consciousness and development of seizures. Since no specific LA antidote is available, symptomatic countermeasures need to be taken immediately. If signs of cardiac inhibition predominate, epinephrine must be given intravenously. If CNS toxicity is present, anticonvulsant drugs have to be administered (e.g., diazepam i.v.).

A. Local anesthetics and pH value

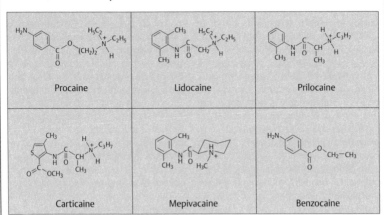

Procaine

Lidocaine

Prilocaine

Carticaine

Mepivacaine

Benzocaine

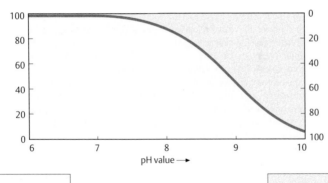

← [H⁺] Proton concentration

pH value →

Active form cationic-amphiphilic

Membrane-permeable lipophilic form

Poor

Ability to penetrate lipophilic barriers and cell membranes

Good

□ Opioid Analgesics—Morphine Type

Sources of opioids. *Morphine* is an opium alkaloid (p. 4). Besides morphine, opium contains alkaloids devoid of analgesic activity, e. g., the spasmolytic papaverine. All semisynthetic derivatives (hydromorphone) and fully synthetic derivatives (pentazocine, pethidine = meperidine, *l*-methadone, and fentanyl) that possess the analgesic effect of morphine are collectively referred to as *opiates* and *opioids*, respectively. The high analgesic effectiveness of xenobiotic opioids derives from their affinity for receptors normally acted upon by endogenous opioids (enkephalins, β-endorphin, dynorphins; **A**). Opioid receptors occur on nerve cells. They are found in various brain regions and the spinal medulla, as well as in intramural nerve plexuses that regulate the motility of the alimentary and urogenital tracts. There are several types of opioid receptors, designated μ, δ, κ, which mediate the various opioid effects, and all belong to the superfamily of G-protein coupled receptors (p. 66).

Endogenous opioids are peptides that are cleaved from the precursors, proenkephalin, pro-opiomelanocortin, and prodynorphin. All contain the amino acid sequence of the pentapeptides [Met]- or [Leu]-enkephalin (**A**). The effects of the opioids can be abolished by antagonists (e. g., naloxone; **A**), with the exception of buprenorphine.

Mode of action of opioids. Most neurons react to opioids with a hyperpolarization, reflecting an increase in K^+ conductance. Ca^{2+} influx into nerve terminals during excitation is decreased, leading to a decreased release of transmitters and decreased synaptic activity (**A**). Depending on the cell population affected, this synaptic inhibition translates into a depressant or excitant effect (**B**).

Effects of opioids (B). The analgesic effect results from actions at the level of the spinal cord (inhibition of nociceptive impulse transmission) and the brain (disinhibition of the descending antinociceptive system, attenuation of impulse spread, and inhibition of pain perception). Attention and ability to concentrate are impaired. There is a **mood change**, the direction of which depends on the initial condition. Aside from the relief associated with the abatement of strong pain, there is a feeling of **detachment** (floating sensation) and a sense of well-being (**euphoria**), particularly after intravenous injection and, hence, rapid build-up of drug levels in the brain. The desire to reexperience this state by renewed administration of drug may become overpowering: *development of psychological dependence.*

The attempt to quit repeated use of the drug results in withdrawal signs of both physical (e. g., cardiovascular disturbances) and psychological (e. g., restlessness, anxiety, depression) nature.

Opioids meet the criteria of drugs producing dependence, that is, a psychological and physiological need to continue use of the drug as well as the compulsion to increase the dose.

For these reasons, prescription of opioids is subject to special rules (Controlled Substances Act, USA; Narcotic Control Act, Canada; etc). Certain opioid analgesics such as codeine and tramadol may be prescribed in the usual manner, because of their lesser potential for abuse and development of dependence. Differences among opioids in efficacy and liability to cause dependence probably reflect differing patterns of affinity and intrinsic activity at individual receptor subtypes, as well as genetic variation of opioid receptors. A given substance does not necessarily act as an agonist or antagonist at each subtype; instead, it may behave as an agonist at one subtype and as a partial agonist/antagonist at another, or even as a pure antagonist (p. 212). In particular, the addictive potential is determined by kinetic properties; only with rapid drug entry into the brain can the euphoriant "rush" be experienced. All high-potency opioids pose the risk of *respiratory depression* (paralysis of the respiratory center) after overdosage. The maximally

A. Action of endogenous and exogenous opioids at opioid receptors

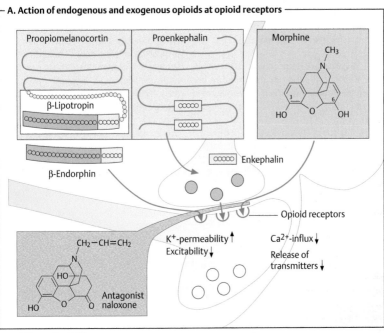

Proopiomelanocortin

β-Lipotropin

β-Endorphin

Proenkephalin

Enkephalin

Morphine

CH$_3$

N

3

HO   O   OH

6

Opioid receptors

K$^+$-permeability ↑
Excitability ↓

Ca^{2+}-influx ↓

Release of
transmitters ↓

CH$_2$−CH=CH$_2$

N

HO

HO   O   O

Antagonist
naloxone

B. Effects of opioids

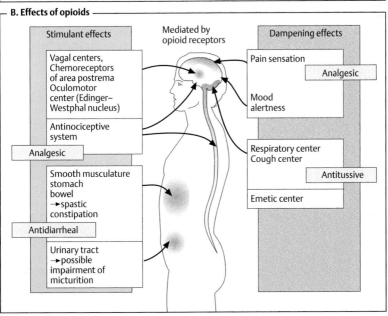

Stimulant effects

Mediated by
opioid receptors

Dampening effects

Vagal centers,
Chemoreceptors
of area postrema
Oculomotor
center (Edinger–
Westphal nucleus)

Pain sensation

Analgesic

Antinociceptive
system

Analgesic

Mood
alertness

Smooth musculature
stomach
bowel
→spastic
constipation

Respiratory center
Cough center

Antitussive

Antidiarrheal

Emetic center

Urinary tract
→possible
impairment of
micturition

possible extent of respiratory depression is thought to be less for partial agonists/antagonists (pentazocine, nalbuphine).

The *cough-suppressant* (*antitussive*) effect produced by inhibition of the cough reflex is independent of the effects on nociception or respiration (antitussives: *codeine, noscapine*).

Stimulation of chemoreceptors in the area postrema (p. 342) results in *vomiting*, particularly after *first-time administration* or in the *ambulant* patient. The emetic effect disappears with *repeated use* because a direct *inhibition of the emetic center* then predominates.

Opioids elicit *pupillary narrowing* (*miosis*) by stimulating the parasympathetic portion (Edinger–Westphal nucleus) of the oculomotor nucleus.

The peripheral effects concern the *motility and tonus of gastrointestinal smooth muscle*; segmentation is enhanced but propulsive peristalsis is inhibited. The tonus of sphincter muscles is markedly raised (spastic constipation). The antidiarrhetic effect is used therapeutically (*loperamide*, p. 180). Gastric emptying is delayed (pyloric spasm) and drainage of bile and pancreatic juice is impeded because the sphincter of Oddi contracts. Likewise, bladder function is affected; specifically *bladder emptying* is impaired owing to an increased tone of the vesicular sphincter.

Kinetics of opioids. The endogenous opioids (e.g., metenkephalin, leuenkephalin, β-endorphin) cannot be used therapeutically because, owing to their peptide nature, they are rapidly degraded or excluded from passage through the blood–brain barrier, thus preventing access to their sites of action even after parenteral administration (**A**). *Morphine* can be given orally or parenterally, as well as epidurally or intrathecally in the spinal cord. Fentanyl is of such potency and high tissue penetrability as to permit application in the form of a patch (transdermal delivery system) (**A**). In opiate abuse, drug ("stuff," "junk," "smack," "jazz," "China white"; mostly heroin = diacetylmorphine) is injected intravenously ("mainlining") to achieve the fastest possible rate of rise in brain concentration. Evidently, psychic effects ("kick," "buzz," "rush") are especially intense with this route of delivery. The user may also resort to other more unusual routes: opium is smoked; heroin can be taken as snuff (**B**).

Metabolism (C). Like other opioids bearing a free hydroxyl group, morphine is conjugated to glucuronic acid and excreted renally. Glucuronidation of the OH group at position 6, unlike that at position 3, does not affect affinity for the receptors.

Tolerance. With repeated administration of opioids, their CNS effects undergo habituation (adaptation). In the course of therapy, progressively larger doses are thus needed to achieve the same degree of pain relief. The peripheral effects are less altered by the development of tolerance, so that persistent constipation during prolonged use may force a discontinuation of analgesic therapy however urgently needed. Frequently laxatives must be prescribed.

Morphine antagonists and partial agonists. The effects of opioids can be abolished by the antagonists naloxone or naltrexone (**A**), irrespective of the receptor type involved. Given by itself, neither has any effect in normal subjects; however, in opioid-dependent subjects, both precipitate acute withdrawal signs. Because of its rapid presystemic elimination, naloxone is only suitable for parenteral use. Naltrexone is metabolically more stable and can be given orally. Naloxone is effective as antidote in the treatment of opioid-induced respiratory paralysis. Since it is more rapidly eliminated than most opioids, repeated doses may be needed. Naltrexone may be used as adjunct in withdrawal therapy.

A. Opioids: mode of application and bioavailability

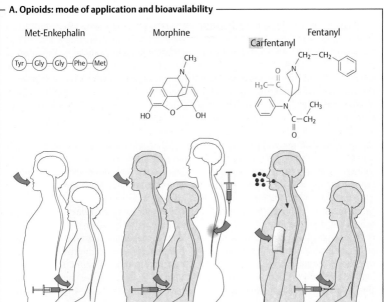

Met-Enkephalin

Tyr—Gly—Gly—Phe—Met

Morphine

Carfentanyl

Fentanyl

B. Application and rate of disposition

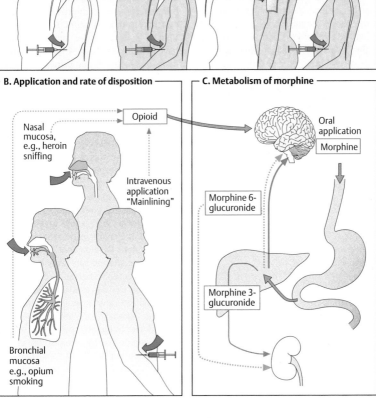

Opioid

Nasal mucosa, e.g., heroin sniffing

Intravenous application "Mainlining"

Bronchial mucosa e.g., opium smoking

C. Metabolism of morphine

Oral application

Morphine

Morphine 6-glucuronide

Morphine 3-glucuronide

Buprenorphine behaves like a partial agonist/antagonist at μ-receptors. **Pentazocine** is an antagonist at μ-receptors and an agonist at κ-receptors (**A**). Both are classified as "low-ceiling" opioids (**B**), because neither is capable of eliciting the maximal analgesic effect obtained with morphine or meperidine. Intoxication with buprenorphine cannot be reversed with antagonists, because the drug dissociates too slowly from the opioid receptors. **Tramadol** is a moderately potent opioid with supposedly less potential for abuse. Its dosage (oral or parenteral) is about 10 times that of morphine (i.e., 50–100 mg; maximum 400 mg/day). Respiratory depression is unlikely to occur at this dose level. The mechanism of its analgesic effect is complex and extends beyond agonism at opioid receptors. Tramadol is a racemate. The (+)-enantiomer has preferential affinity for μ-receptors and is more potent in this regard than the (–)-enantiomer. The O-desmethyl metabolite possesses still higher affinity. Moreover, transport systems for the neuronal reuptake of norepinephrine and serotonin are inhibited—actually with inverse enantioselectivity. The most prominent adverse effect is vomiting (~10% of cases). Tramadol cannot alleviate craving for morphine in addicts but can reinitiate physical dependence.

Fentanyl merits special mention, being ~20-times more potent than morphine. It is administered in the form of a skin patch (transdermal delivery system) for chronic pain management. Specific effectiveness is greatly augmented by introduction into the molecule of a side chain (see p. 211**A**), leading to **carfentanyl**. Carfentanyl has a potency 5000 times that of morphine and a long duration of action. The drug is approved for veterinary tranquilization of large animals. In aqueous solution it can be applied as an aerosol. Its action can be surmounted by morphine antagonists; however, unusually high doses are required.

Uses. Two conditions must be distinguished:

(1) Acute severe pain after trauma (accidents), myocardial infarction, etc. and life-threatening pulmonary edema requiring inhibition of the respiratory center. For these indications, administration of morphine (intravenously or subcutaneously) in sufficient amounts is appropriate. With short-term use, development of tolerance or dependence is of no concern.

(2) Severe chronic pain, especially in cancer patients. In these cases, the aim is to establish a constant plasma level of opioid for a prolonged period. Drug must be given *before* the appearance of pain, not after the patient has begun to suffer from intolerable pain. Like some of the other opioids (hydromorphone, meperidine, pentazocine, codeine), morphine is rapidly eliminated; its duration of action is about 4 hours. To achieve continuous analgesia, these substances would have to be given every 4 hours. For treatment of severe chronic pain states, use of morphine (or oxycodone) in **controlled release form** is the most advantageous regimen because (a) the slow rise in serum levels avoids the subjective "rush" sensation and, hence, the development of "addiction" (psychological dependence); (b) the effect is prolonged; (c) under this condition, an increased proportion of morphine is converted to the 6-glucuronide and contributes to the central effect; and (d) the patient can independently control intake of morphine (i.e., next sustained-release tablet before severe pain re-emerges). If a cancer patient has reached a terminal state, development of tolerance is quite acceptable and can easily be compensated. In a moribund person, a certain degree of euphoria, possibly associated with diminished vigilance, appears ethically acceptable.

Under special conditions (oral route unavailable; intolerable peripheral side effects), opioids may be administered by continuous infusion (pump) or applied near the spinal cord under control by the patient. The advantage is much lower dosage (300-fold) and constant therapeutic level; the disadvantage is the need for a catheter.

A. Opioids: μ- and κ-receptor ligands

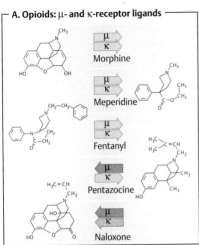

μ
κ
Morphine

μ
κ
Meperidine

μ
κ
Fentanyl

μ
κ
Pentazocine

μ
κ
Naloxone

B. Opioids: dose-response relationship

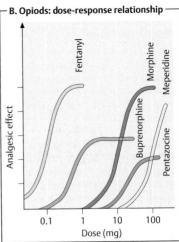

Analgesic effect

Fentanyl

Morphine

Meperidine

Buprenorphine

Pentazocine

Dose (mg)

0.1   1   10   100

C. Enantioselective effects of tramadol

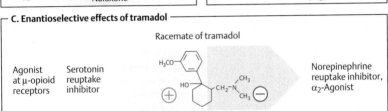

Racemate of tramadol

Agonist
at μ-opioid
receptors

Serotonin
reuptake
inhibitor

Norepinephrine
reuptake inhibitor,
α₂-Agonist

D. Morphine and methadone during chronic intake

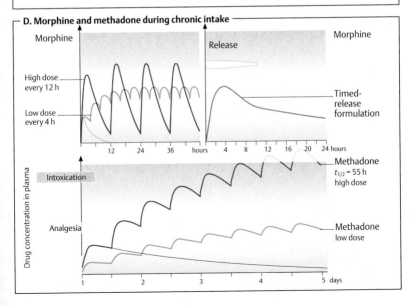

Morphine

High dose
every 12 h

Low dose
every 4 h

12   24   36   hours

Release

Morphine

Timed-
release
formulation

4   8   12   16   20   24 hours

Drug concentration in plasma

Intoxication

Analgesia

Methadone
t₁/₂ = 55 h
high dose

Methadone
low dose

1   2   3   4   5 days

□ General Anesthesia and General Anesthetic Drugs

General anesthesia is a state of drug-induced reversible inhibition of central nervous function, during which surgical procedures can be carried out in the absence of consciousness, responsiveness to pain, defensive or involuntary movements, and significant autonomic reflex responses (**A**).

The required level of anesthesia depends on the intensity of the pain-producing stimuli, i.e., the degree of nociceptive stimulation. The skillful anesthetist, therefore, dynamically adapts the plane of anesthesia to the demands of the surgical situation. Originally, anesthesia was achieved with a single anesthetic agent (e.g., diethyl ether, first successfully demonstrated in 1846 by W. T. G. Morton, Boston). To suppress defensive reflexes, such a "monoanesthesia" necessitates a dosage in excess of that needed to cause unconsciousness, thereby increasing the risk of paralyzing vital functions, such as cardiovascular homeostasis (**B**). Modern anesthesia employs a combination of different drugs to achieve the goals of surgical anesthesia (**balanced anesthesia**). This approach reduces the hazards of anesthesia. In (**C**) are listed examples of drugs that are used concurrently or sequentially as anesthesia adjuncts. Neuromuscular blocking agents are covered elsewhere in more detail. Recall that "curarization" of the patient necessitates artificial ventilation. However, the use of neuromuscular blockers is making an essential contribution to risk reduction in modern anesthesia. In the following, some special methods of anesthesia are considered before presentation of the anesthetic agents.

Neuroleptanalgesia can be considered a special form of combination anesthesia: the short-acting opioid analgesic *fentanyl* is combined with a strongly sedating and affect-blunting neuroleptic. Because of major drawbacks, including insufficient elimination of consciousness and extrapyramidal motor disturbances, this procedure has become obsolete.

In **regional anesthesia** (spinal anesthesia) with a local anesthetic (p. 202), nociceptive conduction is interrupted. Since consciousness is preserved, this procedure does not fall under the definition of anesthesia.

According to their mode of application, **general anesthetics** in the narrow sense are divided into inhalational (gaseous, volatile) and injectable agents.

Inhalational anesthetics are administered in and, for the most part, eliminated via respired air. They serve especially to maintain anesthesia (p. 216)

Injectable anesthetics (p. 218) are frequently employed for induction. Intravenous injection and rapid onset of action are clearly more agreeable to the patient than is breathing a stupefying gas. The effect of most injectable anesthetics is limited to a few minutes. This allows brief procedures to be carried out or preparation of the patient for inhalational anesthesia (intubation). Administration of the volatile anesthetic must then be titrated in such a manner as to counterbalance the waning effect of the injectable agent. Increasing use is now being made of injectable, instead of inhalational, anesthetics during prolonged combined anesthesia (e.g., propofol; total intravenous anaesthesia—TIVA).

A. Goals of surgical anesthesia

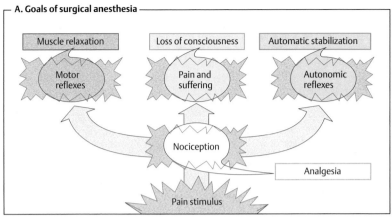

B. Traditional monoanesthesia vs. modern balanced anesthesia

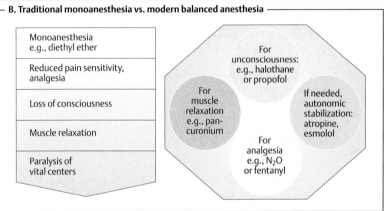

C. Regimen for balanced anesthesia

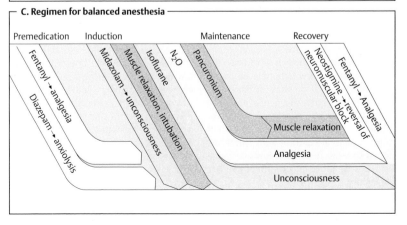

□ Inhalational Anesthetics

The mechanism of action of inhalational anesthetics is not known in detail. In the first instance, the diversity of chemical structures (inert gas xenon; hydrocarbons; halogenated hydrocarbons) possessing anesthetic activity appeared to argue against the involvement of specific sites of action. The *correlation between anesthetic potency and lipophilicity* of anesthetic drugs (**A**) pointed to a nonspecific uptake into the hydrophobic interior of the plasmalemma, with a resultant impairment of neuronal function. Meanwhile, several lines of evidence support an interaction with membrane proteins; among these ligand-gated ion channel proteins assume special importance. Experimental studies favor the idea that anesthetics enhance the effectiveness of inhibitory GABA and glycine receptors, while attenuating responsiveness to stimulation of excitatory glutamate receptors.

Anesthetic potency can be expressed in terms of the minimal alveolar concentration (MAC) at which 50% of patients remain immobile following a defined painful stimulus (skin incision). Whereas the poorly lipophilic nitrous oxide must be inhaled in high concentrations, much smaller concentrations are required in the case of the more lipophilic halothane.

The **rates of onset and cessation** of action vary widely among different inhalational anesthetics and also depend on the degree of lipophilicity. In the case of nitrous oxide, elimination from the body is rapid when the patient is ventilated with normal air. Owing to the high partial pressure in blood, the driving force for transfer of the drug into expired air is large and, since tissue uptake is minor, the body can be quickly cleared of nitrous oxide. In contrast, with halothane, partial pressure in blood is low and tissue uptake is high, resulting in a much slower elimination.

Given alone, *nitrous oxide* (N_2O, "laughing gas") is incapable of producing anesthesia of sufficient depth for surgery, even when taking up 80% of the inspired air volume (O_2 20% vol. is necessary!). It has good analgesic efficacy that can be exploited when it is used in conjunction with other anesthetics. As a gas, N_2O can be administered directly; it is not metabolized appreciably and is cleared entirely by exhalation (**B**).

Halothane (boiling point [BP] 50°C), *enflurane* (BP 56°C), *isoflurane* (BP 48°C) and the newer substances, *desflurane* and *sevoflurane*, have to be vaporized by special devices. Part of the administered halothane (up to 20%) is converted into hepatotoxic metabolites (**B**). Liver damage may result from halothane anesthesia. With a single exposure, the risk involved is unpredictable; however, the risk increases with the frequency of exposure and the shortness of the interval between successive exposures (estimated incidence 1 in 35 000 procedures).

Degradation products of enflurane or isoflurane (fraction biotransformed < 2%) probably do not play any role in anesthetic action.

Halothane exerts a hypotensive effect (vasodilation and negative inotropic effect). Enflurane and isoflurane cause less circulatory depression. Halothane sensitizes the myocardium to catecholamines. This effect is much less pronounced with enflurane and isoflurane. Unlike halothane, enflurane and isoflurane have a muscle-relaxant effect that is additive with that of nondepolarizing neuromuscular blockers.

Desflurane is a close structural relative of isoflurane, but has low lipophilicity and a low rate of biotransformation (0.02%). This permits rapid induction and recovery as well as good control of anesthetic depth. The newest member of this group, *sevoflurane*, is similarly fast-acting and convenient to control but has a higher rate of biotransformation (up to 5%) and lower incidence of laryngospasm and cough.

A. Lipophilicity, potency and elimination of N₂O and halothane

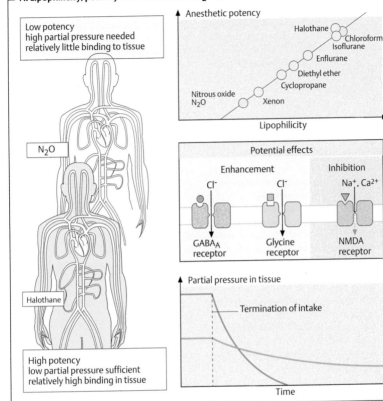

Low potency
high partial pressure needed
relatively little binding to tissue

N₂O

Halothane

High potency
low partial pressure sufficient
relatively high binding in tissue

Anesthetic potency

Halothane
Chloroform
Isoflurane
Enflurane
Diethyl ether
Cyclopropane
Nitrous oxide
N₂O   Xenon

Lipophilicity

Potential effects

Enhancement		Inhibition
Cl^-	Cl^-	Na^+, Ca^{2+}
GABA$_A$ receptor	Glycine receptor	NMDA receptor

Partial pressure in tissue

Termination of intake

Time

B. Elimination routes of different volatile anesthetics

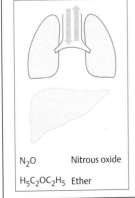

N₂O   Nitrous oxide

H₅C₂OC₂H₅   Ether

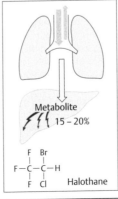

Metabolite
15 – 20%

$$F-\overset{F}{\underset{F}{C}}-\overset{Br}{\underset{Cl}{C}}-H$$ Halothane

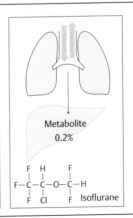

Metabolite
0.2%

$$F-\overset{F}{\underset{F}{C}}-\overset{H}{\underset{Cl}{C}}-O-\overset{F}{\underset{F}{C}}-H$$ Isoflurane

□ Injectable Anesthetics

Substances from different chemical classes suspend consciousness when given intravenously and can be used as injectable anesthetics (**A**). Like inhalational agents, most of these drugs affect consciousness only and are devoid of analgesic activity (exception: ketamine). The effect appears to arise from an interaction with ligand-gated ion channels. Channels mediating neuronal excitation (NMDA receptor, see below) are blocked, while the function of channels dampening excitation (GABA$_A$ receptor, p.222; and, for three drugs, additionally also the glycine receptor) is enhanced allosterically.

Most injectable anesthetics are characterized by a short duration of action. The rapid cessation of action is largely due to **redistribution**: after intravenous injection, brain concentration climbs rapidly to effective anesthetic levels because of the high cerebral blood flow; the drug then distributes evenly in the body, i.e., concentration rises in the periphery, but falls in the brain—redistribution and cessation of anesthesia (**A**). Thus, the effect subsides before the drug has left the body. A second injection of the same drug would encounter "presaturated" body compartments and thus be difficult to predict in terms of effect intensity. Only etomidate and propofol may be given by infusion over a longer period to maintain unconsciousness. If no additional inhalational agent is employed, the procedure is referred to as *total intravenous anesthesia* (*TIVA*).

Thiopental and *methohexital* belong to the barbiturates, which, depending on dose, produce sedation, sleepiness, or anesthesia. Barbiturates lower pain threshold and thereby facilitate defensive reflex movements; they also depress central inspiratory drive. Barbiturates are frequently used for induction of anesthesia.

Ketamine has analgesic activity that persists up to 1 hour after injection, well beyond the initial period of unconsciousness (~15 minutes only). On regaining consciousness, the patient may experience a disconnection between outside reality and inner mental state (*dissociative anesthesia*). Frequently there is memory loss for the duration of the recovery period; however, adults in particular complain about distressing dreamlike experiences. These can be counteracted by administration of a benzodiazepine (e.g., midazolam). The CNS effects of ketamine arise, in part, from an interference with excitatory glutamatergic transmission via ligand-gated cation channels of the NMDA subtype, at which ketamine acts as a channel blocker. The nonnatural excitatory amino acid *N*-methyl D-aspartate (NMDA) is a selective agonist at this receptor. Ketamine can induce release of catecholamines with a resultant increase in heart rate and blood pressure.

Propofol has a remarkably simple structure resembling that of phenol disinfectants. Because the substance is water-insoluble, an injectable emulsion is prepared by means of soy oil, phosphatide, and glycerol. The effect has a rapid onset and decays quickly, being experienced by the patient as fairly pleasant. The intensity of the effect can be well controlled during prolonged administration. Possible adverse reactions include hypotension and respiratory depression, and a potentially fatal syndrome of bronchospasm, hypotension, and erythema.

The anesthetic effect of (+)-etomidate subsides within a few minutes owing to redistribution of the drug. Etomidate can provoke myoclonic movements that can be prevented by premedication with a benzodiazepine or an opioid. Because it has little effect on the autonomic nervous system, it is suitable for induction in combination anesthesia. Etomidate inhibits cortisol synthesis in subanesthetic doses and can therefore be used in the long-term treatment of adrenocortical overactivity (Cushing disease).

Midazolam is a rapidly metabolized benzodiazepine (p.224) that is used for induction of anesthesia. The longer-acting *lorazepam* is preferred as an adjunctive anesthetic in prolonged cardiac surgery with cardiopulmonary bypass; its amnesiogenic effect is pronounced.

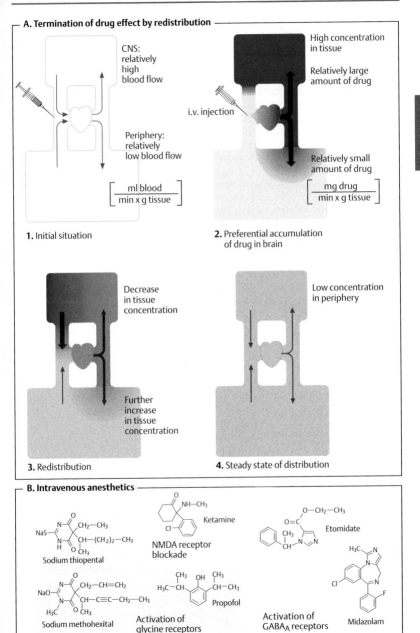

A. Termination of drug effect by redistribution

CNS: relatively high blood flow

Periphery: relatively low blood flow

$$\left[\frac{ml\ blood}{min \times g\ tissue}\right]$$

1. Initial situation

High concentration in tissue

Relatively large amount of drug

i.v. injection

Relatively small amount of drug

$$\left[\frac{mg\ drug}{min \times g\ tissue}\right]$$

2. Preferential accumulation of drug in brain

Decrease in tissue concentration

Further increase in tissue concentration

3. Redistribution

Low concentration in periphery

4. Steady state of distribution

B. Intravenous anesthetics

Sodium thiopental

Ketamine
NMDA receptor blockade

Etomidate

Sodium methohexital

Propofol
Activation of glycine receptors

Activation of GABA$_A$ receptors

Midazolam

☐ Sedatives, Hypnotics

During sleep, the brain generates a patterned rhythmic activity that can be monitored by means of the electroencephalogram (EEG). Internal sleep cycles recur 4–5 times per night, each cycle being interrupted by a **r**apid **e**ye **m**ovement (REM) sleep phase (**A**). The REM stage is characterized by EEG activity similar to that seen in the waking state, rapid eye movements, vivid dreams, and occasional twitches of individual muscle groups against a background of generalized atonia of skeletal musculature. Normally, the REM stage is entered only after a preceding non-REM cycle. Frequent interruption of sleep will, therefore, decrease the REM portion. Shortening of REM sleep (normally ~25% of total sleep duration) results in increased irritability and restlessness during the daytime. With undisturbed night rest, REM deficits are compensated by increased REM sleep on subsequent nights (**B**).

Hypnotic drugs can shorten REM sleep phases (**B**). With repeated ingestion of a hypnotic on several successive days, the proportion of time spent in REM vs. non-REM sleep returns to normal despite continued drug intake. Withdrawal of the hypnotic drug results in REM rebound, which tapers off only over many days (**B**). Since REM stages are associated with vivid dreaming, sleep with excessively long REM episodes is experienced as unrefreshing. Thus, the attempt to discontinue use of hypnotics may result in the impression that refreshing sleep calls for a hypnotic, probably promoting **hypnotic drug dependence**.

Benzodiazepines and benzodiazepine-like substances are the hypnotics of greatest therapeutic importance. They display a positive allosteric action at the GABA$_A$ receptor (p. 222). The formerly popular barbiturates have become obsolete because of their narrow margin of safety (respiratory arrest after overdosage). Barbiturates can also activate GABA$_A$ receptors allosterically; however, this action does not occur at benzodiazepine binding sites. At high dosage, barbiturates can apparently produce an additional direct GABA agonist effect.

Depending on their blood levels, both benzodiazepines and barbiturates produce **calming** and **sedative** effects. At higher dosage, both groups **promote the onset** of sleep or **induce** it (**C**). At low doses, benzodiazepines have a predominantly **anxiolytic** effect.

Unlike barbiturates, **benzodiazepine derivatives** administered orally lack a general anesthetic action; cerebral activity is not globally inhibited (the virtual impossibility of respiratory paralysis negates suicidal misuse) and autonomic functions, such as blood pressure, heart rate, or body temperature, are unimpaired. Thus, benzodiazepines possess a therapeutic margin considerably wider than that of barbiturates.

Zolpidem (an imidazopyridine), **zaleplone** (a pyrazolopyrimidine) and **zopiclone** (a cyclopyrrolone) are hypnotics that, despite their different chemical structure, can bind to the benzodiazepine site on the GABA$_A$ receptor (p. 222). However, their effects do not appear to be identical to those of benzodiazepines. Thus, compared with benzodiazepines, zolpidem exerts a weaker effect on sleep phases, supposedly carries a lower risk of dependence, and appears to have less anxiolytic activity. Heterogeneity of GABA$_A$ receptors may explain these differences in activity. GABA$_A$ receptors consist of five subunits that exist in several subtypes.

Antihistaminics are popular as **nonprescription** (over-the-counter) sleep remedies (e. g., diphenhydramine, doxylamine, p. 118), in which case their sedative side effect is used as the principal effect. The hypnotic effect is weak; adverse effects (e. g., atropine-like) and corresponding contraindications need to be taken into account.

A. Succession of different sleep phases during night rest

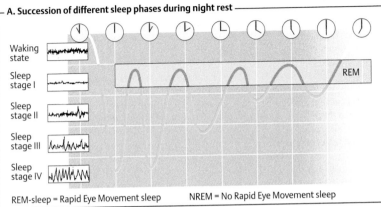

Waking state

Sleep stage I

Sleep stage II

Sleep stage III

Sleep stage IV

REM

REM-sleep = Rapid Eye Movement sleep NREM = No Rapid Eye Movement sleep

B. Influence of hypnotics on sleep phases

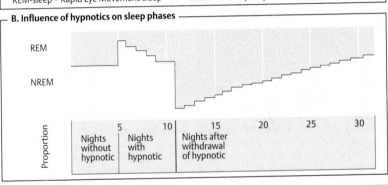

REM

NREM

Proportion

| 5 | 10 | 15 | 20 | 25 | 30 |

Nights without hypnotic

Nights with hypnotic

Nights after withdrawal of hypnotic

C. Concentration dependence of effects

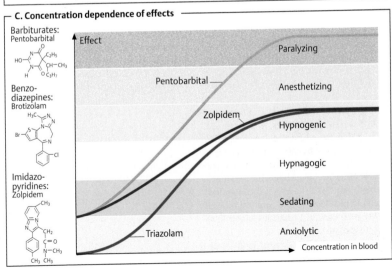

Barbiturates: Pentobarbital

Benzodiazepines: Brotizolam

Imidazopyridines: Zolpidem

Effect

Paralyzing

Pentobarbital

Anesthetizing

Zolpidem

Hypnogenic

Hypnagogic

Sedating

Triazolam

Anxiolytic

Concentration in blood

□ Benzodiazepines

Balanced CNS activity requires inhibitory and excitatory mechanisms. Spinal and cerebral inhibitory interneurons chiefly utilize γ-aminobutyric acid (GABA) as transmitter substance, which decreases the excitability of target cells via **GABA$_A$ receptors**. Binding of GABA to the receptor leads to opening of a chloride (Cl^-)ion channel, chloride influx, neuronal hyperpolarization, and decreased excitability. The pentameric subunit assembly making up the receptor/ion channel contains a high-affinity binding site for benzodiazepines, in addition to the GABA binding locus. Binding of benzodiazepine agonists allosterically enhances binding of GABA and its action on the channel. The prototypical benzodiazepine is diazepam. Barbiturates also possess an allosteric binding site on the Cl^--channel protein; their effect is to increase the channel mean open-time during GABA stimulation.

Benzodiazepines exhibit a broad spectrum of activity: they exert sedating, sleep-inducing, anxiolytic, myorelaxant, and anticonvulsant effects and can be used for induction of anesthesia. Of special significance for the use of benzodiazepines is their wide margin of safety. At therapeutic dosages, neither central respiratory control nor cardiovascular regulation are affected. By virtue of these favorable properties, benzodiazepines have proved themselves for a variety of indications. At low dosage, they calm restless or agitated patients and allay anxiety, though without solving problems. Use of benzodiazepines as sleep remedies is widespread. Here, preference is given to substances that are completely eliminated during the night hours (tetracyclic compounds such as triazolam, brotizolam, alprazolam). For longer-lasting anxiolytic therapy, compounds should be selected that are eliminated slowly and ensure a constant blood level (e. g., diazepam).

In psychosomatic reactions, benzodiazepines can exert an uncoupling effect. They are therefore of great value in hyperacute disease states (e. g., myocardial infarction, p. 320) or severe accidents. Status epilepticus is a necessary indication for parenteral administration (p. 190); however, benzodiazepines can also be used for the long-term treatment of certain forms of epilepsy, if necessary in combination with other anticonvulsants. Rapidly eliminated benzodiazepines are suitable for the intravenous induction of anesthesia.

Use of benzodiazepines may lead to personality changes characterized by flattening of affect. Subjects behave with indifference and fail to react adequately. Any tasks requiring prompt and target-directed action—not only driving a motor vehicle—should be left undone.

Benzodiazepine Antagonist

The drug **flumazenil** binds with high affinity to the benzodiazepine receptor but lacks any agonist activity. Consequently, the receptor is occupied and unavailable for binding of benzodiazepine agonists. Flumazenil is a specific antidote and is used with success for reversal of benzodiazepine toxicity or to terminate benzodiazepine sedation. When patients suffering from benzodiazepine dependence are given flumazenil, withdrawal symptoms are precipitated.

Flumazenil is eliminated relatively rapidly with a $t_{1/2}$ of ~ 1 hour. Therefore, the required dose of 0.2–1.0 mg i.v. must be repeated a corresponding number of times when toxicity is due to long-acting benzodiazepines.

A. Action of benzodiazepines

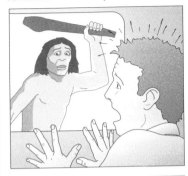

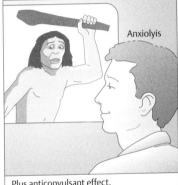

Anxiolyis

Plus anticonvulsant effect, sedation, muscle relaxation

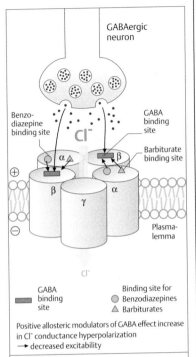

GABAergic neuron

Benzodiazepine binding site

GABA binding site

Barbiturate binding site

Cl^-

Benzodiazepine binding site

GABA binding site

α

β

β

γ

α

Plasmalemma

Cl^-

GABA binding site

Binding site for
○ Benzodiazepines
△ Barbiturates

Positive allosteric modulators of GABA effect increase in Cl^- conductance hyperpolarization
→ decreased excitability

GABA$_A$ receptor with allosteric binding sites

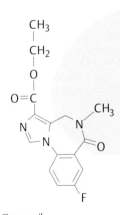

Flumazenil
Benzodiazepine antagonist

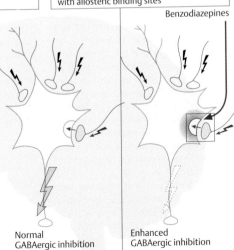

Benzodiazepines

Normal
GABAergic inhibition

Enhanced
GABAergic inhibition

□ Pharmacokinetics of Benzodiazepines

A typical metabolic pathway for benzodiazepines, as exemplified by the drug diazepam, is shown in panel (**A**): first the methyl group on the nitrogen atom at position 1 is removed, with a concomitant or subsequent hydroxylation of the carbon at position 3. The resulting product is the drug oxazepam. These intermediary metabolites are biologically active. Only after the hydroxyl group (position 3) has been conjugated to glucuronic acid is the substance rendered inactive and, as a hydrophilic molecule, readily excreted renally. The metabolic degradation of desmethyldiazepam (nordiazepam) is the slowest step ($t_{1/2}$ = 30–100 hours). This sequence of metabolites encompasses other benzodiazepines that may be considered precursors of desmethyldiazepam, e.g., prazepam and chlordiazepoxide (the first benzodiazepine = Librium®). A similar metabolite pattern is seen in benzodiazepines in which an $-NO_2$ group replaces the chlorine atom on the phenyl ring and in which the phenyl substituent on carbon 5 carries a fluorine atom (e.g., flurazepam). With the exception of oxazepam, all these substances are long-acting. Oxazepam represents those benzodiazepines that are **inactivated in a single metabolic step**; nevertheless, its half-life is still as long as 8 ± 2 hours. Substances with a short half-life result only from introduction of an additional nitrogen-containing ring (see **A**) bearing a methyl group that can be rapidly hydroxylated. Midazolam, brotizolam, and triazolam are members of such tetracyclic benzodiazepines; the latter two are used as hypnotics, whereas midazolam given intravenously is employed for anesthesia induction.

Another possible way of obtaining compounds with an intermediate duration of action is to replace the chlorine atom in diazepam with an NO_2 residue (rapidly reduced to an amine group with immediate acetylation) or with a bromine atom (which causes ring cleavage in the organism). In these cases, biological inactivation again consists of a one-step reaction.

Dependence potential. Prolonged regular use of benzodiazepines can lead to physical dependence. With the long-acting substances marketed initially, this problem was less obvious in comparison with other dependence-producing drugs, because of the delayed appearance of withdrawal symptoms (the decisive criterion for dependence). Symptoms manifested during withdrawal include restlessness, irritability, nervousness, anxiety, insomnia, and, occasionally or in susceptible patients, convulsions. These symptoms are hardly distinguishable from those considered indications for the use of benzodiazepines. Benzodiazepine withdrawal reactions are more likely to occur after abrupt cessation of prolonged or excessive dosage and are more pronounced in shorter-acting substances, but may also be evident after discontinuance of therapeutic dosages administered for no longer than 1–2 weeks.

Administration of a benzodiazepine antagonist would abruptly provoke abstinence signs. Benzodiazepines exhibit cross-dependence with ethanol and can thus be used in the management of delirium tremens. There are indications that substances with intermediate elimination half-lives have the highest abuse potential. Withdrawal of benzodiazepines should be done gradually and cautiously. A long-acting substance such as diazepam is the drug of choice for controlled tapering of withdrawal.

A. Biotransformation of benzodiazepines

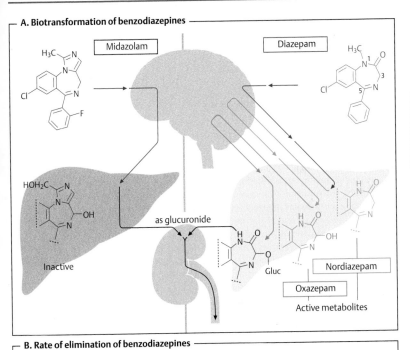

Midazolam

Diazepam

as glucuronide

Inactive

Nordiazepam

Oxazepam

Active metabolites

B. Rate of elimination of benzodiazepines

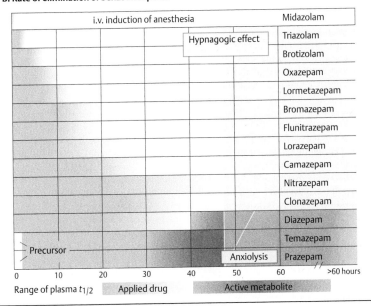

i.v. induction of anesthesia — Midazolam

Hypnagogic effect

Triazolam

Brotizolam

Oxazepam

Lormetazepam

Bromazepam

Flunitrazepam

Lorazepam

Camazepam

Nitrazepam

Clonazepam

Diazepam

Temazepam

Precursor

Anxiolysis — Prazepam

0   10   20   30   40   50   60   >60 hours

Range of plasma $t_{1/2}$ Applied drug   Active metabolite

□ Therapy of Depressive Illness

The term "depression" is used for a variety of states that are characterized by downswings in mood varying from slight to most severe. The principal types are:

- Endogenous depression, ranging from its severe form (major depression) to lighter cases (minor depression)
- Dysthymia (neurotic depression)
- Reactive depression as (overshooting) reaction to psychic insults or somatic illness

Endogenous depression generally follows a phasic course with intervals of normal mood. When mood swings do not change direction, unipolar depression is said to be present. Bipolar illness designates an alternation between depressive states and manic episodes. Besides devitalizing melancholia with its attendant burden of suffering, the behavior of patients in depression may vary from strongly inhibited to anxious, agitated, guilt-ridden, presuicidal, and so on. Depressive states are frequently associated with somatic symptoms; the patients project their mood disturbance into a physical ailment. Accordingly, many depressive patients initially visit a family physician or internist.

The pharmacotherapy of depression is a difficult undertaking. At the outset, it is necessary to determine the type of depression. For instance, in neurotic depression, psychotherapy may be sufficient. A reactive mood disorder calls for attempts to establish the causal link. In either condition, temporary use of antidepressants may be warranted. The proper indication for thymoleptics is endogenous depression. However, even for this endogenous psychosis, it is difficult to evaluate the effectiveness of this drug class. One fundamental reason is the lack of experimental animal models of depression: the efficacy of drugs cannot be tested in experiments on animals. Moreover, depression is periodic in nature; spontaneous remission nearly always occurs. Intensive psychological support may also sometimes be effective in improving the condition of patients. According to some estimates, one-third of therapeutic success in moderately severe depression can be attributed to a placebo effect, one-third to intensive support, and the remaining one-third to use of antidepressant agents. In severe depression, pharmacotherapy may achieve somewhat more favorable results. Because objective documentation of therapeutic success is extraordinarily difficult, it is hardly surprising that no specific antidepressant has proved superior in comparison with others. About 30% of patients are resistant to currently available drug treatments. A workable general rule would be to prescribe tricyclic compounds (and venlafaxine) for severe depression, and selective serotonin reuptake inhibitors (SSRI) for moderately severe to mild cases. No scientifically convincing evidence is available for the "alternative" phytomedicinal, St. John's wort (*Hypericum perforatum*), although drug interactions are well documented.

It would be a major therapeutic error to administer a drive-enhancing drug such as amphetamine to a depressed patient with psychomotor inhibition (**A**). Suicide would be an expected consequence.

The antidepressant effect of thymoleptics manifests after a prolonged latency; usually 1–3 weeks pass before subjective or objective improvement becomes noticeable (**A**). In contrast, somatic effects are immediately evident; specifically, the interference with neuronal transmitter/modulator systems (norepinephrine, serotonin, acetylcholine, histamine, dopamine). Reuptake of released serotonin, norepinephrine, or both is impaired (→ elevated concentration in synaptic cleft) and/or receptors are blocked (example in **A**). These effects are demonstrable in animal studies and are the cause of acute adverse effects.

The importance of these phenomena for the antidepressant effect remains unclear. Presumably, adaptation of receptor systems to altered concentrations or actions of transmitter/modulator substances plays a role.

A. Effect of antidepressants

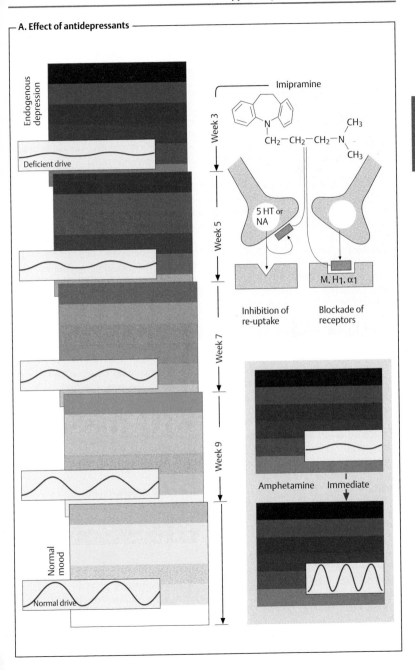

Imipramine

Week 3
Week 5
Week 7
Week 9

Endogenous depression

Deficient drive

5 HT or NA

Inhibition of re-uptake

M, H1, α1

Blockade of receptors

Normal mood

Normal drive

Amphetamine   Immediate

The thymoleptic mechanism of action remains to be elucidated.

Antidepressants can be divided into four groups:

1. Tricyclic antidepressants (A), such as desipramine, amitriptyline, and many analogue substances, possess a hydrophobic ring system. The central 7-membered ring increases the annelation angle between the outer flanking rings. This moiety can also be tetracyclic (e.g., maprotiline). The ring system bears a side chain with a secondary or tertiary amine that can be protonated depending on its pK_a value. These substances can thus take on an amphiphilic character, permitting insertion into lipid membranes and enrichment in cellular structures. The basic structure of tricyclic antidepressants also explains their affinity for receptors and transmitter transport mechanisms. Receptor blockade is the chief cause of the adverse effects in this drug group, including: tachycardia, inhibition of glandular secretion (dry mouth), constipation, difficulty in micturition, blurred vision, and orthostatic hypotension (**A** upper). A sedative action probably arising from antagonism at CNS H_1 histamine receptors, as obtained with amitriptyline, can be desirable.

2. Selective serotonin reuptake inhibitors (SSRI). These substances (e.g., fluoxetine) also possess a protonatable nitrogen atom and, instead of a larger ring system, contain simpler aromatic moieties. They also have amphiphilic character. Because their affinity for receptors is much less (no blockade of acetylcholine or norepinephrine receptors), acute adverse effects are less marked than those of tricyclic thymoleptics. Blockade of reuptake is confined to serotonin (5-HT). Antidepressant potency is equal to or slightly inferior to that of tricyclics. Fluoxetine has a long duration of action. Together with its active metabolite, it is eliminated with a half-life of several days. The SSRI group includes several other substances such as citalopram, paroxetine, sertraline and fluvoxamine. Besides depression, these substances are also marketed for various other psychiatric indications, including anxiety disorders, posttraumatic stress, and obsessive-compulsive disorder.

Labeling of most drugs in this group was recently revised to include a warning statement concerning a worsening of depression and treatment-emergent suicidality in both adult and pediatric patients.

3. Inhibitors of monoamine oxidase A (thymeretics). Moclobemide is the only representative of this group. It produces a reversible inhibition of MAO$_A$, which is responsible for inactivation of the amines norepinephrine, dopamine, and serotonin (**A**). Enzyme inhibition results in an increased concentration of these neurotransmitters in the synaptic cleft. Moclobemide is less effective as an antidepressant than as a psychomotor stimulant. It is indicated only in depressions with extreme psychomotor slowing and is contraindicated in patients at risk of suicide.

Tranylcypromine causes irreversible inhibition of the two isozymes MAO$_A$ and MAO$_B$. Therefore, presystemic elimination in the liver of biogenic amines, such as tyramine, that are ingested in food (e. g., in aged cheese and Chianti) is impaired (with danger of a diet-induced hypertensive crisis). The compound is obsolete in some countries.

4. Atypical antidepressants represent a heterogeneous group comprising agents that interfere only weakly or not at all with monoamine reuptake (trazodone, nefazodone, bupropion, mirtazapine), preferentially block reuptake of norepinephrine (reboxetine), or act as dual inhibitors of 5-HT and norepinephrine reuptake (venlafaxine, milnacipran, duloxetine). Venlafaxine appears to be as effective as tricyclic antidepressants in severe depression.

A. Antidepressants: activity profiles

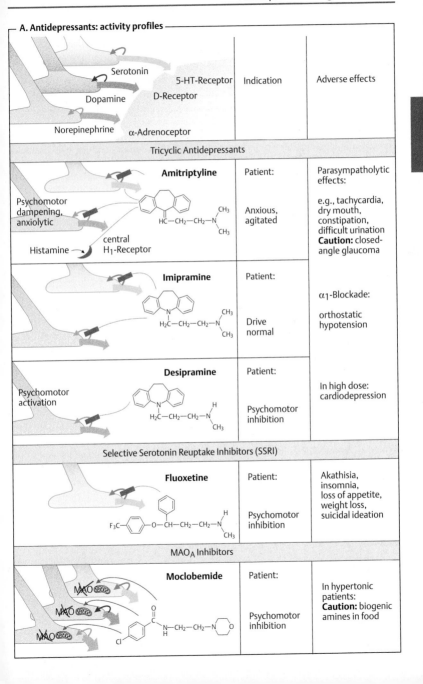

		Indication	Adverse effects
Serotonin	5-HT-Receptor		
Dopamine	D-Receptor		
Norepinephrine	α-Adrenoceptor		

Tricyclic Antidepressants

	Amitriptyline	Patient:	Parasympatholytic effects:
Psychomotor dampening, anxiolytic	HC—CH₂—CH₂—N(CH₃)₂	Anxious, agitated	e.g., tachycardia, dry mouth, constipation, difficult urination **Caution:** closed-angle glaucoma
Histamine — central H₁-Receptor			

	Imipramine	Patient:	α₁-Blockade: orthostatic hypotension
	H₂C—CH₂—CH₂—N(CH₃)₂	Drive normal	

	Desipramine	Patient:	In high dose: cardiodepression
Psychomotor activation	H₂C—CH₂—CH₂—N(H)(CH₃)	Psychomotor inhibition	

Selective Serotonin Reuptake Inhibitors (SSRI)

	Fluoxetine	Patient:	Akathisia, insomnia, loss of appetite, weight loss, suicidal ideation
	F₃C—⟨⟩—O—CH—CH₂—CH₂—N(H)(CH₃)	Psychomotor inhibition	

MAO_A Inhibitors

	Moclobemide	Patient:	In hypertonic patients: **Caution:** biogenic amines in food
MAO	Cl—⟨⟩—C(O)—N(H)—CH₂—CH₂—N⟨O⟩	Psychomotor inhibition	

□ Mania

The manic phase is characterized by exaggerated elation, flight of ideas, and a pathologically increased psychomotor drive. This is symbolically illustrated in (**A**) by a disjointed structure and aggressive color tones. The patients are overconfident, continuously active, show progressive incoherence of thought and loosening of associations, and act irresponsibly (financially, sexually, etc.).

Lithium. Lithium is the lightest of the alkali metal atoms (**A**), of which family sodium and potassium have special significance for the organism. Lithium ions (Li$^+$) distribute nearly evenly in the extracellular and intracellular fluid compartments and thus build up only a small concentration gradient across the cell membrane. The lithium ion cannot be transported by the membranal Na$^+$/K$^+$-ATPase. Intracellularly, lithium ions interfere in transduction mechanisms. For instance, they reduce the hydrolysis of inositol phosphate, leading to a reduced sensitivity to transmitter of nerve cells. In addition, the metabolism of transmitters is thought to be altered in the presence of lithium ions. These and other biochemical findings observed after administration of lithium do not provide a satisfactory explanation for the therapeutic effect of this "simple" pharmaceutical, particularly so because the somatic disturbance underlying mania remains unknown. As in endogenous depression, it is surmised that imbalances between different transmitter systems are at fault. Remarkably, Li$^+$ ions do not exert psychotropic effects in healthy humans, although they elicit the typical adverse effects.

Indications for lithium therapy.

1. Acute treatment of manic phase; therapeutic response develops only in the course of several days (**A**).
2. Long-term administration (6–12 months until full effect reached) for the prophylaxis of both manic and depressive phases of bipolar illness (**A**).
3. Adjunctive therapy in severe therapy-resistant depressions.

Lithium therapy of acute mania is difficult because of the **narrow margin of safety** and because the patient being treated lacks insight. Therapeutic levels should be closely monitored and kept between 0.8 and 1.2 mM in fasting morning blood samples. For prevention of relapse, slightly lower blood levels of 0.6–0.8 mM are recommended. Adverse effects that occur at therapeutic serum concentration during long-term intake of lithium salts include renal (diabetes insipidus) and endocrine manifestations (goiter and/or hypothyroidism, glucose intolerance, hyperparathyroidism, sexual dysfunction). At concentrations > 1.2–1.5 mM, signs of mild toxicity are evident, including a fine hand tremor, weakness, fatigue, and abdominal complaints. As blood levels rise further, decreased ability to concentrate, agitation, confusion, and cerebellar signs are noted. In the most severe cases of poisoning, seizures may occur and the patient may lapse into a comatose state. During lithium therapy, fluctuations in blood level are quasi expected because changes in dietary daily intake of NaCl or fluid losses (diarrhea, diuretics) can markedly alter renal elimination of lithium. Lithium therapy thus requires special diligence on the part of the physician and cooperation on the part of the patient or his or her relatives.

A. Effect of lithium salts in mania

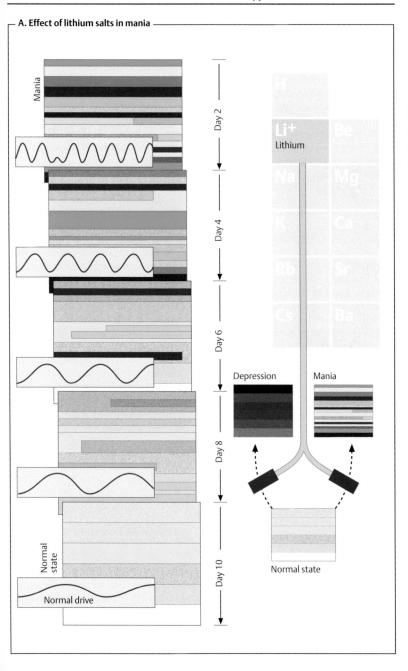

☐ Therapy of Schizophrenia

Schizophrenia is an endogenous psychosis of episodic character; in most cases, recovery is incomplete (residual defects, burned-out end stage). The different forms of schizophrenic illness will not be considered here. From a therapeutic perspective, it is relevant to differentiate between

- Positive signs including delusions, hallucinations, disorganized speech, behavior disturbance; and
- Negative signs, such as social isolation, affective flattening, avolition, poverty of speech, and anhedonia

since both symptom complexes respond differently to antipsychotic drugs.

Neuroleptics

After neuroleptic treatment of a psychotic episode is initiated, the antipsychotic effect proper manifests following a latent period. Acutely, psychomotor damping with anxiolysis and distancing is noted. Tormenting paranoid ideas and hallucinations lose their subjective importance (**A**, dimming of flashy colors); initially, however, the psychotic process persists but then wanes gradually over the course of several weeks.

Complete normalization often cannot be achieved. Even though a "cure" is unrealizable, these changes signify success because (a) the patient obtains relief from the torment of psychotic personality changes; (b) care of the patient is facilitated; and (c) return into a familiar community environment is accelerated. Neuroleptic therapy utilizes different drug classes, namely phenothiazines, butyrophenones, and the atypical neuroleptics.

The **phenothiazines** were developed from the H_1-antihistamine promethazine: prototype chlorpromazine and congeners with a tricyclic ring system and a side chain containing a protonatable nitrogen atom. Phenothiazines exhibit affinity for various receptors and exert corresponding antagonistic actions. Blockade of dopamine receptors, specifically in the mesolimbic prefron-

tal system, appears important for the antipsychotic effect. The latency of the antipsychotic effect suggests that adaptive processes induced by receptor blockade play a role in the therapeutic response. Besides affinity for D_2 dopamine receptors, neuroleptics also exhibit varying affinity to other receptors, including M-ACh receptors, α_1-adrenoceptors, and histamine H_1 and 5-HT receptors. Antagonism at these receptors contributes to the adverse effects. Affinity profiles of "classical" neuroleptics (phenothiazine and butyrophenone derivatives) differ significantly from those of newer atypical drugs (see p. 235**B**), in which affinity for 5-HT receptors predominates.

Neuroleptics *do not have anticonvulsant* activity. Because they *inhibit the thermoregulatory center*, neuroleptics can be employed for controlled hypothermia ("artificial hibernation").

Chronic use of neuroleptics can on occasion give rise to *hepatic damage* associated with cholestasis. A very rare, but dramatic, adverse effect is the *malignant neuroleptic syndrome* (skeletal muscle rigidity, hyperthermia, stupor), which can have a fatal outcome in the absence of intensive countermeasures (including treatment with dantrolene).

With other phenothiazines (e. g., fluphenazine with a piperazine side chain substituent), antagonism at other receptor types tends to recede into the background vis-à-vis the blockade of D_2 dopamine receptors. In panel (**B**) on p. 235 the D_2 receptor affinity of the drugs concerned is defined as ++, while the differences in absolute affinity for the other receptors are ignored.

The **butyrophenones** (prototype haloperidol) were introduced after the phenothiazines. With these agents, blockade of D_2 receptors predominates entirely (p. 235**B**). Antimuscarinic and antiadrenergic effects are attenuated. The "extrapyramidal" motor disturbances that result from D_2 receptor blockade are, however, preserved and constitute the clinically most important adverse reactions that often limit therapy.

A. Effects of neuroleptics in schizophrenia

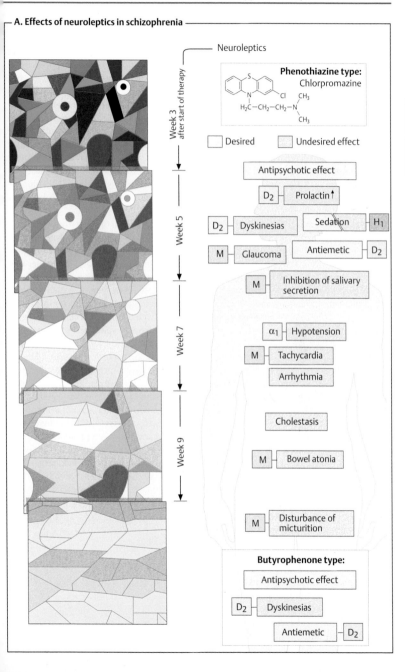

Neuroleptics

Phenothiazine type:
Chlorpromazine

Week 3 after start of therapy

| Desired | Undesired effect |

Antipsychotic effect

D₂ — Prolactin ↑

D₂ — Dyskinesias

Sedation — H₁

M — Glaucoma

Antiemetic — D₂

Week 5

M — Inhibition of salivary secretion

α₁ — Hypotension

M — Tachycardia

Arrhythmia

Week 7

Cholestasis

M — Bowel atonia

Week 9

M — Disturbance of micturition

Butyrophenone type:

Antipsychotic effect

D₂ — Dyskinesias

Antiemetic — D₂

Early dyskinesias occur immediately after neuroleptization and are manifested by involuntary abnormal movements in the head neck and shoulder region. After treatment of several weeks to months, a *parkinsonian syndrome* (pseudoparkinsonism) (p. 188) or *akathisia* (motor restlessness) may develop. All these disturbances can be treated by administration of antiparkinsonian drugs of the anticholinergic type, such as biperiden. As a rule, these disturbances disappear after withdrawal of neuroleptic medication. *Tardive dyskinesia* may become evident after chronic neuroleptization for several years, particularly when the drug is discontinued. Its postulated cause is a hypersensitivity of the dopamine receptor system. The condition is exacerbated by administration of anticholinergics.

The butyrophenones carry an increased risk of adverse motor reactions because they lack anticholinergic activity and, hence, are prone to upset the balance between striatal cholinergic and dopaminergic activity.

Atypical neuroleptics differ in structure and pharmacological properties from the aforementioned drug groups. Extrapyramidal motor reactions are absent or less prevalent. The antipsychotic effect involves not only the positive but also the negative symptoms. In the case of *clozapine*, it was assumed at first that the drug acted as a selective antagonist at D_4 dopamine receptors. Subsequently, however, the drug was recognized as a high-affinity ligand and antagonist at other receptors (**B**). Clozapine can be used when other neuroleptics have to be discontinued because of extrapyramidal motor reactions. Clozapine may cause agranulocytosis, necessitating close hematological monitoring. It produces marked *sedation.*

Olanzapine is structurally related to clozapine; thus far the risk of agranulocytosis appears to be low or absent.

Risperidone differs in structure from the aforementioned drugs; it possesses relatively lower affinity for all "non–D_2-receptors." *Ziprasidone* shows high affinity for 5-HT_{2A} receptors. Remarkably, this new substance also stimulates 5-HT_{1A} receptors, which translates into an antidepressant effect. Ziprasidone particularly influences negative symptoms, its effect on positive symptoms reportedly being equivalent to that of classical neuroleptics. Adverse effects due to blockade of M-ACh, H_1 and α_1-receptors are comparatively weak. Central disturbances (giddiness, ataxia, etc.) may occur. Moreover, QT interval prolongation has been observed; concurrent administration of QT-prolonging drugs must therefore be avoided.

Uses. Management of acute psychotic phases requires high-potency neuroleptics. In highly agitated patients, i.v. injection of haloperidol may be necessary. The earlier therapy is started, the better is the clinical outcome. Most schizophrenic patients require maintenance therapy for which a low dosage can be selected. For stabilization and prevention of relapse, atypical neuroleptics are especially suited since they improve negative symptoms in responsive patients. The patients need good care and, if possible, integration into a suitable milieu. Difficulties arise because patients do not take their prescribed medication (N.B.: counseling of both patient and caregivers). To circumvent lack of compliance, depot preparations have been developed, e.g., fluphenazine decanoate (i.m. every 2 weeks) and haloperidol decanoate (i.m. every 4 weeks), which yield stable blood levels for the period indicated.

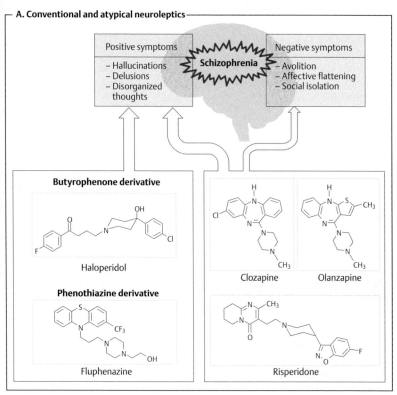

A. Conventional and atypical neuroleptics

Positive symptoms
- Hallucinations
- Delusions
- Disorganized thoughts

Schizophrenia

Negative symptoms
- Avolition
- Affective flattening
- Social isolation

Butyrophenone derivative

Haloperidol

Phenothiazine derivative

Fluphenazine

Clozapine

Olanzapine

Risperidone

B. Receptor affinity profile with reference to D₂-dopamine receptor

	D_2	MACh	α_1	H_1	5-HT_{2A}	5-HT_{1A}
Chlorpromazine	++	+	+++	++	+++	–
Fluphenazine	++	–	+	+	+	–
Haloperidol	++	+	+	+	+	–
Clozapine	++	+++	+++	+++	+++	–
Olanzapine	++	++	++	+++	+++	–
Risperidone	++	–	++	++	++	–
Ziprasidone	++	+	+	+	+++	!++!

The receptor affinities of each drug are compared in relation to its D_2-receptor affinity, arbitrarily set at (++); antagonistic effects, except for ziprasidone (5-HT_{1A} agonism)

□ Psychotomimetics (Psychedelics, Hallucinogens)

Psychotomimetics are able to elicit psychic changes like those manifested in the course of a psychosis, such as **illusionary distortion of perception** and **hallucinations**. This experience may be dreamlike in character; its emotional or intellectual transposition appears incomprehensible to the outsider.

A psychotomimetic effect is pictorially recorded in the series of portraits drawn by an artist under the influence of lysergic acid diethylamide (LSD). As the intoxicated state waxes and wanes wavelike, he reports seeing the face of the portrayed subject turn into a grimace, phosphoresce bluish-purple, and fluctuate in size as if viewed through a moving zoom lens, creating the illusion of abstruse changes in proportion and grotesque motion sequences. The diabolic caricature is perceived as threatening.

Illusions also affect the senses of hearing and smell; sounds (tones) are "experienced" as floating beams and visual impressions as odors ("synesthesia"). Intoxicated individuals see themselves temporarily from the outside and pass judgment on themselves and their condition. The boundary between self and the environment becomes blurred. An elating sense of being one with the other and the cosmos sets in. The sense of time is suspended; there is neither present nor past. Objects are seen that do not exist, and experiences are felt that transcend explanation, hence the term "psychedelic" (Greek *delosis* = revelation) implying expansion of consciousness.

The contents of such illusions and hallucinations can occasionally become extremely threatening (a "bad trip" or "bum trip"); the individual may feel provoked to turn violent or to commit suicide. Intoxication is followed by a phase of intense fatigue, feelings of shame, and humiliating emptiness.

The mechanism of the psychotogenic effect remains unclear. LSD and some natural hallucinogens such as *psilocin*, *psilocybin* (from fungi), *bufotenin* (the cutaneous gland secretion of a toad), and *mescaline* (from the Mexican cactus *Anhalonium lewinii*—peyote) bear structural resemblance to 5HT (p.120) and chemically synthesized amphetamine-derived hallucinogens (4-methyl-2,5-dimethoxyamphetamine, 3,4-dimethoxyamphetamine, 2,5-dimethoxy-4-ethylamphetamine) that are thought to interact with the agonist recognition site of the $5-HT_{2A}$ receptor. Conversely, most of the psychotomimetic effects are annulled by *neuroleptics* having $5-HT_{2A}$ antagonist activity (e.g., clozapine, risperidone). The structures of other agents such as *tetrahydrocannabinol* (from the hemp plant, *Cannabis sativa*—hashish, marihuana), *muscimol* (from the fly agaric, *Amanita muscaria*), or *phencyclidine* (formerly used as injectable general anesthetic) do not reveal a similar connection. Hallucinations may also occur as adverse effects after intake of other substances, e.g., *scopolamine* (medieval witches' ointment) and other centrally-active parasympatholytics. Naturally occurring hallucinogens are employed by priests (shamans) of nature religions to achieve a **trance state**. Synthetic LSD was popular among artists in the 1960s; "psychedelic art" denotes pictorial representation of experiential spaces and hallucinatory signs that elude rational comprehension.

In addition, other drugs that do not act as primary hallucinogens, such as methylenedioxyamphetamine derivatives (e.g., 3,4-dimethylene-dioxymethamphetamine, "Ecstasy") and cocaine pose a health risk. The acute intoxication is associated with a misperception of reality, a period of exhaustion follows. After prolonged use, dependence develops associated with intellectual degradation and physical decay. Withdrawal therapy is very difficult. Marihuana frequently serves as an entry-level recreational substance for hard drugs.

Psychotomimetics are devoid of therapeutic value; however, since their use leads to toxic effects and permanent damage, their manufacture and commercial distribution are prohibited (Schedule I, Controlled Drugs).

A. Psychotomimetic effect of LSD in a portrait artist

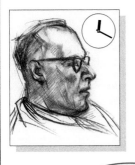
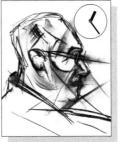
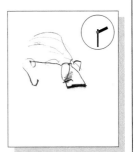
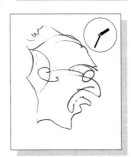
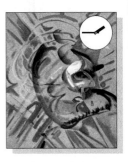
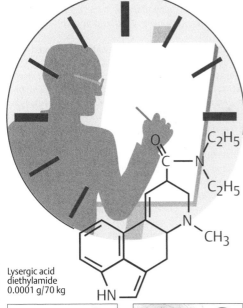

Lysergic acid
diethylamide
0.0001 g/70 kg

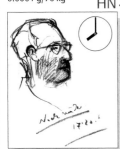
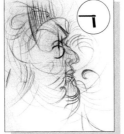
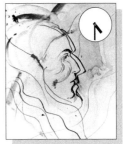

□ Hypothalamic and Hypophyseal Hormones

The endocrine system is controlled by the brain. **Nerve cells of the hypothalamus** synthesize and release messenger substances that regulate adenohypophyseal (AH) hormone release or that are themselves secreted into the body as hormones. The latter comprise the so-called **neurohypophyseal (NH) hormones**.

The axonal processes of hypothalamic neurons project to the neurohypophysis, where they store the *nonapeptides vasopressin* (= antidiuretic hormone, ADH) and *oxytocin* and release them on demand into the blood. Therapeutically (ADH, p.168, oxytocin, p.130), these peptide hormones are given parenterally or via the nasal mucosa.

The **hypothalamic releasing hormones** are *peptides*. They reach their target cells in the AH lobe by way of a portal vascular route consisting of two serially connected capillary beds. The first of these lies in the hypophyseal stalk, the second corresponds to the capillary bed of the AH lobe. Here, the hypothalamic hormones diffuse from the blood to their target cells, whose activity they control. Hormones released from the AH cells enter the blood, in which they are distributed to peripheral organs (**1**).

Nomenclature of releasing hormones.

(RH – releasing hormone; RIH – release-inhibiting hormone.)

GnRH, gonadotropin-RH = gonadorelin: stimulates the release of FSH (follicle-stimulating hormone) and LH (luteinizing hormone).

TRH, thyrotropin-RH (protirelin): stimulates the release of **TSH** (thyroid-stimulating hormone = thyrotropin).

CRH, corticotropin-RH: stimulates the release of ACTH (adrenocorticotropic hormone = corticotropin).

GRH, growth hormone-RH = somatorelin: stimulates the release of GH (growth hormone = STH, somatotropic hormone).

GRIH = somatostatin: inhibits release of STH (and also other peptide hormones including insulin, glucagon and gastrin).

PRIH inhibits the release of prolactin and is identical with dopamine.

Therapeutic control of AH cells. GnRH is used in *hypothalamic infertility in women* to stimulate FSH and LH secretion and to induce ovulation. For this purpose, it is necessary to mimic the physiological intermittent release ("pulsatile," approximately every 90 minutes) by means of a programmed infusion pump.

Gonadorelin superagonists are GnRH analogues that bind with very high avidity to GnRH receptors of AH cells. As a result of the nonphysiological uninterrupted receptor stimulation, initial augmentation of FSH and LH output is followed by a prolonged decrease. *Buserelin, leuprorelin, goserelin*, and *triptorelin* are used to shut down gonadal function in this manner ("chemical castration," e.g., in advanced prostatic carcinoma). **Gonadorelin receptor antagonists**, such as cetrorelix and ganirelix, block the GnRH receptors of AH cells and thus cause cessation of gonadotropin release (**2**).

The **dopamine D_2 agonists**, bromocriptine and cabergoline (p.116), inhibit prolactin-releasing AH cells (indications: suppression of lactation, prolactin-producing tumors). Excessive, but not normal, growth hormone release can also be inhibited (indication: acromegaly).

Octreotide is a somatostatin analogue; it is used in the treatment of somatostatin-secreting pituitary tumors.

Growth hormone requires mediation by somatomedins for many of its actions. These are chiefly formed in the liver, including the important somatomedin C (= insulin-like growth factor 1, IGF-1). *Pegvisomant* is a newly developed antagonist at the GH receptor and inhibits the production of IGF-1.

A. Hypothalamic and hypophyseal hormones

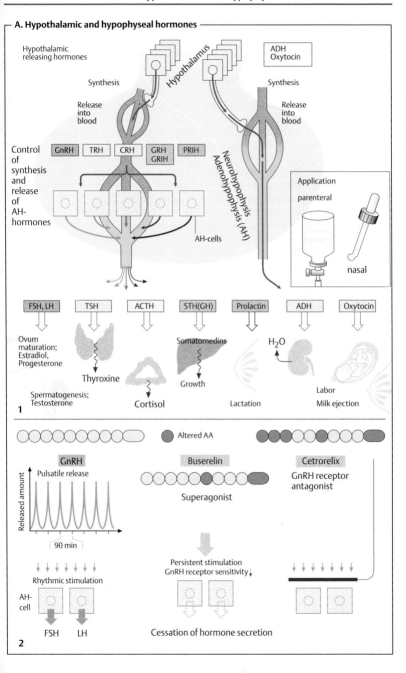

Hypothalamic releasing hormones

ADH
Oxytocin

Synthesis

Hypothalamus

Synthesis

Release into blood

Release into blood

Control of synthesis and release of AH-hormones

GnRH | TRH | CRH | GRH GRIH | PRIH

Neurohypophysis
Adenohypophysis

AH-cells

AH-cells (AH)

Application parenteral

nasal

FSH, LH | TSH | ACTH | STH(GH) | Prolactin | ADH | Oxytocin

Ovum maturation; Estradiol, Progesterone

Thyroxine

Somatomedins

H_2O

Spermatogenesis; Testosterone

Cortisol

Growth

Lactation

Labor

Milk ejection

1

Altered AA

GnRH

Pulsatile release

Released amount

90 min

Buserelin

Superagonist

Cetrorelix

GnRH receptor antagonist

Persistent stimulation
GnRH receptor sensitivity↓

Rhythmic stimulation

AH-cell

FSH LH

Cessation of hormone secretion

2

□ Thyroid Hormone Therapy

Thyroid hormones accelerate metabolism. Their release (**A**) is regulated by the hypophyseal glycoprotein TSH, whose release, in turn, is controlled by the hypothalamic tripeptide TRH. Secretion of TSH declines as the blood level of thyroid hormones rises; by means of this negative feedback mechanism, hormone production is "automatically" adjusted to demand.

The thyroid releases predominantly thyroxine (T_4). However, the active form appears to be triiodothyronine (T_3); T_4 is converted in part to T_3, receptor affinity in target organs being 10-fold higher for T_3. The effect of T_3 develops more rapidly and has a shorter duration than does that of T_4. Plasma elimination $t_{1/2}$ for T_4 is about 7 days; that for T_3, however, is only 1.5 days. Conversion of T_4 to T_3 releases iodide; 150 µg T_4 contains 100 µg of iodine.

For therapeutic purposes, T_4 is chosen, although T_3 is the active form and better absorbed from the gut. With T_4 administration, more constant blood levels can be achieved because T_4 degradation is so slow. Since T_4 absorption is maximal from an empty stomach, T_4 is taken about half an hour before breakfast.

Replacement therapy of hypothyroidism. Whether primary, i. e., caused by thyroid disease, or secondary, i. e., resulting from TSH deficiency, hypothyroidism is treated by oral administration of T_4. Since too rapid activation of metabolism entails the hazard of cardiac overload (angina pectoris, myocardial infarction), therapy is usually started with low doses and gradually increased. The final maintenance dose required to restore a euthyroid state depends on individual needs (~ 150 µg/day).

Thyroid suppression therapy of euthyroid goiter (B). The cause of goiter (struma) is usually a dietary deficiency of iodine. Owing to increased TSH action, the thyroid is activated to raise utilization of the little iodine available to a level at which hypothyroidism is averted. Accordingly, the thyroid increases in size. In addition, intrathyroid depletion of iodine stimulates growth.

Because of the negative feedback regulation of thyroid function, thyroid activation can be inhibited by administration of T_4 doses equivalent to the endogenous daily output (~ 150 µg/day). Deprived of stimulation, the inactive thyroid regresses in size.

If a euthyroid goiter has not persisted for too long, increasing iodine supply (with potassium iodide tablets) can also be effective in reversing overgrowth of the gland.

In older patients with goiter due to iodine deficiency, there is a risk of provoking hyperthyroidism by increasing iodine intake (p. 243**B**). During chronic maximal stimulation, thyroid follicles can become independent of TSH stimulation ("autonomic tissue" containing TSH receptor mutants with spontaneous "constitutive activity"). If the iodine supply is increased, thyroid hormone production increases while TSH secretion decreases owing to feedback inhibition. The activity of autonomic tissue, however, persists at a high level; thyroxine is released in excess, resulting in iodine-induced hyperthyroidism.

Iodized salt prophylaxis. Goiter is endemic in regions where soils are deficient in iodine. Use of iodized table salt allows iodine requirements (150–300 µg/day) to be met and effectively prevents goiter.

A. Thyroid hormones – release, effects, degradation

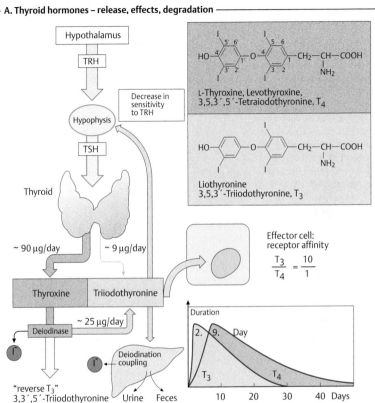

Hypothalamus

TRH

Decrease in sensitivity to TRH

Hypophysis

TSH

Thyroid

HO—$4'$—O—CH$_2$—CH—COOH
$5'$ $6'$ 5 6
$3'$ $2'$ 3 2
$1'$ 1
NH$_2$

L-Thyroxine, Levothyroxine, 3,5,3′,5′-Tetraiodothyronine, T$_4$

HO—O—CH$_2$—CH—COOH
NH$_2$

Liothyronine
3,5,3′-Triiodothyronine, T$_3$

Effector cell:
receptor affinity

$$\frac{T_3}{T_4} = \frac{10}{1}$$

~ 90 µg/day   ~ 9 µg/day

Thyroxine | Triiodothyronine

Deiodinase

~ 25 µg/day

I$^-$

"reverse T$_3$"
3,3′,5′-Triiodothyronine

Deiodination coupling

I$^-$

Urine   Feces

Duration

2.   9. Day

T$_3$ T$_4$

10   20   30   40   Days

B. Endemic goiter and its treatment with thyroxine

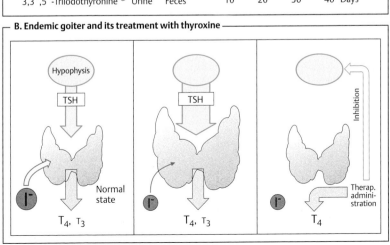

Hypophysis

TSH

I$^-$ Normal state

T$_4$, T$_3$

TSH

I$^-$

T$_4$, T$_3$

Inhibition

I$^-$

Therap. administration

T$_4$

☐ Hyperthyroidism and Antithyroid Drugs

Thyroid overactivity in Graves disease (**A**) results from formation of IgG antibodies that bind to and activate TSH receptors. Consequently, there is overproduction of hormone with cessation of TSH secretion. Graves disease can abate spontaneously after 1–2 years; therefore, initial therapy consists in reversible suppression of thyroid activity by means of antithyroid drugs. In other forms of hyperthyroidism, such as hormone-producing (morphologically benign) thyroid adenoma, the preferred therapeutic method is removal of tissue, either by surgery or by administration of iodine-131 (^{131}I) in sufficient dosage. Radioiodine is enriched in thyroid cells and destroys tissue within a sphere of a few millimeters by emitting β-particles (electrons) during its radioactive decay.

Antithyroid drugs inhibit thyroid function. Release of thyroid hormone (**C**) is preceded by a chain of events. A membrane Na^+/I^- symporter actively accumulates iodide in thyroid cells (the required energy comes from a Na^+/K^+-ATPase located in the basolateral membrane region); this is followed by oxidation to iodine, iodination of tyrosine residues in thyroglobulin, conjugation of two diiodotyrosine groups, and formation of T_4 moieties. These reactions are catalyzed by thyroid peroxidase, which is localized in the apical border of the follicular cell membrane. T_4-containing thyroglobulin is stored inside the thyroid follicles in the form of thyrocolloid. Upon endocytotic uptake, colloid undergoes lysosomal enzymatic hydrolysis, enabling thyroid hormone to be released as required. A "thyrostatic" effect can result from inhibition of synthesis or release. When synthesis is arrested, the antithyroid effect develops after a delay, as stored colloid continues to be utilized.

Antithyroid drugs for long-term therapy (C). **Thiourea-derivatives** (thioamides) inhibit peroxidase and, hence, hormone synthesis. To restore a euthyroid state, two therapeutic principles can be applied in Graves disease: (a) monotherapy with a thioamide, with gradual dose reduction as the disease abates; (b) administration of high doses of a thioamide, with concurrent administration of thyroxine to offset diminished hormone synthesis. Adverse effects of thioamides are rare, but the possibility of agranulocytosis has to be kept in mind.

Perchlorate, given orally as the sodium salt, inhibits the iodide pump. Adverse reactions include aplastic anemia. Compared with thioamides, its therapeutic importance is low.

Short-term thyroid suppression (C). Iodine in high dosage (> 6000 µg/day) exerts a transient "thyrostatic" effect in hyperthyroid, but usually not in euthyroid, individuals. Since release is also blocked, the effect develops more rapidly than does that of thioamides.

Clinical applications include preoperative suppression of thyroid secretion according to *Plummer* with *Lugol's* solution (5% iodine + 10% potassium iodide, 50–100 mg iodine/day for a maximum of 10 days). In thyrotoxic crisis, Lugol's solution is given together with thioamides and β-blockers. *Adverse effects*: allergies. *Contraindications*: iodine-induced thyrotoxicosis.

Lithium ions inhibit thyroxine release. Lithium salts can be used instead of iodine for rapid thyroid suppression in iodine-induced thyrotoxicosis. Regarding administration of lithium in manic-depressive illness, see p. 230.

A. Graves' disease

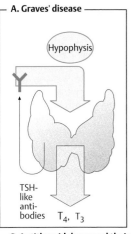

Hypophysis

TSH-like antibodies

T_4, T_3

B. Iodine hyperthyroidosis in endemic goiter

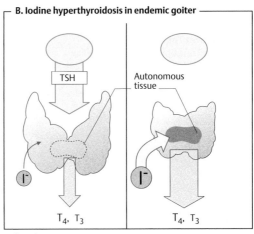

TSH

Autonomous tissue

I^-

T_4, T_3

I^-

T_4, T_3

C. Antithyroid drugs and their modes of action

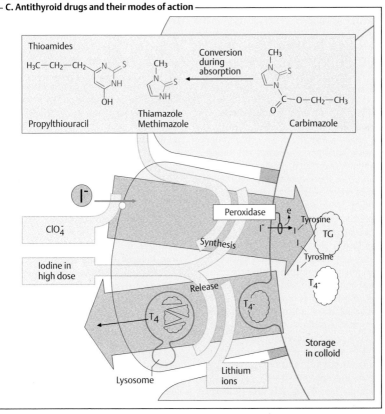

Thioamides

$H_3C-CH_2-CH_2$

Conversion during absorption

CH_3

Propylthiouracil

Thiamazole
Methimazole

Carbimazole

ClO_4^-

Peroxidase

Tyrosine

I^-

TG

Iodine in high dose

Synthesis

Tyrosine

T_4^-

Release

T_4

T_4^-

Storage in colloid

Lysosome

Lithium ions

□ Glucocorticoid Therapy

I. Replacement Therapy

The adrenal cortex (AC) produces the *glucocorticoid cortisol* (hydrocortisone) in the zona fasciculata and the *mineralocorticoid aldosterone* in the zona glomerulosa. Both steroid hormones are vitally important in adaptation responses to stress situations, such as disease, trauma, or surgery. Cortisol secretion is stimulated by hypophyseal ACTH; aldosterone secretion by angiotensin II in particular (p. 128). In AC failure (*primary adrenocortical insufficiency*; Addison disease), both *cortisol* and *aldosterone* must be replaced; when ACTH production is deficient (*secondary adrenocortical insufficiency*), *cortisol alone* needs to be replaced. Cortisol is effective when given orally (30 mg/day, 2/3 a.m., 1/3 p.m.). In stress situations, the dose is raised 5- to 10-fold. Aldosterone is poorly effective via the oral route; instead, the mineralocorticoid fludrocortisone (0.1 mg/day) is given.

II. Pharmacodynamic Therapy with Glucocorticoids (A)

In unphysiologically high concentrations, cortisol or other glucocorticoids suppress all phases (exudation, proliferation, scar formation) of the inflammatory reaction, i. e., the organism's defensive measures against foreign or noxious matter. This effect is mediated by multiple components, all of which involve alterations in gene transcription (p. 64) Thus, synthesis of the anti-inflammatory protein lipocortin (macrocortin) is stimulated. Lipocortin inhibits the enzyme phospholipase A_2. Consequently, release of arachidonic acid is diminished, along with the formation of inflammatory mediators of the prostaglandin and leukotriene series (pp. 196, 200). Conversely, glucocorticoids inhibit synthesis of several proteins that participate in the inflammatory process, including interleukins (p. 304) and other cytokines, phospholipase A_2 (p. 196), and cyclooxygenase-2 (p. 200). At very high dosage, non-genomic effects via membrane-bound receptors may also contribute.

Desired effects. As *antiallergics, immunosuppressants,* or *anti-inflammatory* drugs, glucocorticoids display excellent efficacy against "undesired" inflammatory reactions, such as allergy, rheumatoid arthritis, etc.

Unwanted effects. With *short-term use*, glucocorticoids are practically free of adverse effects, even at the highest dosage. **Long-term use** is likely to cause changes mimicking the signs of **Cushing syndrome** (endogenous overproduction of cortisol). Sequelae of the anti-inflammatory action are lowered resistance to infection and delayed wound healing. Sequelae of exaggerated glucocorticoid action are (a) increased gluconeogenesis and release of glucose, insulin-dependent conversion of glucose to triglycerides (adiposity mainly noticeable in the face, neck, and trunk), and "steroid-diabetes" if insulin release is insufficient; (b) increased protein catabolism with atrophy of skeletal musculature (thin extremities), osteoporosis, growth retardation in infants, and skin atrophy. Sequelae of the intrinsically weak, but now manifest, mineralocorticoid action of cortisol are salt and fluid retention, hypertension, edema; and KCl loss with danger of hypokalemia. Psychic changes, chiefly in the form of euphoric or manic mood swings, also need to be taken into account during chronic intake of glucocorticoids.

Measures for attenuating or preventing drug-induced Cushing syndrome. (**a**) *Use of cortisol derivatives with less* (e. g., prednisolone) or *negligible mineralocorticoid activity* (e. g., triamcinolone, dexamethasone). Glucocorticoid activity of these congeners is more pronounced. Glucocorticoid, anti-inflammatory, and feedback-inhibitory (p. 246) actions on the hypophysis are correlated. An exclusively anti-inflammatory congener does not exist. The "glucocorticoid"-related Cushinglike symptoms cannot be avoided. The table opposite lists relative

A. Glucocorticoids: principal and adverse effects

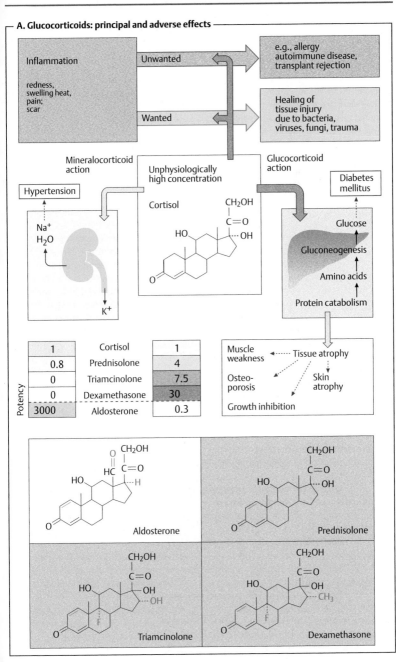

Potency		
1	Cortisol	1
0.8	Prednisolone	4
0	Triamcinolone	7.5
0	Dexamethasone	30
3000	Aldosterone	0.3

activity (potency) with reference to cortisol, whose mineralocorticoid and glucocorticoid activities are assigned a value of 1.0. All listed glucocorticoids are effective orally.

(**b**) *Local application.* This enables therapeutically effective concentrations to be built up at the site of application without a corresponding systemic exposure. Glucocorticoids that are subject to rapid biotransformation and inactivation following diffusion from the site of action are the preferred choice. Thus, inhalational administration employs glucocorticoids with a high presystemic elimination such as beclomethasone dipropionate, budesonide, flunisolide, or fluticasone propionate (p. 14). Adverse effects, however, also occur locally: e. g., with inhalational use, oropharyngeal candidiasis (thrush) and hoarseness; with cutaneous use, skin atrophy, striae, telangiectasias and steroid acne; and with ocular use, cataracts and increased intraocular pressure (glaucoma).

(**c**) *Lowest dosage possible.* For long-term medication, a just-sufficient dose should be given. However, in attempting to lower the dose to the minimally effective level, it is necessary to take into account that administration of exogenous glucocorticoids will suppress production of endogenous cortisol owing to activation of an inhibitory feedback mechanism. In this manner, a very low dose could be "buffered," so that unphysiologically high glucocorticoid activity and the anti-inflammatory effect are both prevented.

Effect of glucocorticoid administration on adrenocortical cortisol production (A). Release of cortisol depends on stimulation by hypophyseal ACTH, which in turn is controlled by hypothalamic corticotropin-releasing hormone (CRH). In both in the hypophysis and hypothalamus there are cortisol receptors through which cortisol can exert a feedback inhibition of ACTH or CRH release. By means of these cortisol "sensors," the regulatory centers can monitor whether the actual blood level of the hormone corresponds to the "set-point." If the blood level exceeds the set-point, ACTH output is decreased and thus also the cortisol production. In this way, cortisol level is maintained within the required range. The regulatory centers respond to synthetic glucocorticoids as they do to cortisol. Administration of exogenous cortisol or any other glucocorticoid reduces the amount of endogenous cortisol needed to maintain homeostasis. Release of CRH and ACTH declines ("inhibition of higher centers by exogenous glucocorticoid") and, hence, cortisol secretion ("adrenocortical suppression"). After weeks of exposure to unphysiologically high glucocorticoid doses, the cortisol-producing portions of the adrenal cortex shrink ("adrenocortical atrophy"). Aldosterone-synthesizing capacity remains unaffected, however. When glucocorticoid medication is suddenly withheld, the atrophic cortex is unable to produce sufficient cortisol and a potentially life-threatening cortisol deficiency may develop. Therefore, glucocorticoid therapy should always be tapered off by gradual reduction of the dosage.

Regimens for prevention of adrenocortical atrophy. Cortisol secretion is high in the early morning and low in the late evening (circadian rhythm). Accordingly, sensitivity to feedback inhibition must be high in the late evening.

(a) *Circadian administration*: The daily dose of glucocorticoid is given in the morning. Endogenous cortisol production will already have begun, the regulatory centers being relatively insensitive to inhibition. In the early morning hours of the next day, CRF/ACTH release and adrenocortical stimulation will resume.

(b) *Alternate day therapy*: Twice the daily dose is given on alternate mornings. On the "off" day, endogenous cortisol production is allowed to occur.

The disadvantage with either regimen is a recrudescence of disease symptoms during the glucocorticoid-free interval.

A. Cortisol release and its modification by glucocorticoids

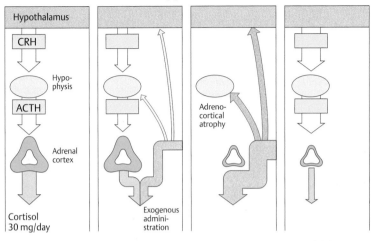

Hypothalamus			
CRH			
Hypo-physis		Adreno-cortical atrophy	
ACTH			
Adrenal cortex			
Cortisol 30 mg/day	Exogenous admini-stration		

Cortisol production under normal conditions

Decrease in cortisol production with cortisol dose < daily production

Cessation of cortisol production with cortisol dose > daily production

Cortisol deficiency after abrupt cessation of administration

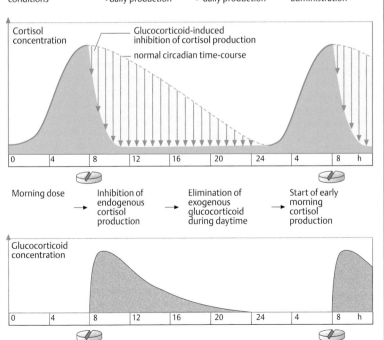

Cortisol concentration

Glucocorticoid-induced inhibition of cortisol production

normal circadian time-course

Morning dose → Inhibition of endogenous cortisol production → Elimination of exogenous glucocorticoid during daytime → Start of early morning cortisol production

Glucocorticoid concentration

□ Androgens, Anabolic Steroids, Antiandrogens

Androgens are masculinizing substances. The endogenous male gonadal hormone is the steroid **testosterone** from the interstitial Leydig cells of the testis. Testosterone secretion is stimulated by hypophyseal luteinizing hormone (LH), whose release is controlled by hypothalamic GnRH (gonadorelin, p. 238). Release of both hormones is subject to feedback inhibition by circulating testosterone. Reduction of testosterone to dihydrotestosterone occurs in most target organs (e. g., the prostate gland); the latter possesses higher affinity for androgen receptors. Rapid intrahepatic degradation (plasma $t_{1/2} \sim 15$ minutes) yields androsterone among other metabolites (17-ketosteroids) that are eliminated as conjugates in the urine. Because of rapid hepatic metabolism, testosterone is unsuitable for oral use. Although it is well absorbed, it undergoes virtually complete presystemic elimination.

Testosterone (T.) derivatives for clinical use. Because of its good tissue penetrability, testosterone is well suited for percutaneous administration in the form of a patch (transdermal delivery system, p. 18). *T. esters for i. m. depot injection are T. propionate* and *T. heptanoate* (or *enanthate*). These are given in oily solution by deep intramuscular injection. Upon diffusion of the ester from the depot, esterases quickly split off the acyl residue to yield free T. With increasing lipophilicity, esters will tend to remain in the depot, and the duration of action therefore lengthens. A *T. ester for oral use is the undecanoate.* Owing to the fatty acid nature of undecanoic acid, this ester is absorbed into the lymph, enabling it to bypass the liver and enter the general circulation via the thoracic duct. *17-α Methyltestosterone* is effective by the oral route owing to its increased metabolic stability, but because of the hepatotoxicity of C17-alkylated androgens (cholestasis, tumors) its use should be avoided.

Orally active *mesterolone* is 1-α-methyldihydrotestosterone.

Indication: for hormone replacement in deficiency of endogenous T. production.

Anabolics are testosterone derivatives (e. g., clostebol, metenolone, nandrolone, stanozolol) that are used in debilitated patients, and are misused by athletes, because of their protein anabolic effect. They act via stimulation of androgen receptors and, thus, also display androgenic actions (e. g., virilization in females, suppression of spermatogenesis).

Inhibitory Principles

GnRH superagonists (p. 238), such as buserelin, leuprolin, goserelin, and triptorelin, are used in patients with metastasizing prostate cancer to inhibit production of testosterone which promotes tumor growth. Following a transient stimulation, gonadotropin release subsides within a few days and testosterone levels fall as low as after surgical removal of the testes.

Androgen receptor antagonists. The antiandrogen *cyproterone* is a competitive antagonist of testosterone. By virtue of an additional progestin action, it decreases secretion of gonadotropins. *Indications:* in the male, dampening of sexual drive in hypersexuality, prostatic cancer; in the female, treatment of virilization phenomena, if necessary, with concomitant utilization of the gestagen contraceptive effect.

Flutamide and *bicalutamide* are structurally different androgen receptor antagonists lacking progestin activity.

Finasteride and **dutasteride** inhibit 5α-reductase, the enzyme responsible for converting T. to dihydrotestosterone (DHT). Thus, androgenic stimulation is reduced in those tissues where DHT is the active species (e. g., the prostate). T.-dependent tissues and functions are not or hardly affected: e. g., skeletal musculature, feedback inhibition of gonadotropin release, or libido. Both can be used in benign prostatic hyperplasia to shrink the gland and to improve micturition.

A. Testosterone

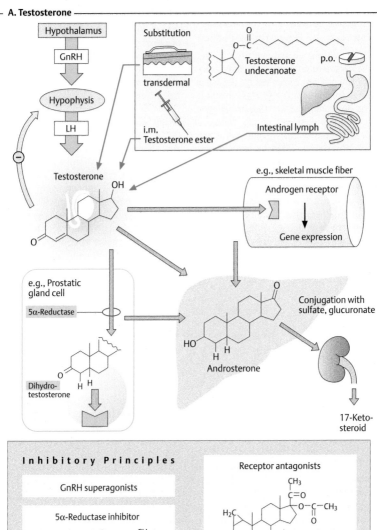

□ Follicular Growth and Ovulation, Estrogen and Progestin Production

Follicular maturation and ovulation, as well as the associated production of female gonadal hormones, are controlled by the hypophyseal gonadotropins FSH (follicle-stimulating hormone) and LH (luteinizing hormone). In the first half of the menstrual cycle, FSH promotes growth and maturation of ovarian tertiary follicles that respond with accelerating synthesis of estradiol. Estradiol stimulates endometrial growth and increases the permeability of cervical mucus for sperm cells. When the estradiol blood level approaches a predetermined set-point, FSH release is inhibited owing to feedback action on the anterior hypophysis. Since follicle growth and estrogen production are correlated, hypophysis and hypothalamus can "monitor" the follicular phase of the ovarian cycle through their estrogen receptors. Immediately prior to ovulation, when the nearly mature tertiary follicles are producing a high concentration of estradiol, the control loop switches to positive feedback. LH secretion transiently surges to peak levels and triggers ovulation. Within hours after ovulation, the tertiary follicle develops into the corpus luteum, which then also releases progesterone in response to LH. This initiates the secretory phase of the endometrial cycle and lowers the permeability of cervical mucus. Nonruptured follicles continue to release estradiol under the influence of FSH. After two weeks, production of progesterone and estradiol subsides, causing the secretory endometrial layer to be shed (menstruation).

The natural hormones are unsuitable for oral application because they are subject to presystemic hepatic elimination. Estradiol is converted via estrone to estriol; by conjugation, all three can be rendered water-soluble and amenable to renal excretion. The major metabolite of progesterone is pregnanediol, which is also conjugated and eliminated renally.

Estrogen preparations. Depot preparations for i.m. injection are oily solutions of esters of estradiol (3- or 17-OH group). The hydrophobicity of the acyl moiety determines the rate of absorption, hence the duration of effect. Released ester is hydrolyzed to yield free estradiol.

Orally used preparations. *Ethinylestradiol* (*EE*) is more stable metabolically, passes the liver after oral intake and mimics estradiol at estrogen receptors. *Mestranol* itself is inactive; however, cleavage of the C3 methoxy group again yields EE. In oral contraceptives, one of the two agents forms the estrogen component (p. 252). *(Sulfate-) Conjugated estrogens* (excretory products) can be extracted from equine urine and are used in the therapy of climacteric complaints. Their effectiveness is a matter of debate. Estradiol **transdermal delivery systems** are available.

Progestin preparations. Depot formulations for i.m. injection are *17-α-hydroxyprogesterone caproate* and *medroxyprogesterone acetate*. **Preparations for oral use** are derivatives of ethinyltestosterone = ethisterone (e. g., norethisterone, dimethisterone, lynestrenol, desogestrel, gestoden), or of 17α-hydroxyprogesterone acetate (e. g., chlormadinone acetate or cyproterone acetate).

Indications for estrogens and progestins include hormonal contraception (p. 252); hormone replacement, as in postmenopausal women for prophylaxis of osteoporosis; bleeding anomalies; menstrual and severe climacteric complaints.

Adverse effects. After long-term intake of estrogen/progestin preparations, increased risks have been reported for breast cancer, coronary heart disease, stroke, and thromboembolism. Although the incidence of bone fractures also decreases, the risk–benefit relationship is unfavorable. Concerning the adverse effects of oral contraceptives, see p. 252.

A. Estradiol, progesterone, and derivatives

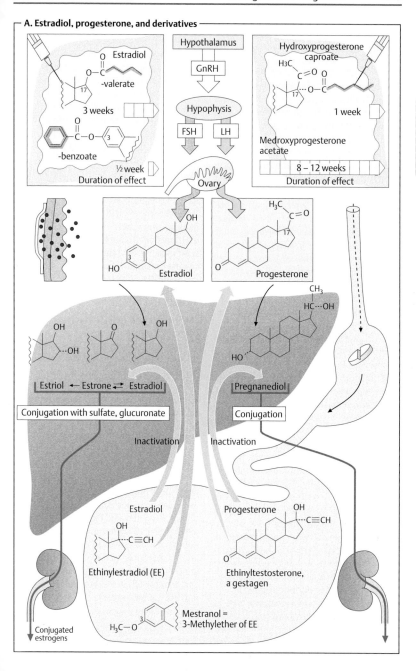

☐ Oral Contraceptives

Inhibitors of ovulation. Negative feedback control of gonadotropin release can be utilized to inhibit the ovarian cycle. **Administration of exogenous estrogens** (ethinylestradiol or mestranol) during the first half of the cycle permits **FSH production** to be suppressed (as it is by administration of progestins alone). Owing to the reduced FSH stimulation of tertiary follicles, **maturation of follicles and hence ovulation are prevented**. In effect, the regulatory brain centers are deceived, as it were, by the elevated estrogen blood level, which signals normal follicular growth and a decreased requirement for FSH stimulation. If estrogens alone are given during the first half of the cycle, endometrial and cervical responses, as well as other functional changes, will occur in the normal fashion. By adding a progestin (p. 250) during the second half of the cycle, the secretory phase of the endometrium and associated effects can be elicited. Discontinuance of hormone administration would be followed by menstruation.

The physiological time course of estrogen-progesterone release is simulated in the so-called **biphasic (sequential) preparations** (A). In **monophasic preparations**, estrogen and progestin are taken concurrently. Early administration of progestin reinforces the inhibition of CNS regulatory mechanisms, prevents both normal endometrial growth and conditions for ovum implantation, and decreases penetrability of cervical mucus to sperm cells. The two latter effects also act to prevent conception. According to the staging of progestin administration, one distinguishes (A): one-, two-, and three-stage preparations. Even with one-stage preparations, "withdrawal bleeding" occurs when hormone intake is discontinued (if necessary, by substituting dummy tablets).

Unwanted effects. An increased risk of thromboembolism is attributed to the estrogen component in particular but is also associated with certain progestins (gestoden and desogestrel). The risk of myocardial infarction, stroke, and benign liver tumors is elevated. Nonetheless, the absolute prevalence of these events is low. Predisposing factors (family history, cigarette smoking, obesity, and age) have to be taken into account. The overall risk of malignant tumors does not appear to be increased. In addition, hypertension, fluid retention, cholestasis, nausea, and chest pain, are reported.

Minipill. Continuous low-dose administration of progestin alone can prevent pregnancy. Ovulations are not suppressed regularly; the effect is then due to progestin-induced alterations in cervical and endometrial function. Because of the need for constant intake at the same time of day, a lower success rate, and relatively frequent bleeding anomalies, these preparations are now rarely employed.

"Morning-after" pill. This refers to administration of a high dose of estrogen and progestin, preferably within 12–24 hours, but no later than 72 hours after coitus. The mechanism of action is unclear.

Stimulation of ovulation. Gonadotropin secretion can be increased by *pulsatile delivery of GnRH* (p. 238). Regarding clomifene, see p. 254; whereas this substance can be given orally, the gonadotropins presented below must be given parenterally. HMG is human menopausal gonadotropin extracted from the urine of postmenopausal women. Owing to the cessation of ovarian function, gonadotropins show elevated blood levels and pass into urine in utilizable quantities. HMG (menotropins) consists of FSH and LH. HCG is human chorionic gonadotropin; it is obtained from the urine of pregnant women and acts like LH. Recombinant FSH (follitropin) and LH are available.

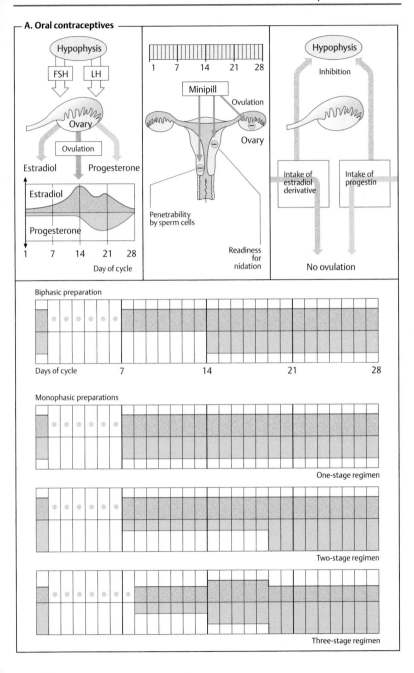

A. Oral contraceptives

Hypophysis

FSH LH

Ovary

Ovulation

Estradiol Progesterone

Estradiol

Progesterone

1 7 14 21 28

Day of cycle

1 7 14 21 28

Minipill

Ovulation

Ovary

Penetrability by sperm cells

Readiness for nidation

Hypophysis

Inhibition

Intake of estradiol derivative

Intake of progestin

No ovulation

Biphasic preparation

Days of cycle 7 14 21 28

Monophasic preparations

One-stage regimen

Two-stage regimen

Three-stage regimen

☐ Antiestrogen and Antiprogestin Active Principles

Selective estrogen receptor modulators (SERMs) (A). Estrogen receptors belong to the group of transcription-regulating receptors (p. 64). The female gonadal hormone estradiol is an agonist at these receptors. Several drugs are available that can produce estrogen-*antagonistic* effects. Interestingly, these are associated with estrogen-*agonistic* effects in certain tissues. A tentative explanation derives from the idea that each ligand induces a specific conformation of the estrogen receptor. The ligand–estrogen receptor complexes combine with co-activators or repressors at specified gene sequences. The pattern of co-regulators differs from tissue to tissue, allowing each SERM to generate a tissue-specific activity. It is of therapeutic significance that the patterns of estrogenic and antiestrogenic effects differ in a substance-specific manner among the drugs of this class.

It is useful to compare the activity profile of a SERM with that of estradiol, particularly in relation to effects seen postmenopausally. During chronic administration of estradiol, the risk of endometrial cancer rises; co-administration of a progestin prevents this effect. Breast cancers occur more frequently, likewise thromboembolic diseases. Estradiol effectively alleviates climacteric hot flashes and sweating. After chronic treatment it reduces the incidence of osteoporotic bone fractures by preventing the loss of an estrogen-dependent portion of bone mass. Nonetheless, estrogens can no longer be recommended for this purpose because of the unfavorable benefit–risk constellation (p. 330).

Clomifene is a stilbene derivative used orally for the therapy of female infertility. Owing to its antagonistic action at estrogen receptors in the adenohypophysis, feedback inhibition by estradiol of gonadotropin secretion is suppressed. The resulting increase in release of FSH induces augmented maturation of oocyte follicles. For instance, clomifene can be used for the treatment of luteal phase defects associated with disturbances of follicular maturation or the treatment of polycystic ovary syndrome. Since its use is confined to a few selected days during the ovarian cycle, chronic effects need not be considered.

Tamoxifen is a stilbene derivative that is used in metastasizing breast cancer to block the estrogenic stimulus for tumor cell growth. As a mixed estrogenic antagonist/partial agonist, tamoxifen promotes rather than ameliorates climacteric complaints; at the same time it displays agonistic features that are of concern as a potential risk factor when use of the drug for the prophylaxis of breast cancer is being considered.

Raloxifene is approved for use in the treatment and prophylaxis of osteoporosis. As shown in the table opposite, it has other beneficial as well as adverse effects.

The estrogen receptor antagonist **fulvestrant** is devoid of agonist activities and, given as a monthly injection may be used to delay progression of breast cancer. It causes downregulation and degradation of the estrogen receptor protein.

Progestin receptor antagonist (B). Approximately one week after conception, the embryo implants itself into the endometrium in the form of the blastocyst. By secreting human chorionic gonadotropin (HCG, mainly LH), the trophoblast maintains the corpus luteum and secretion of progesterone and thereby prevents menstrual bleeding. *Mifepristone* is an antagonist at progestin receptors and prevents maintenance of the endometrium during early pregnancy. Consequently, it acts as an abortifacient in early pregnancy. Its use has provoked medical debates (comparison of adverse reactions to mifepristone vs. surgical intervention) and aroused ethical-ideological conflicts.

A. Selective estrogen receptor modulators (SERM)

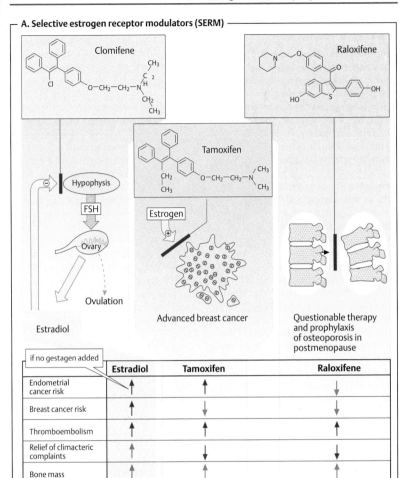

Clomifene

Raloxifene

Tamoxifen

Hypophysis

FSH

Ovary

Ovulation

Estradiol

Estrogen

Advanced breast cancer

Questionable therapy and prophylaxis of osteoporosis in postmenopause

if no gestagen added	Estradiol	Tamoxifen	Raloxifene
Endometrial cancer risk	↑	↑	↓
Breast cancer risk	↑	↓	↓
Thromboembolism	↑	↑	↑
Relief of climacteric complaints	↑	↓	↓
Bone mass	↑	↑	↑

B. Gestagen receptor antagonist

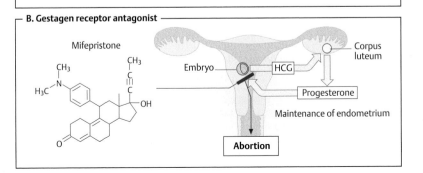

Mifepristone

Embryo

HCG

Corpus luteum

Progesterone

Maintenance of endometrium

Abortion

□ Aromatase Inhibitors

Aromatase inhibitors constitute an additional antiestrogenic principle that is based upon inhibition of estrogen formation. They are used chiefly in the *therapy of advanced breast cancer* when the tumor has become insensitive to estrogen and the patient has completed menopause. However, one agent in this class (anastrozole) was recently licensed for use in early breast cancer.

Aromatase. The enzyme converts androgens such as testosterone and androstenedione into the estrogens estradiol and estrone. This reaction involves cleavage of the methyl group at C10 and aromatization of ring A. Aromatase is a cytochrome P450-containing enzyme (isozyme CYP19). During the female *reproductive phase*, the major portion of circulating estrogens originates from the ovaries, where estradiol is synthesized in the granulosa cells of the maturing tertiary follicles. Theca cells surrounding the granulosa cells supply androgen precursors. FSH stimulates formation of estrogens by inducing the synthesis of aromatase in granulosa cells. An isoform of the enzyme 17β-hydroxysteroid dehydrogenase (17β-HSD 1) catalyzes the conversion of androstenedione to testosterone and of estrone to estradiol. After menopause, *ovarian function* ceases. However, estrogens do not disappear completely from the blood because they continue to enter the circulation from certain other tissues, in particular the subcutaneous adipose tissue, which produces estrone. In hormone-dependent breast cancers, tumor growth is thereby promoted. In addition, breast cancer cells themselves may be capable of producing estrogens via aromatase.

Aromatase inhibitors serve to eliminate extraovarian synthesis of estrogens in breast cancer patients. This can be achieved effectively only in postmenopause because, as an FSH-dependent enzyme, ovarian aromatase is subject to feedback regulation of female gonadal hormones. A drop in blood estradiol concentration would lead to increased release of FSH with a compensatory increase in synthesis of aromatase and estrogens.

Two groups of inhibitors can be distinguished on the basis of chemical structure and mechanism of action. *Steroidal inhibitors* (formestane, exemestane) attach to the androgen binding site on the enzyme and in the form of intermediary products give rise to an irreversible inhibition of the enzyme. *Nonsteroidal inhibitors* (anastrozole, letrozole) attach to a different binding site of the enzyme; via their triazole ring they interact reversibly with the heme iron of cytochrome P450.

Among the *adverse effects*, climacteric-like complaints predominate, reflecting the decline in estrogen levels. Unlike the SERMs, tamoxifen, which is used for the same indication, aromatase inhibitors do not promote endometrial growth and do not increase the risk of thromboembolic complications.

A. Aromatase inhibitors

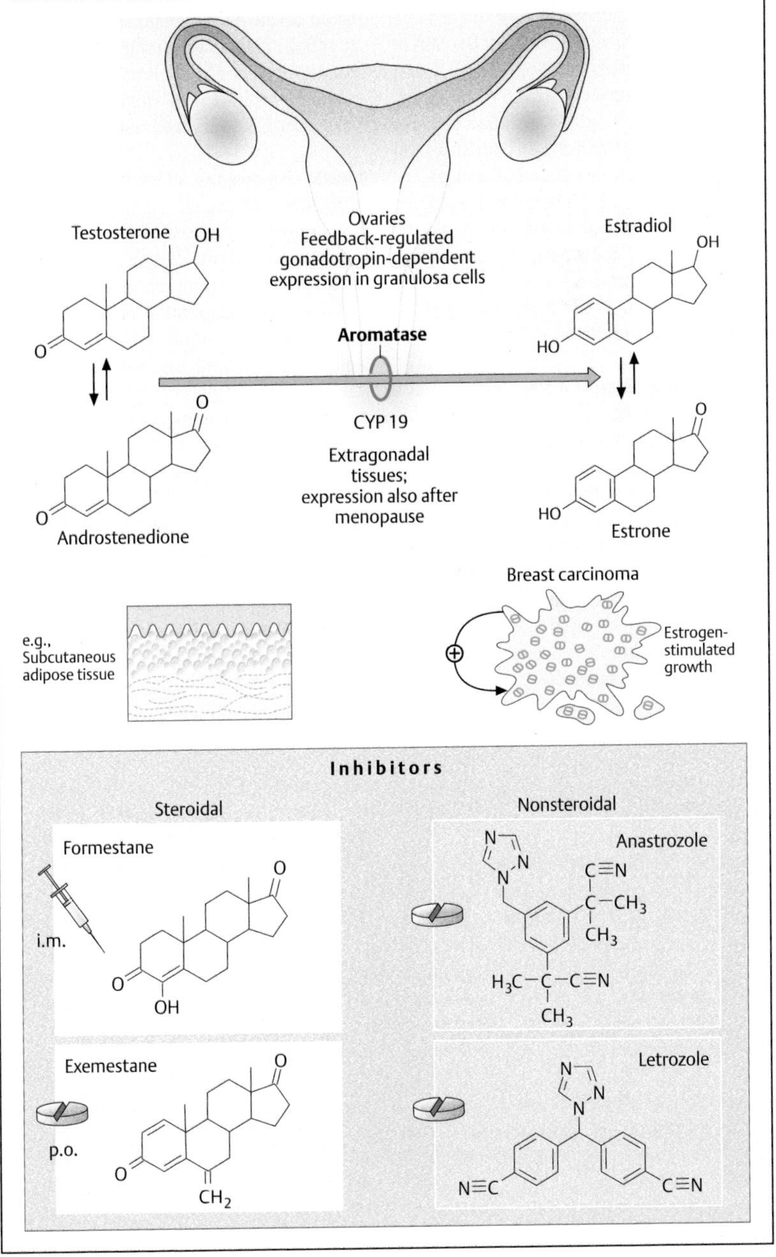

Testosterone

Ovaries
Feedback-regulated
gonadotropin-dependent
expression in granulosa cells

Estradiol

Aromatase

CYP 19

Extragonadal
tissues;
expression also after
menopause

Androstenedione

Estrone

Breast carcinoma

e.g.,
Subcutaneous
adipose tissue

Estrogen-
stimulated
growth

Inhibitors

Steroidal

Nonsteroidal

Formestane

i.m.

Anastrozole

$C \equiv N$

CH_3

CH_3

$H_3C - C - C \equiv N$

CH_3

OH

Exemestane

p.o.

Letrozole

CH_2

$N \equiv C$

$C \equiv N$

☐ Insulin Formulations

Insulin is synthesized in the B- (or β-) cells of the pancreatic islets of Langerhans. It is a protein (MW 5800) consisting of two peptide chains linked by two disulfide bridges; the A chain has 21 and the B chain 30 amino acids. Upon ingestion of carbohydrates, insulin is released into the blood and promotes uptake and utilization of glucose in specific organs, namely, the heart, adipose tissue, and skeletal muscle.

Insulin is used in the **replacement therapy** of **diabetes mellitus**.

Sources of therapeutic insulin preparations (A). *Porcine insulin* differs from human insulin by one B-chain amino acid. Owing to the slightness of this difference, its biological activity is similar to that of human hormone.

Human insulin is produced by two methods: biosynthetically from porcine insulin, by exchanging the wrong amino acid; or by gene technology involving synthesis in *E. coli* bacteria.

Recombinant insulin is produced to modify pharmacokinetic properties (see below). It is important in these insulin analogues that specificity for the insulin receptor is preserved (e.g., also toward the receptor for IGF-1 = somatomedin C, which promotes proliferation of cells; p. 238).

Control of delivery from injection site into blood (B). As a peptide, insulin is unsuitable for oral administration (owing to destruction by gastrointestinal proteases) and thus needs to be given parenterally. Usually, insulin preparations are injected subcutaneously. The duration of action depends on the rate of absorption from the injection site.

Variations in Dosage Form
Insulin solution. Dissolved insulin is dispensed as a clear neutral solution known as regular (R) insulin or crystalline zinc insulin. In emergencies, such as hyperglycemic coma,

it can be given intravenously (mostly by infusion because i.v. injections have too short an action; plasma $t_{\frac{1}{2}} \sim 9$ minutes). With the usual subcutaneous application, the effect is evident within 15–20 minutes, reaches a peak after ~3 hours, and lasts for ~6 hours.

Insulin suspensions. When it is injected as a suspension of insulin-containing particles, dissolution and release of the hormone in subcutaneous tissue is retarded (**extended-action insulins**). Suitable particles can be obtained by precipitation of apolar, poorly water-soluble complexes consisting of anionic insulin and cationic partners, e.g., the polycationic protein protamine. In the presence of zinc ions, insulin crystallizes; crystal size determines the rate of dissolution. Intermediate-acting insulin preparations (*NPH* or *isophane*; *Lente*) act for 18–26 hours, slow-acting preparations (*protamine zinc, ultralente*) for up to 36 hours.

Variation in Amino Acid Sequence
Rapidly acting insulin analogues. After injection of a regular insulin solution, insulin molecules exist at the injection site in the form of hexameric aggregates. Only after disintegration into monomers can rapid diffusion into the bloodstream occur. In *insulin lispro*, two amino acids are exchanged, resulting in a diminished propensity toward aggregate formation. Thus, diffusion from the injection site is faster, with rapid onset and short duration of action. *Insulin aspart* has similar properties. Fast-acting insulins are injected immediately before a meal, whereas regular insulin requires a 15–30 minute interval between injection and food intake.

Long-acting insulin analogues. The more extensive alteration of amino acids in *insulin glargine* changes the electric charge of the molecule. At pH 4 of the injectate, it is dissolved; however, at the pH of tissue it is poorly water-soluble and precipitates. Resolubilization and diffusion into the bloodstream take about one day.

A. Human insulin

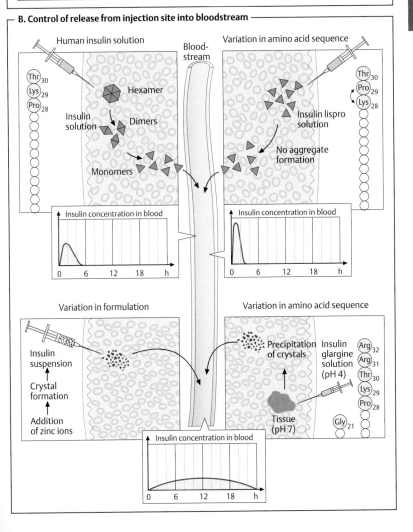

B. Control of release from injection site into bloodstream

□ Treatment of Insulin-dependent Diabetes Mellitus

Pathogenesis and complications (A). Type I diabetes mellitus typically manifests in childhood or adolescence (juvenile onset diabetes mellitus); it is caused by the destruction of insulin-producing B cells in the pancreas. A genetic predisposition together with a precipitating factor (viral infection) could start an autoimmune reaction against B-cells. Replacement of insulin (daily dose ~40 U, equivalent to ~1.6 mg) becomes necessary.

Therapeutic objectives. (1) prevention of life-threatening hyperglycemic (diabetic) coma; (2) prevention of diabetic sequelae arising from damage to small and large blood vessels, precise "titration" of the patient being essential to avoid even short-term spells of pathological hyperglycemia; (3) prevention of insulin overdosage leading to life-threatening hypoglycemic shock (CNS disturbance due to lack of glucose).

Therapeutic principles. In healthy subjects, the amount of insulin is "automatically" matched to carbohydrate intake, hence to blood glucose concentration. The critical secretory stimulus is the rise in plasma glucose level. Food intake and physical activity (increased glucose uptake into musculature, decreased insulin demand) are accompanied by corresponding changes in insulin secretion.

Methods of insulin replacement (B). In the diabetic, insulin can be administered as it is normally secreted. For instance, administration of a long-acting insulin in the late evening generates a basal level, whereas a fast acting insulin is used before meals. The dose needed is determined on the basis of the actual blood glucose concentration measured by the patient and the meal-dependent demand. This regimen (so-called *intensified insulin therapy*) provides the patient with much flexibility in planning daily activities. A well-educated, cooperative, and compe-

tent patient is a precondition. In other cases, a fixed-dosage schedule (*conventional insulin therapy*) will be needed, e.g., with morning and evening injections of a combination insulin (a mixture of regular insulin plus insulin suspension) in constant respective dosage (**A**). To avoid hypoglycemia or hyperglycemia, dietary carbohydrate (CH) intake must be synchronized with the time course of insulin absorption from the s.c. depot: diet control! Caloric intake is to be distributed (50% CH, 30% fat, 20% protein) in small meals over the day so as to achieve a steady CH supply—snacks, late night meal. Rapidly absorbable CH (sweets, cakes) must be avoided (hyperglycemic peaks) and replaced with slowly digestible ones.

Undesirable Effects
Hypoglycemia is heralded by warning signs: tachycardia, unrest, tremor, pallor, profuse sweating. Some of these are due to the release of glucose-mobilizing epinephrine. *Counter-measures:* glucose administration, rapidly absorbed CH orally (diabetics should always have a suitable preparation within reach) or 10–20 g glucose i.v. in case of unconsciousness; if necessary, injection of glucagon, the pancreatic hyperglycemic hormone.

Allergic reactions are rare; locally, redness may occur at the injection site and atrophy of adipose tissue; *lipodystrophy*). A possible local *lipohypertrophy* can be avoided by alternating injection sites.

Even with optimal control of blood sugar, s. c. administration of insulin cannot fully replicate the physiological situation. In healthy subjects, absorbed glucose and insulin released from the pancreas simultaneously reach the liver in high concentrations, whereby effective presystemic elimination of both substances is achieved. In the diabetic, s.c. injected insulin is uniformly distributed in the body. Since insulin concentration in blood supplying the liver cannot rise, less glucose is extracted from portal blood. A significant amount of glucose enters extrahepatic tissues, where it has to be utilized.

A. Diabetes mellitus type I: pathogenesis and complications

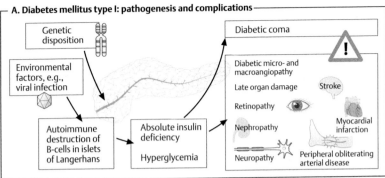

Genetic disposition

Environmental factors, e.g., viral infection

Autoimmune destruction of B-cells in islets of Langerhans

Absolute insulin deficiency

Hyperglycemia

Diabetic coma

Diabetic micro- and macroangiopathy

Late organ damage

Retinopathy

Nephropathy

Neuropathy

Stroke

Myocardial infarction

Peripheral obliterating arterial disease

B. Methods of insulin replacement

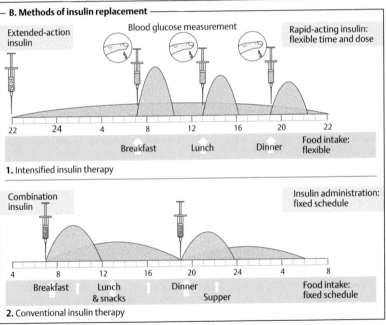

Extended-action insulin

Blood glucose measurement

Rapid-acting insulin: flexible time and dose

22 24 4 8 12 16 20 22

Breakfast   Lunch   Dinner   Food intake: flexible

1. Intensified insulin therapy

Combination insulin

Insulin administration: fixed schedule

4 8 12 16 20 24 4 8

Breakfast   Lunch & snacks   Dinner   Supper   Food intake: fixed schedule

2. Conventional insulin therapy

C. Presystemic and systemic insulin action in healthy and diabetic subjects

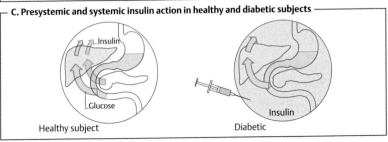

Insulin

Glucose

Healthy subject

Insulin

Diabetic

□ Treatment of Maturity-Onset (Type II) Diabetes Mellitus

In overweight adults, a diabetic metabolic condition may develop (type II or *non-insulin-dependent diabetes*) when there is a relative insulin deficiency—enhanced demand cannot be met by a diminishing insulin secretion.

The cause of **increased insulin requirement** is an **insulin resistance** of target organs. The decrease in the effectiveness of insulin is due to a reduction in the density of insulin receptors in target tissues and a decreased efficiency of signal transduction of insulin-receptor complexes. Conceivably, obesity with increased storage of triglycerides causes a decrease in insulin sensitivity of target organs. The loss in sensitivity can be compensated by enhancing insulin concentration. In panel (**A**), this situation is represented schematically by the decreased receptor density. In the obese patient, the maximum binding possible (plateau of curve) is displaced downward, indicative of the reduction in receptor numbers. At low insulin concentrations, correspondingly less binding of insulin occurs, compared with the control condition (normal weight). For a given metabolic effect (say, utilization of carbohydrates contained in a piece of cake), a certain number of receptors must be occupied. As shown by the binding curves (dashed lines), this can still be achieved with a reduced receptor number; although only at a higher concentration of insulin.

Development of adult diabetes (B). A subject with normal body weight (left) ingests a specified amount of carbohydrate; to maintain blood glucose concentration within the physiological range, the necessary amount of insulin is released into the blood. Compared with a normal subject, the overweight patient with insulin resistance requires a continually elevated output of insulin (orange curves) to avoid an excessive rise of blood glucose levels (green curves) during an equivalent carbohydrate load. When **the insulin secretory capacity of the pancreas decreases**, this is first noted as a rise in blood glucose during glucose loading (latent diabetes mellitus). As insulin secretory capacity declines further, not even the fasting blood level can be maintained (manifest, overt diabetes).

Treatment. Caloric restriction to restore body weight to normal is associated with an increase in insulin responsiveness, even before a normal weight is reached. Moreover, physical activity is important because it enhances peripheral utilization of glucose. When changes in lifestyle are insufficient in correcting the diabetic condition, therapy with oral antidiabetics is indicated (p. 264). **Therapy of first choice is weight reduction, not administration of drugs!**

A **metabolic syndrome** is said to be present when at least three of the following five risk factors can be identified in a patient:
1. Elevated blood glucose levels
2. Elevated blood lipid levels
3. Obesity
4. Lowered HDL levels
5. Hypertension

Overweight and resistance to insulin appear to play pivotal roles in the pathophysiological process. The resulting hyperinsulinemia induces a rise in systemic arterial blood pressure and probably also a hyperglyceridemia associated with an unfavorable LDL/HDL quotient. This combination of risk factors lowers life expectancy and calls for therapeutic intervention. The metabolic syndrome has a high prevalence; in industrialized countries, up to 20% of adults are believed to suffer from it.

A. Insulin concentration and binding in normal and overweight subjects

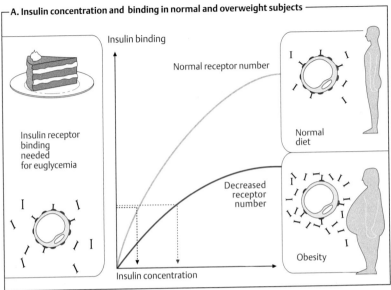

Insulin binding

Normal receptor number

Insulin receptor binding needed for euglycemia

Normal diet

Decreased receptor number

Obesity

Insulin concentration

B. Development of maturity-onset diabetes

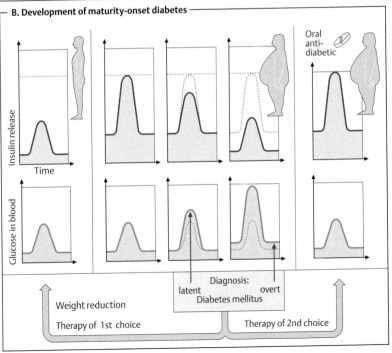

Oral anti-diabetic

Insulin release

Time

Glucose in blood

Diagnosis:
latent   overt
Diabetes mellitus

Weight reduction

Therapy of 1st choice

Therapy of 2nd choice

□ Oral Antidiabetics

In principle, the blood concentration of glucose represents a balance between influx into the bloodstream (chiefly from liver and intestines) and egress from blood into consuming tissues and organs. In (**A**), drugs available for lowering an elevated level of glucose are grouped schematically in relation to these two processes.

Metformin is a **biguanide derivative** that can normalize an elevated blood glucose level, provided that insulin is present. The mechanism underlying this effect is not completely understood. Decreased glucose release from the liver appears to play an essential part. Metformin does not increase release of insulin and therefore does not promote hyperinsulinemia. The risk of hypoglycemia is relatively less common. Triglyceride concentrations can decrease. Metformin has proved itself as a monotherapeutic in obese type II diabetics. It can be combined with other oral antidiabetics as well as insulin. Frequent adverse effects include anorexia, nausea, and diarrhea. Overproduction of lactic acid (lactate acidosis) is a rare, potentially fatal reaction. It is contraindicated in renal insufficiency and therefore should be avoided in elderly patients.

Oral antidiabetics of the *sulfonylurea* type increase the release of insulin from pancreatic B-cells. They inhibit *ATP-gated K⁺ channels* and thereby cause depolarization of the B-cell membrane. Normally, these channels are closed when intracellular levels of glucose, and hence of ATP, increase. This drug class includes tolbutamide (500–2000 mg/day) and glyburide (glibenclamide) (1.75–10.5 mg/day). In some patients, it is not possible to stimulate insulin secretion from the outset; in others, therapy fails later. Matching of dosage of the oral antidiabetic and caloric intake is necessary. Hypoglycemia is the most important unwanted effect. Enhancement of the hypoglycemic effect can result from drug interactions: displacement of antidiabetic drug from plasma protein binding sites, for example, by sulfonamides or acetylsalicylic acid.

Repaglinide possesses the same mechanism of action as the sulfonylureas but differs in chemical structure. After oral administration, the effect develops rapidly and fades away quickly. Therefore, repaglinide can be taken immediately before a meal.

"Glitazone" is an appellation referring to thiazolidinedione derivatives such as *rosiglitazone* and *pioglitazone*. These substances augment the insulin sensitivity of target tissues. They are agonists at the peroxisome proliferator-activated receptor of the γ subtype (PPARγ), a transcription-regulating receptor. As a result, they (a) promote the maturation of preadipocytes into adipocytes, (b) increase insulin sensitivity, and (c) enhance cellular glucose uptake. Besides fat tissue, skeletal muscle is also affected.

Rosiglitazone and pioglitazone are approved only for combination therapy when adequate glycemic control cannot be achieved with either metformin or a sulfonylurea alone. A combination with insulin is contraindicated. Adverse effects include weight gain and fluid retention (thus contraindication for any stage of congestive heart failure). Hepatic function requires close monitoring (withdrawal of troglitazone because of fatal liver failure).

Acarbose is an inhibitor of α-glucosidase (localized in the brush border of intestinal epithelium), which liberates glucose from disaccharides. It *retards* breakdown of carbohydrates, and hence absorption of glucose. Owing to increased fermentation of carbohydrates by gut bacteria, flatulence and diarrhea may develop. Miglitol has a similar effect but is absorbed from the intestine.

A. Oral antidiabetics

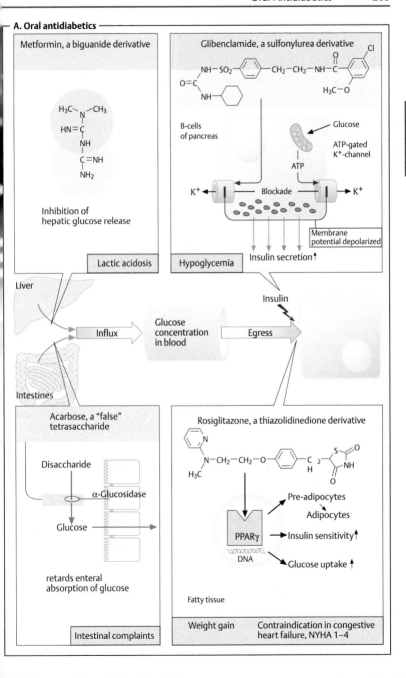

Metformin, a biguanide derivative

Inhibition of hepatic glucose release

Lactic acidosis

Glibenclamide, a sulfonylurea derivative

B-cells of pancreas

Glucose

ATP-gated K⁺-channel

ATP

K⁺ ← Blockade → K⁺

Membrane potential depolarized

Hypoglycemia

Insulin secretion↑

Liver

Insulin

Influx → Glucose concentration in blood → Egress

Intestines

Acarbose, a "false" tetrasaccharide

Disaccharide

α-Glucosidase

Glucose

retards enteral absorption of glucose

Intestinal complaints

Rosiglitazone, a thiazolidinedione derivative

Pre-adipocytes

Adipocytes

PPARγ → Insulin sensitivity↑

DNA

Glucose uptake ↑

Fatty tissue

Weight gain

Contraindication in congestive heart failure, NYHA 1–4

□ Drugs for Maintaining Calcium Homeostasis

At rest, the intracellular concentration of free calcium ions (Ca^{2+}) is kept at 0.1 μm (see p. 132 for mechanisms involved). During excitation, a transient rise of up to 10 μm elicits contraction in muscle cells (electromechanical coupling) and secretion in glandular cells (electrosecretory coupling). The cellular content of Ca^{2+} is in equilibrium with the extracellular Ca^{2+} concentration (~ 1000 μm), as is the plasma protein-bound fraction of calcium in blood. Ca^{2+} may crystallize with phosphate to form hydroxyapatite, the mineral of bone. Osteoclasts are phagocytes that mobilize Ca^{2+} by resorption of bone. Slight changes in extracellular Ca^{2+} concentration can alter organ function: thus, excitability of skeletal muscle increases markedly as Ca^{2+} is lowered (e. g., in hyperventilation tetany). Three hormones are available to the body for maintaining a constant extracellular Ca^{2+} concentration.

Vitamin D hormone is derived from *vitamin D* (*cholecalciferol*). Vitamin D can also be produced in the body; it is formed in the skin from dehydrocholesterol during irradiation with UV light. When there is lack of solar radiation, dietary intake becomes essential, cod liver oil being a rich source. Metabolically active vitamin D hormone results from two successive hydroxylations: in the liver at position 25 ($\rightarrow$calcifediol) and in the kidney at position 1 ($\rightarrow$calcitriol = vitamin D hormone). 1-Hydroxylation depends on the level of calcium homeostasis and is stimulated by parathormone and a fall in plasma levels of Ca^{2+} and phosphate. Vitamin D hormone promotes enteral absorption and renal reabsorption of Ca^{2+} and phosphate. As a result of the increased Ca^{2+} and phosphate concentration in blood, there is an increased tendency for these ions to be deposited in bone in the form of hydroxyapatite crystals. In vitamin D deficiency, bone mineralization is inadequate (rickets, osteomalacia). **Therapeutic use** aims at *replacement*. Mostly, vitamin D is given; in liver disease, calcifediol may be indicated, in renal disease, calcitriol. Effectiveness, as well as rate of onset and cessation of action increase in the order vitamin D < 25-OH-vitamin D < 1,25-di-OH vitamin D. **Overdosage** may induce hypercalcemia with deposits of calcium salts in tissues (particularly in kidney and blood vessels): calcinosis.

The polypeptide **parathormone** is released from the parathyroid glands when the plasma Ca^{2+} level falls. It *stimulates osteoclasts* to increase bone resorption; in the kidneys it promotes calcium reabsorption while phosphate excretion is enhanced. As blood phosphate concentration diminishes the tendency of Ca^{2+} to precipitate as bone mineral decreases. By stimulating the formation of vitamin D hormone, parathormone has an indirect effect on the enteral uptake of Ca^{2+} and phosphate. In parathormone deficiency, vitamin D can be used as a substitute that, unlike parathormone, is effective orally. *Teriparatide* is a recombinant shortened parathormone derivative containing the portion required for binding to the receptor. It can be used in the therapy of postmenopausal osteoporosis and promotes bone formation. While this effect seems paradoxical in comparison with hyperparathyroidism, it obviously arises from the special mode of administration: the once daily s.c. injection generates a quasi-pulsatile stimulation. Additionally, adequate intake of calcium and vitamin D must be ensured.

The polypeptide **calcitonin** is secreted by thyroid C-cells during imminent hypercalcemia. It lowers elevated plasma Ca^{2+} levels by *inhibiting osteoclast activity*. Its uses include hypercalcemia and osteoporosis. Remarkably, calcitonin injection may produce a sustained *analgesic* effect that alleviates pain associated with bone diseases (Paget disease, osteoporosis, neoplastic metastases) or Sudek syndrome.

Hypercalcemia can be treated by (1) administering 0.9% NaCl solution plus furosemide (if necessary) $\rightarrow$ renal excretion ↑; (2) the osteoclast inhibitors calcitonin and clodronate (a biphosphonate) $\rightarrow$ bone Ca mobilization↓; (3) glucocorticoids.

A. Calcium homeostasis of the body

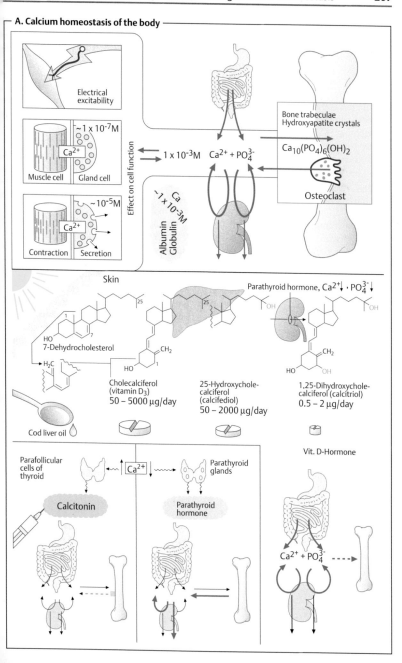

Electrical excitability

Muscle cell | Gland cell $\sim 1 \times 10^{-7}M$

Ca^{2+}

$1 \times 10^{-3}M \quad Ca^{2+} + PO_4^{3-}$

Contraction | Secretion $\sim 10^{-5}M$

Ca^{2+}

Effect on cell function

$\sim 1 \times 10^{-3}M$ Ca

Albumin Globulin

Bone trabeculae
Hydroxyapatite crystals

$Ca_{10}(PO_4)_6(OH)_2$

Osteoclast

Skin

Parathyroid hormone, $Ca^{2+}\downarrow$, $PO_4^{3-}\downarrow$

HO   7-Dehydrocholesterol

H_2C

Cholecalciferol
(vitamin D_3)
50 – 5000 μg/day

25-Hydroxychole-
calciferol
(calcifediol)
50 – 2000 μg/day

1,25-Dihydroxychole-
calciferol (calcitriol)
0.5 – 2 μg/day

Cod liver oil

Parafollicular
cells of
thyroid

$Ca^{2+}\downarrow$

Parathyroid
glands

Calcitonin

Parathyroid
hormone

Vit. D-Hormone

$Ca^{2+} + PO_4^{3-}$

□ Drugs for Treating Bacterial Infections

When bacteria overcome the cutaneous or mucosal barriers and penetrate into body tissues, a bacterial *infection* is present. Frequently the body succeeds in removing the invaders, without outward signs of disease, by mounting an immune response. However, certain pathogens have evolved a sophisticated counterstrategy. Although they are taken up into host cells via the regular phagocytotic pathway, they are able to forestall the subsequent fusion of the phagosome with a lysosome and in this manner can escape degradation. Since the wall of the sheltering vacuole is permeable to nutrients (amino acids, sugars), the germs are able to grow and multiply until the cell dies and the released pathogens can infect new host cells. This strategy is utilized, e.g., by *Chlamydia* and *Salmonella* species, *Mycobacterium tuberculosis*, *Legionella pneumophila*, *Toxoplasma gondii*, and *Leishmania* species. It is easy to see that targeted pharmacotherapy is especially difficult in such cases because the drug cannot reach the pathogen until it has surmounted first the cell membrane and then the vacuolar membrane. If bacteria multiply faster than the body's defenses can destroy them, *infectious disease* develops, with inflammatory signs, e.g., purulent wound infection or urinary tract infection. Appropriate treatment employs substances that injure bacteria and thereby prevent their further multiplication, without harming cells of the host organism (**1**).

Specific damage to bacteria is particularly feasible when a substance interferes with a metabolic process that occurs in bacterial but not in host cells. Clearly this applies to inhibitors of cell wall synthesis, since human or animal cells lack a cell wall. The **points of attack of antibacterial agents** are schematically illustrated in a grossly simplified bacterial cell, as depicted in (**2**).

In the following sections, plasmalemma-damaging polymyxins and tyrothricin are not considered further. Because of their poor tolerability, they are suitable only for topical use.

The effect of antibacterial drugs can be observed in vitro (**3**). Bacteria multiply in a growth medium under controlled conditions. If the medium contains an antibacterial drug, two results can be discerned: (a) bacteria are killed—**bactericidal effect**; or (b) bacteria survive, but do not multiply—**bacteriostatic effect**. Although variations may occur under therapeutic conditions, the different drugs can be classified according to their primary mode of action (color tone in **2** and **3**).

When bacterial growth remains unaffected by an antibacterial drug, bacterial **resistance** is present. This may occur because of certain metabolic characteristics that confer a natural insensitivity to the drug on a particular strain of bacteria (*natural resistance*). Depending on whether a drug affects only few or numerous types of bacteria, the terms **narrow-spectrum** (e.g., penicillin G) or **broad-spectrum** (e.g., tetracyclines) **antibiotic** are applied. Naturally susceptible bacterial strains can be transformed under the influence of antibacterial drugs into resistant ones (*acquired resistance*), when a random genetic alteration (mutation) gives rise to a resistant bacterium. Under the influence of the drug, the susceptible bacteria die off, whereas the mutant multiplies unimpeded. The more frequently a given drug is applied, the more probable the emergence of resistant strains (e.g., hospital strains with multiple resistance)!

Resistance can also be acquired when DNA responsible for nonsusceptibility (so-called *resistance plasmid*) is passed on from other resistant bacteria by conjugation or transduction.

A. Principles of antibacterial therapy

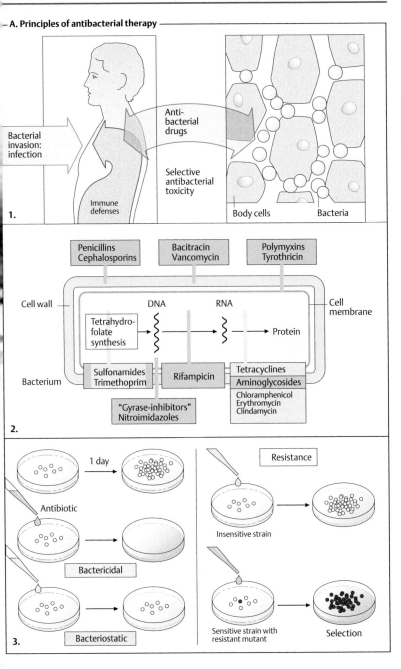

1.

Bacterial invasion: infection

Immune defenses

Anti-bacterial drugs

Selective antibacterial toxicity

Body cells   Bacteria

2.

Penicillins
Cephalosporins

Bacitracin
Vancomycin

Polymyxins
Tyrothricin

Cell wall

Cell membrane

DNA   RNA

Tetrahydro-folate synthesis → Protein

Sulfonamides
Trimethoprim

Rifampicin

Tetracyclines
Aminoglycosides

Chloramphenicol
Erythromycin
Clindamycin

Bacterium

"Gyrase-inhibitors"
Nitroimidazoles

3.

1 day

Antibiotic

Bactericidal

Bacteriostatic

Resistance

Insensitive strain

Sensitive strain with resistant mutant

Selection

□ Inhibitors of Cell Wall Synthesis

In most bacteria, a cell wall surrounds the cell like a rigid shell that protects against noxious outside influences and prevents rupture of the plasma membrane from a high internal osmotic pressure. The structural stability of the cell wall is due mainly to the **murein (peptidoglycan) lattice**. This consists of basic building blocks linked together to form a large macromolecule. Each basic unit contains the two linked aminosugars *N*-acetylglucosamine and *N*-acetylmuramic acid; the latter bears a peptide chain. The building blocks are synthesized in the bacterium, transported outward through the cell membrane, and assembled as illustrated schematically. The enzyme transpeptidase cross-links the peptide chains of adjacent aminosugar chains.

Inhibitors of cell wall synthesis are suitable antibacterial agents because animal, including human, cells lack a cell wall. These agents exert a **bactericidal** action on growing or multiplying germs. Members of this class include β-lactam antibiotics such as the *penicillins* and *cephalosporins*, in addition to *bacitracin* and *vancomycin*.

Penicillins (A). The parent substance of this group is **penicillin G (benzylpenicillin)**. It is obtained from cultures of mold fungi, originally from *Penicillium notatum*. Penicillin G contains the basic structure common to all penicillins, **6-aminopenicillanic acid** (6-APA; p. 273) comprising a thiazolidine and a 4-membered **β-lactam ring**. 6-APA itself lacks antibacterial activity. Penicillins disrupt cell wall synthesis by inhibiting **transpeptidase**. When bacteria are in their growth and replication phase, penicillins are bactericidal; as a result of cell wall defects, the bacteria swell and burst.

Penicillins are generally well tolerated; with penicillin G, the **daily dose** can range from approx. 0.6 g i.m. (= 10^6 international units, 1 Mega IU [MIU]) to 60 g by infusion. The most important **adverse effects** are due to *hypersensitivity* (incidence up to 5%), with manifestations ranging from skin eruptions to anaphylactic shock (in less than 0.05% of patients). Known penicillin allergy is a contraindication for these drugs. Because of an increased risk of sensitization, penicillins must not be used locally. *Neurotoxic effects*, mostly convulsions due to GABA antagonism, may occur if the brain is exposed to extremely high concentrations, e.g., after rapid i.v. injection of a large dose or intrathecal injection.

Penicillin G undergoes rapid renal **elimination** mainly in unchanged form (plasma $t_{1/2} \sim 0.5$ hours). The **duration of the effect** can be prolonged by:

1. *Use of higher doses,* enabling plasma levels to remain above the minimally effective antibacterial concentration.

2. *Combination with probenecid.* Renal elimination of penicillin occurs chiefly via the anion (acid)-secretory system of the proximal tubule (–COOH of 6-APA). The acid probenecid (p. 326) competes for this route and thus retards elimination of penicillin.

3. *Intramuscular administration in depot form.* In its anionic form (–COO⁻) penicillin G forms poorly water-soluble salts with substances containing a positively charged amino group (procaine; clemizole, an antihistaminic; benzathine, dicationic). Depending on the substance, release of penicillin from the depot occurs over a variable interval.

A. Penicillin G: structure and origin; mode of action of penicillins; methods for prolonging duration of action

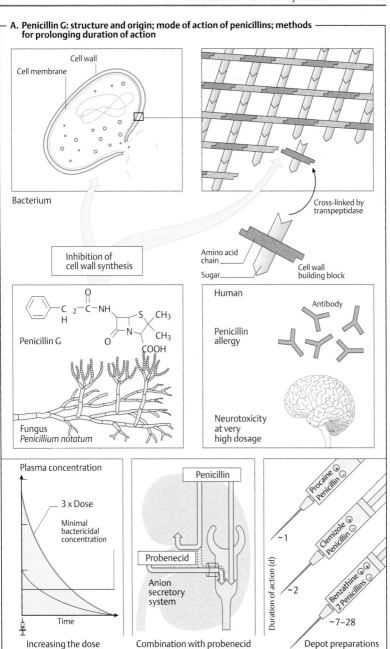

Cell membrane
Cell wall

Bacterium

Cross-linked by transpeptidase

Inhibition of cell wall synthesis

Amino acid chain
Sugar
Cell wall building block

Penicillin G

Fungus
Penicillium notatum

Human

Antibody

Penicillin allergy

Neurotoxicity at very high dosage

Plasma concentration

3 x Dose

Minimal bactericidal concentration

Time

Increasing the dose

Penicillin

Probenecid

Anion secretory system

Combination with probenecid

Procaine ⊕
Penicillin ⊖

Clemizole ⊕
Penicillin ⊖

Benzathine ⊕⊕
2 Penicillins ⊖⊖

Duration of action (d)

~1

~2

~7–28

Depot preparations

Although very well tolerated, **penicillin G** has **disadvantages** (**A**) that limit its therapeutic usefulness: (1) it is inactivated by gastric acid, which cleaves the β-lactam ring, necessitating parenteral administration. (2) The β-lactam ring can also be opened by bacterial enzymes (β-lactamases); in particular, penicillinase, which can be produced by staphylococcal strains, renders them resistant to penicillin G. (3) The antibacterial spectrum is narrow; although it encompasses many Gram-positive bacteria, Gram-negative cocci, and spirochetes, many Gram-negative pathogens are unaffected.

Derivatives with a different substituent on 6-APA possess **advantages** (**B**):

1. **Acid resistance** permits oral administration, provided that enteral absorption is possible. All derivatives shown in (**B**) can be given orally. *Penicillin V* (phenoxymethylpenicillin) exhibits antibacterial properties similar to those of penicillin G.

2. Owing to their **penicillinase resistance**, *isoxazolylpenicillins* (*oxacillin, dicloxacillin, floxacillin*) are suitable for the (oral) treatment of infections caused by penicillinase-producing staphylococci.

3. **Extended-activity spectrum:** The aminopenicillin *amoxicillin* is active against many Gram-negative organisms, e.g., colibacteria or *Salmonella typhi*. It can be protected from destruction by penicillinase by combination with inhibitors of penicillinase (*clavulanic acid, sulbactam, tazobactam*).

The structurally close congener *ampicillin* (no 4-hydroxy group) has a similar activity spectrum. However, because it is poorly absorbed (<50%) and therefore causes more extensive damage to the gut microbial flora (side effect: diarrhea), it should be given only by injection.

A still broader spectrum (including pseudomonad bacteria) is shown by *carboxypenicillins* (carbenicillin, ticarcillin) and acylaminopenicillins (mezclocillin, azlocillin, piperacillin). These substances are neither acid-stable nor penicillinase-resistant.

Cephalosporins (C). These β-lactam antibiotics are also fungal products and have bactericidal activity due to **inhibition of transpeptidase**. Their shared basic structure is 7-aminocephalosporanic acid, as exemplified by *cefalexin* (gray rectangle). Cephalosporins are acid-stable, but many are poorly absorbed. Because they must be given parenterally, most—including those with high activity—are used only in clinical settings. A few, e.g., cefalexin, are suitable for oral use. Cephalosporins are penicillinase-resistant but cephalosporinase-forming organisms do exist. However, some derivatives are also resistant to this β-lactamase. Cephalosporins are broad-spectrum antibacterials. Newer derivatives (e.g., cefotaxime, cefmenoxin, ceftriaxone, ceftazidime) are also effective against pathogens resistant to various other antibacterials. Cephalosporins are mostly well tolerated. All can cause allergic reactions, some also renal injury, alcohol intolerance, and bleeding (vitamin K antagonism).

Other inhibitors of cell wall synthesis. Bacitracin and vancomycin interfere with the transport of peptidoglycans through the cytoplasmic membrane and are only active against Gram-positive bacteria. **Bacitracin** is a polypeptide mixture; it is markedly nephrotoxic and is used only topically. **Vancomycin** is a glycopeptide and the drug of choice for the (oral) treatment of bowel inflammations occurring as a complication of antibiotic therapy (pseudomembranous enterocolitis caused by *Clostridium difficile*). It is not absorbed. Infections with Gram-positive cocci that are resistant against better tolerated drugs can also be treated with vancomycin given systemically. This entails an increased risk of ototoxicity (hearing loss, tinnitus) or vestibular toxicity (vertigo, ataxia, and nystagmus).

A. Disadvantages of penicillin G

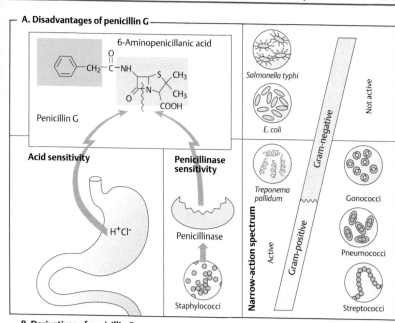

6-Aminopenicillanic acid

Penicillin G

Acid sensitivity

H⁺Cl⁻

Penicillinase sensitivity

Penicillinase

Staphylococci

Salmonella typhi

E. coli

Treponema pallidum

Gonococci

Pneumococci

Streptococci

Narrow-action spectrum

Gram-negative — Not active

Gram-positive — Active

B. Derivatives of penicillin G

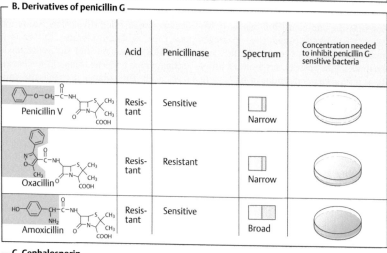

	Acid	Penicillinase	Spectrum	Concentration needed to inhibit penicillin G-sensitive bacteria
Penicillin V	Resistant	Sensitive	Narrow	
Oxacillin	Resistant	Resistant	Narrow	
Amoxicillin	Resistant	Sensitive	Broad	

C. Cephalosporin

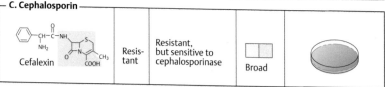

Cefalexin	Resistant	Resistant, but sensitive to cephalosporinase	Broad	

☐ Inhibitors of Tetrahydrofolate Synthesis

Tetrahydrofolic acid (THF) is a coenzyme in the synthesis of purine bases and thymidine. These are constituents of DNA and RNA and are required for cell growth and replication. Lack of THF leads to inhibition of cell proliferation. Formation of THF from dihydrofolate (DHF) is catalyzed by the enzyme dihydrofolate reductase. DHF is made from folic acid, a vitamin that cannot be synthesized in the body but must be taken up from exogenous sources. Most bacteria do not have a requirement for folate, because they are capable of synthesizing it—more precisely DHF—from precursors. Selective interference with bacterial biosynthesis of THF can be achieved with sulfonamides and trimethoprim.

Sulfonamides structurally resemble *p*-aminobenzoic acid (PABA), a precursor in bacterial DHF synthesis. As false substrates, sulfonamides competitively *inhibit* utilization of PABA, and hence *DHF synthesis*. Because most bacteria cannot take up exogenous folate, they are depleted of DHF. Sulfonamides thus possess *bacteriostatic activity* against a *broad spectrum* of pathogens. Sulfonamides are produced by chemical synthesis. The basic structure is shown in (**A**). Residue R determines the pharmacokinetic properties of a given sulfonamide. Most sulfonamides are well absorbed via the enteral route. They are metabolized to varying degrees and eliminated through the kidney. Rates of elimination, hence duration of effect, may vary widely. Some members are poorly absorbed from the gut and are thus suitable for the treatment of bacterial bowel infections. Adverse effects may include allergic reactions, sometimes with severe skin damage (p. 74), and displacement of other plasma protein-bound drugs or bilirubin in neonates (danger of kernicterus, hence contraindication for the last weeks of gestation and in the neonate). Because of the frequent emergence of resistant bacteria, sulfonamides are now rarely used. Introduced in 1935, they were the first broad-spectrum chemotherapeutics.

Trimethoprim inhibits bacterial DHF reductase, the human enzyme being significantly less sensitive than the bacterial one (rarely, bone marrow depression). A 2,4-diaminopyrimidine, trimethoprim has bacteriostatic activity against a broad spectrum of pathogens. It is used mostly as a component of co-trimoxazole.

Co-trimoxazole is a combination of *trimethoprim* and the sulfonamide *sulfomethoxazole*. Since THF synthesis is inhibited at two successive steps, the antibacterial effect of co-trimoxazole is better than that of the individual components. Resistant pathogens are infrequent; a bactericidal effect may occur. Adverse effects correspond to those of the components.

Sulfasalazine. Although originally developed as an antirheumatic agent (p. 332), sulfasalazine (salazosulfapyridine) is used mainly in the treatment of inflammatory bowel disease (ulcerative colitis and terminal ileitis or Crohn disease). Gut bacteria split this compound into the sulfonamide sulfapyridine and *mesalazine* (5-aminosalicylic acid). The latter is probably the antiinflammatory agent (inhibition of prostaglandin and leukotriene synthesis, of chemotactic signals for granulocytes, and of H_2O_2 formation in mucosa), but must be present on the gut mucosa in high concentrations. Coupling to the sulfonamide prevents premature absorption in upper small-bowel segments. The cleaved-off sulfonamide can be absorbed and may produce typical adverse effects (see above). Delayed release (prodrug) formulations of mesalazine without the sulfonamide moiety are available.

A. Inhibitors of tetrahydrofolate synthesis

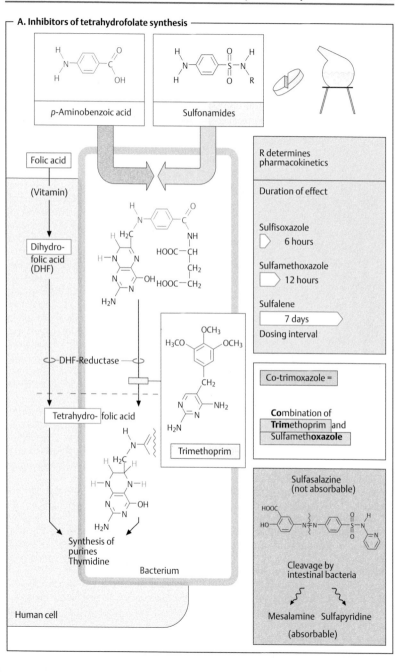

p-Aminobenzoic acid

Sulfonamides

Folic acid

(Vitamin)

Dihydro-folic acid (DHF)

DHF-Reductase

Tetrahydro-folic acid

Trimethoprim

Synthesis of purines
Thymidine

Bacterium

Human cell

R determines pharmacokinetics

Duration of effect

Sulfisoxazole
6 hours

Sulfamethoxazole
12 hours

Sulfalene
7 days
Dosing interval

Co-trimoxazole =

Combination of
Trimethoprim and
Sulfameth**oxazole**

Sulfasalazine
(not absorbable)

Cleavage by intestinal bacteria

Mesalamine   Sulfapyridine

(absorbable)

□ Inhibitors of DNA Function

Deoxyribonucleic acid (DNA) serves as a template for the synthesis of nucleic acids. Ribonucleic acid (RNA) executes protein synthesis and thus permits cell growth. Synthesis of new DNA is a prerequisite for cell division. Substances that inhibit reading of genetic information at the DNA template damage the regulatory center of cell metabolism. The substances listed below are useful as antibacterial drugs because they do not affect human cells.

Gyrase inhibitors. The enzyme gyrase (topoisomerase II) permits the orderly accommodation of a ~ 1000 μm long bacterial chromosome in a bacterial cell of ~ 1 μm. Within the chromosomal strand, double-stranded DNA has a double helical configuration. The former, in turn, is arranged in loops that are shortened by supercoiling. The gyrase catalyzes this operation, as illustrated, by opening, underwinding, and closing of the DNA double strand such that the full loop need not be rotated.

Derivatives of 4-quinolone-3-carboxylic acid (green portion of ofloxacin formula) are inhibitors of bacterial gyrases. They appear to prevent specifically the resealing of opened strands and thereby act bactericidally. These agents are absorbed after oral ingestion. The older drug *nalidixic acid* affects exclusively Gram-negative bacteria and attains effective concentrations only in urine; it is used as a urinary tract antiseptic. *Norfloxacin* has a broader spectrum. *Ofloxacin, ciprofloxacin, enoxacin,* and others, also yield systemically effective concentrations and are used for infections of internal organs.

Besides gastrointestinal problems and allergy, adverse effects particularly involve the CNS (confusion, hallucinations, and seizures). Since they can damage epiphyseal chondrocytes and joint cartilages in laboratory animals, gyrase inhibitors should not be used during pregnancy, lactation, and periods of growth. Tendon damage including rupture may occur in elderly or glucocorticoid-treated patients. In addition, hepatic damage, prolongation of the QT-interval with risk of arrhythmias, and phototoxicity have been observed.

Nitroimidazole derivatives, such as **metronidazole**, damage DNA by complex formation or strand breakage. This occurs in obligate anaerobic bacteria. Under these conditions, conversion to reactive metabolites that attack DNA takes place (e.g., the hydroxylamine shown). The effect is bactericidal. A similar mechanism is involved in the antiprotozoal action on *Trichomonas vaginalis* (causative agent of vaginitis and urethritis) and *Entamoeba histolytica* (causative agent of large-bowel inflammation, amebic dysentery, and hepatic abscesses). Metronidazole is well absorbed via the enteral route; it is also given i.v. or topically (vaginal insert). Because metronidazole is considered potentially mutagenic, carcinogenic, and teratogenic in humans, it should not be used for longer than 10 days, if possible, and should be avoided during pregnancy and lactation. *Timidazole* may be considered equivalent to metronidazole.

Rifampin (rifampicin) inhibits the bacterial enzyme that catalyses DNA template-directed RNA transcription, i.e., DNA-dependent RNA polymerase. Rifampin acts bactericidally against mycobacteria (*Mycobacterium tuberculosis, M. leprae*), as well as many Gram-positive and Gram-negative bacteria. It is well absorbed after oral ingestion. Because resistance may develop with frequent usage, it is restricted to the treatment of tuberculosis and leprosy (p. 282). Rifampin is contraindicated in the first trimester of gestation and during lactation.

Rifabutin resembles rifampin but may be effective in infections resistant to rifampin.

A. Antibacterial drugs acting on DNA

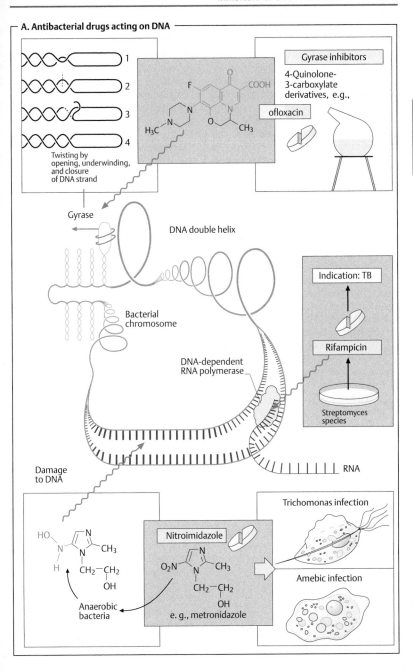

Twisting by opening, underwinding, and closure of DNA strand

Gyrase inhibitors

4-Quinolone-3-carboxylate derivatives, e.g.,

ofloxacin

Gyrase

DNA double helix

Bacterial chromosome

DNA-dependent RNA polymerase

Indication: TB

Rifampicin

Streptomyces species

RNA

Damage to DNA

Nitroimidazole

Trichomonas infection

Amebic infection

Anaerobic bacteria

e.g., metronidazole

□ Inhibitors of Protein Synthesis

Protein synthesis means translation into a peptide chain of a genetic message first transcribed into mRNA. Amino acid (AA) assembly occurs at the ribosome. Delivery of amino acids to mRNA involves different transfer RNA molecules (tRNA), each of which binds a specific AA. Each tRNA bears an "anticodon" nucleobase triplet that is complementary to a particular mRNA coding unit (*codon*, consisting of three nucleobases).

Incorporation of an AA normally involves the following steps (**A**):

1. The ribosome "focuses" two codons on mRNA; one (at the left) has bound its tRNA–AA complex, the AA having already been added to the peptide chain; the other (at the right) is ready to receive the next tRNA–AA complex.
2. After the latter attaches, the AAs of the two adjacent complexes are linked by the action of the enzyme peptide synthetase (peptidyltransferase). Concurrently, AA and tRNA of the left complex disengage.
3. The left tRNA dissociates from mRNA. The ribosome can advance along the mRNA strand and focus on the next codon.
4. Consequently, the right tRNA–AA complex shifts to the left, allowing the next complex to be bound at the right.

These individual steps are susceptible to inhibition by **antibiotics** of different groups. The examples shown originate primarily from *Streptomyces* species, some of the aminoglycosides also being derived from *Micromonospora* bacteria.[1]

1a. Tetracyclines inhibit the binding of tRNA–AA complexes. Their action is bacteriostatic and affects a broad spectrum of pathogens.

1b. Aminoglycosides induce the binding of "wrong" tRNA–AA complexes, resulting in synthesis of false proteins. Aminoglycosides are bactericidal. Their activity spectrum encompasses mainly Gram-negative organisms. Streptomycin and kanamycin are used predominantly in the treatment of tuberculosis.

2. Chloramphenicol inhibits peptide synthetase. It has bacteriostatic activity against a broad spectrum of pathogens. The chemically simple molecule is now produced synthetically.

3. Macrolides suppresses advancement of the ribosome. Their action is predominantly bacteriostatic and is directed mainly against Gram-positive organisms. Intracellular germs such as chlamydias and mycoplasms are also affected. Macrolides are effective orally. The prototype of this group is *erythromycin*. Among other uses, it is suitable as a substitute in allergy or resistance to penicillin. *Clarithromycin, roxithromycin* and *azithromycin* are erythromycin derivatives with similar activity; however, their elimination is slower and, therefore, permits reduction in dosage and less frequent administration. Gastrointestinal disturbances may occur. Because of inhibition of CYP isozymes (CYP3A4) the risk of drug interactions is present. *Telithromycin* is a semisynthetic macrolide with a modified structure ("ketolide"). It has a different pattern of resistance that is attributed to interaction with an additional ribosomal binding site.

Lincosamides. *Clindamycin* has antibacterial activity similar to that of erythromycin. It exerts a bacteriostatic effect mainly on Gram-positive aerobic, as well as on anaerobic pathogens. Clindamycin is a semisynthetic chloro analogue of lincomycin, which derives from a *Streptomyces* species. Taken orally, clindamycin is better absorbed than lincomycin, has greater antibacterial efficacy and is thus preferred. Both penetrate well into bone tissue.

---

[1] A note on spelling: the termination -*mycin* denotes origin from *Streptomyces* species; -*micin* (e. g., gentamicin) denotes origin from *Micromonospora* species.

A. Protein synthesis and modes of action of antibacterial drugs

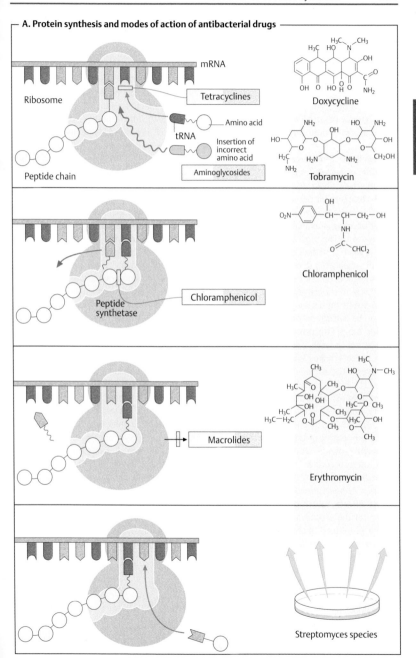

mRNA

Ribosome

Tetracyclines

Amino acid

tRNA

Insertion of incorrect amino acid

Aminoglycosides

Peptide chain

Doxycycline

Tobramycin

Chloramphenicol

Peptide synthetase

Chloramphenicol

Macrolides

Erythromycin

Streptomyces species

4. Oxazolidinones, such as *linezolide*, are a newly discovered drug group (p. 281). They inhibit initiation of synthesis of a new peptide strand at the point where ribosome, mRNA, and the "start-tRNA–AA" complex aggregate. Oxazolidinones exert a bacteriostatic effect on Gram-positive bacteria. Since bone marrow depression has been reported, hematological monitoring is necessary.

Tetracyclines are absorbed from the gastrointestinal tract to differing degrees, depending on the substance, absorption being nearly complete for *doxycycline* and *minocycline*. Intravenous injection is rarely needed (*rolitetracycline* is available only for i.v. administration). The most common unwanted effect is *gastrointestinal upset* (nausea, vomiting, diarrhea, etc.) due to (1) a direct mucosal irritant action of these substances and (2) damage to the natural bacterial gut flora (broad-spectrum antibiotics) allowing colonization by pathogenic organisms, including *Candida* fungi. Concurrent ingestion of antacids or milk would, however, be inappropriate because tetracyclines form insoluble *complexes* with *plurivalent cations* (e. g., Ca^{2+}, Mg^{2+}, Al^{3+}, $Fe^{2+/3+}$) resulting in their inactivation; that is, absorbability, antibacterial activity, and local irritant action are abolished. The ability to chelate Ca^{2+} accounts for the propensity of tetracyclines to accumulate in growing teeth and bones. As a result, there occurs an irreversible yellow-brown *discoloration of teeth* and a reversible *inhibition of bone growth.* Because of these adverse effects, tetracycline should not be given after the second month of pregnancy and not prescribed to children aged 8 years and under. Other adverse effects are increased *photosensitivity* of the skin and *hepatic damage*, mainly after i.v. administration.

Chloramphenicol. The broad-spectrum antibiotic chloramphenicol is completely absorbed after oral ingestion. It undergoes even distribution in the body and readily crosses diffusion barriers such as the blood–brain barrier. Despite these advantageous properties, use of chloramphenicol is only rarely indicated (e. g., in CNS infections) because of the danger of bone marrow damage. *Two types of bone marrow depression* can occur: (1) a dose-dependent, toxic, reversible form manifested during therapy, and (2) a frequently fatal form that may occur after a latency of weeks and is not dose-dependent. Owing to high tissue penetrability, the danger of bone marrow depression must be taken into account even after local use (e. g., eye drops).

Aminoglycoside antibiotics consist of glycoside-linked amino sugars (cf. gentamicin C_{1a}, a constituent of the gentamicin mixture). They contain numerous hydroxyl groups and amino groups that can bind protons. Hence, these compounds are highly polar, poorly membrane permeable and not absorbed enterally. *Neomycin* and *paromomycin* are given orally in order to eradicate intestinal bacteria (prior to bowel surgery or for reducing NH_3 formation by gut bacteria in hepatic coma). Aminoglycosides for the treatment of serious infections must be injected (e. g., *gentamicin, tobramycin, amikacin, netilmicin, sisomycin*). In addition, local inlays of a gentamicin-releasing carrier can be used in infections of bone or soft tissues. Aminoglycosides gain access to the bacterial interior via bacterial *transport systems.* In the kidney, they enter the cells of the proximal tubules via an uptake system for oligopeptides. Tubular cells are susceptible to damage (*nephrotoxicity*, mostly reversible). In the inner ear, sensory cells of the vestibular apparatus and Corti's organ may be injured (*ototoxicity*, in part irreversible).

A. Aspects of the therapeutic use of tetracyclines, chloramphenicol, and aminoglycosides

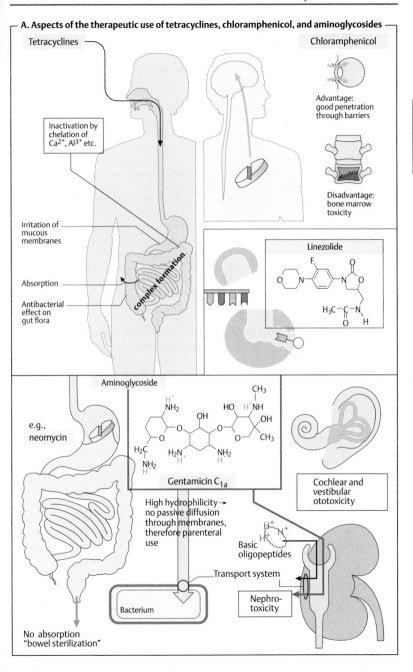

Tetracyclines

Chloramphenicol

Advantage: good penetration through barriers

Disadvantage: bone marrow toxicity

Inactivation by chelation of Ca^{2+}, Al^{3+} etc.

Irritation of mucous membranes

Absorption

Antibacterial effect on gut flora

complex formation

Linezolide

Aminoglycoside

e.g., neomycin

H_2C NH_2 H

Gentamicin C_{1a}

High hydrophilicity → no passive diffusion through membranes, therefore parenteral use

Cochlear and vestibular ototoxicity

Basic oligopeptides

Transport system

Bacterium

Nephro-toxicity

No absorption "bowel sterilization"

□ Drugs for Treating Mycobacterial Infections

In the past 100 years, advances in hygiene have led to a drastic decline in **tubercular** diseases in central Europe. Infection with *Mycobacterium tuberculosis* could be diagnosed increasingly earlier and in most cases be cured by a systematic long-term therapy (6–12 months) with effective chemotherapeutics. Worldwide, however, tuberculosis has remained one of the most threatening diseases. In developing countries, long-term combination therapy is scarcely realizable. Therapeutic success is thwarted by a lack of adequate (medical) infrastructure and financial resources, and insufficient compliance of patients; as a result, millions of persons die annually of tuberculosis infections. The insufficient treatment entails an additional bad consequence: more and more mycobacterial strains develop resistance and cannot be adequately treated. Patients suffering from immune deficiency are affected more severely by infections with *M. tuberculosis*.

Antitubercular drugs (1)

Drugs of choice are isoniazid, rifampin, and ethambutol, along with streptomycin and pyrazinamide. Less well tolerated, second-line agents include *p*-aminosalicylic acid, cycloserine, viomycin, kanamycin, amikacin, capreomycin, and ethionamide.

Isoniazid is bactericidal against growing *M. tuberculosis*. Its mechanism of action remains unclear. In the bacterium it is converted to isonicotinic acid, which is membrane impermeable and hence likely to accumulate intracellularly. Isoniazid is rapidly absorbed after oral administration. In the liver, it is inactivated by acetylation. Notable adverse effects are peripheral neuropathy, optic neuritis preventable by administration of vitamin B_6 (pyridoxine), and liver damage.

Rifampin. Source, antibacterial activity, and routes of administration are described on p. 276. Although mostly well tolerated, this drug may cause several adverse effects including hepatic damage, hypersensitivity with flulike symptoms, disconcerting but harmless red/orange discoloration of body fluids, and enzyme induction (failure of oral contraceptives). Concerning rifabutin, see p. 276.

Pyrazinamide exerts a bactericidal action by an unknown mechanism. It is given orally. Pyrazinamide may impair liver function; hyperuricemia results from inhibition of renal urate elimination.

Streptomycin must be given i.v. like other aminoglycoside antibiotics (p. 280). It damages the inner ear and the labyrinth. Its nephrotoxicity is comparatively minor

Ethambutol. The cause of ethambutol's specific antitubercular action is unknown. It is given orally. It is generally well tolerated, but may cause dose-dependent reversible disturbances of vision (red/green blindness, visual field defects).

Antileprotic drugs (2)

Rifampin is frequently given in combination with one or both of the following two agents.

Dapsone is a sulfone that, like sulfonamides, inhibits dihydrofolate synthesis (p. 274). It is bactericidal against susceptible strains of *M. leprae*. Dapsone is given orally. The most frequent adverse effect is methemoglobinemia with accelerated erythrocyte degradation (hemolysis).

Clofazimine is a dye with bactericidal activity against *M. leprae* and anti-inflammatory properties. It is given orally but is incompletely absorbed. Because of its high lipophilicity, it accumulates in adipose and other tissues and leaves the body only rather slowly ($t_{1/2}$ ~70 days). Red-brown skin pigmentation is an unwanted effect, particularly in fair-skinned patients.

A. Drugs used to treat infections with mycobacteria (1. tuberculosis, 2. leprosy)

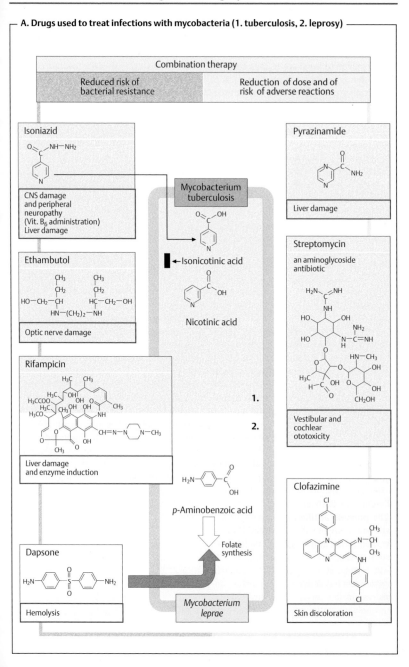

Combination therapy

Reduced risk of bacterial resistance

Reduction of dose and of risk of adverse reactions

Isoniazid

CNS damage and peripheral neuropathy (Vit. B₆ administration) Liver damage

Ethambutol

Optic nerve damage

Rifampicin

Liver damage and enzyme induction

Dapsone

Hemolysis

Mycobacterium tuberculosis

← Isonicotinic acid

Nicotinic acid

p-Aminobenzoic acid

Folate synthesis

Mycobacterium leprae

Pyrazinamide

Liver damage

Streptomycin

an aminoglycoside antibiotic

Vestibular and cochlear ototoxicity

Clofazimine

Skin discoloration

1.

2.

□ Drugs Used in the Treatment of Fungal Infections

Infections due to fungi are usually confined to the skin or mucous membranes: local or superficial mycosis. However, in immune deficiency states, internal organs may also be affected: systemic or deep mycosis.

Mycoses are most commonly due to *dermatophytes*, which affect the skin, hair, and nails following external infection, and to *Candida albicans*, a yeast organism normally found on body surfaces, which may cause infections of mucous membranes, less frequently of the skin or internal organs when natural defenses are impaired (immunosuppression, or damage of microflora by broad-spectrum antibiotics).

Imidazole derivatives inhibit synthesis of ergosterol, an integral constituent of cytoplasmic membranes of fungal cells. Fungi stop growing (fungistatic effect) or die (fungicidal effect). The spectrum of affected fungi is very broad. Because they are poorly absorbed and poorly tolerated systemically, most imidazoles are suitable only for topical use (*clotrimazole, econazole, oxiconazole* and other *azoles*). *Fluconazole* and *itroconazole* are newer orally effective **triazole** derivatives. Owing to its hydroxyl group, fluconazole is sufficiently water-soluble to allow formulation as an injectable solution. Both substances are slowly eliminated (plasma $t_{1/2}$ ~30 hours). The topically active **allyl amine** *naftidine* and the **morpholine** *amorolfine* also inhibit ergosterol synthesis, albeit at a different step. Both are for topical use.

The **polyene antibiotics** amphotericin B and nystatin are of bacterial origin. They insert themselves into fungal cell membranes (probably next to ergosterol molecules) and cause formation of hydrophilic channels. *Amphotericin B* is active against most organisms responsible for systemic mycoses. Because polyene antimycotics are nonabsorbable, it must be given by infusion, which is, however, poorly tolerated (chills, fever, CNS disturbances, impaired renal function, and phlebitis at the infusion site). Applied topically to skin or mucous membranes, amphotericin B is useful in the treatment of candidal mycosis. Because of the low rate of enteral absorption, oral administration in intestinal candidiasis can be considered a topical treatment. Likewise, *nystatin* is only used topically (e.g., oral cavity, gastrointestinal tract) against candidiasis.

Flucytosine is converted in candidal fungi to 5-fluorouracil by the action of a specific fungal cytosine deaminase. As an antimetabolite, this compound disrupts DNA and RNA synthesis (p. 300), resulting in a fungicidal effect. Given orally, flucytosine is rapidly absorbed. It is often combined with amphotericin B to allow dose reduction of the latter.

Caspofungin is a cyclic polypeptide that inhibits synthesis of the fungal cell wall. It can be used in systemic mycoses due to aspergillus fungi when amphotericin B or itroconazole cannot be employed. It is given by infusion and causes various adverse effects.

Griseofulvin originates from molds and has activity only against dermatophytes. It presumably acts as a spindle poison to inhibit fungal mitosis. Although targeted against local mycoses, griseofulvin must be used systemically. It is incorporated into newly-formed keratin. "Impregnated" in this manner, keratin becomes unsuitable as a fungal nutrient. The time required for the eradication of dermatophytes corresponds to the renewal period of skin, hair, or nails. Griseofulvin may cause uncharacteristic adverse effects. Because of its cumbersome application, this antimycotic is becoming obsolete.

A. Antifungal drugs

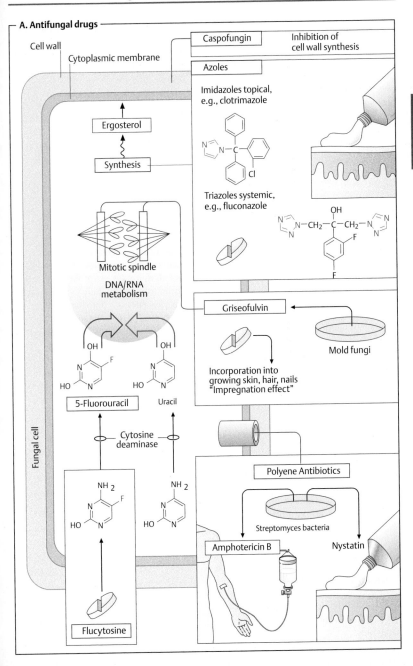

Cell wall

Cytoplasmic membrane

Caspofungin — Inhibition of cell wall synthesis

Azoles

Imidazoles topical, e.g., clotrimazole

Triazoles systemic, e.g., fluconazole

Ergosterol

Synthesis

Mitotic spindle

DNA/RNA metabolism

Griseofulvin

Mold fungi

Incorporation into growing skin, hair, nails "Impregnation effect"

5-Fluorouracil

Uracil

Cytosine deaminase

Polyene Antibiotics

Streptomyces bacteria

Amphotericin B

Nystatin

Fungal cell

Flucytosine

□ Chemotherapy of Viral Infections

Viruses essentially consist of genetic material (nucleic acids) and a capsular envelope made up of proteins, often with a coat of a phospholipid (PL) bilayer with embedded proteins. They lack a metabolic system and depend on the infected cell for their growth and replication. Targeted therapeutic suppression of viral replication requires selective inhibition of those metabolic processes that specifically serve viral replication in infected cells.

Viral replication as exemplified by _herpes simplex_ viruses (A).

1. The viral particle attaches to the host cell membrane (_adsorption_) via envelope glycoproteins that make contact with specific structures of the cell membrane.
2. The viral coat fuses with the plasmalemma of host cells and the nucleocapsid (nucleic acid plus capsule) enters the cell interior (_penetration_).
3. The capsule opens ("uncoating") near the nuclear pores and viral DNA moves into the cell nucleus. The genetic material of the virus can now direct the cell's metabolic system.
4a. _Nucleic acid synthesis_: The genetic material (DNA in this instance) is replicated and RNA is produced for the purpose of _protein synthesis._
4b. The proteins are used as "viral enzymes" catalyzing viral multiplication (e.g., DNA polymerase and thymidine kinase), as capsomers, or as coat components, or are incorporated into the host cell membrane.
5. Individual components are assembled into new virus particles (_maturation_).
6. Release of daughter viruses results in spread of virus inside and outside the organism.

With herpesviruses, replication entails host cell destruction and development of disease symptoms.

Antiviral mechanisms (A). The organism can disrupt viral replication with the aid of cytotoxic T-lymphocytes that recognize and destroy virus-producing cells (presenting viral proteins on their surface, p. 304) or by means of antibodies that bind to and inactivate extracellular virus particles. Vaccinations are designed to activate **specific immune defenses**.

Interferons (IFN) are glycoproteins that, among other products, are released from virus-infected cells. In neighboring cells, interferon stimulates the production of "antiviral proteins." These inhibit the synthesis of viral proteins by (preferential) destruction of viral DNA or by suppressing its translation. Interferons are not directed against a specific virus, but have a broad spectrum of antiviral action that is, however, species-specific. Thus, interferon for use in humans must be obtained from cells of human origin, such as leukocytes (IFN-α), fibroblasts (IFN-β), or lymphocytes (IFN-γ). Interferons are used in the treatment of certain viral diseases, as well as malignant neoplasias and autoimmune diseases; e.g., IFN-α for the treatment of chronic hepatitis C and hairy cell leukemia; and IFN-β in severe herpes virus infections and multiple sclerosis.

Virustatic antimetabolites are "false" DNA building blocks (**B**) or nucleosides. A nucleoside (e.g., thymidine) consists of a nucleobase (e.g., thymine) and the sugar deoxyribose. In antimetabolites, one of the components is defective. In the body, the abnormal nucleosides undergo bioactivation by attachment of three phosphate residues (p. 289).

Idoxuridine and congeners are incorporated into DNA with deleterious results. This also applies to the synthesis of human DNA. Therefore, idoxuridine and analogues are suitable only for topical use (e.g., in herpes simplex keratitis).

A. Virus multiplication and modes of action of antiviral agents

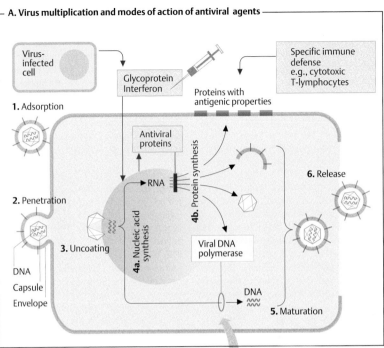

B. Chemical structure of virustatic antimetabolites

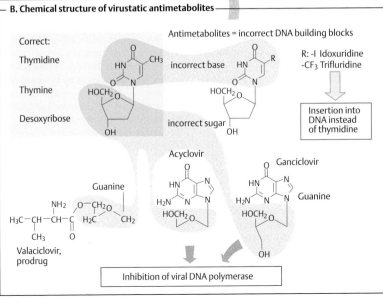

Among virustatic antimetabolites, **aciclovir** (**A**) has both specificity of the highest degree and optimal tolerability because it undergoes bioactivation only in infected cells, where it preferentially inhibits viral DNA synthesis. (1) A virally coded thymidine kinase (specific to herpes simplex and varicella-zoster viruses) performs the initial phosphorylation step; the remaining two phosphate residues are attached by cellular kinases. (2) The polar phosphate residues render aciclovir triphosphate membrane-impermeable and cause it to accumulate in infected cells. (3) Aciclovir triphosphate is a preferred substrate of viral DNA polymerase; it inhibits enzyme activity and, following its incorporation into viral DNA, induces strand breakage because it lacks the 3′-OH group of deoxyribose that is required for the attachment of additional nucleotides. The high therapeutic value of aciclovir is evident in severe infections with herpes simplex viruses (e.g., encephalitis, generalized infection) and varicella-zoster viruses (e.g., severe herpes zoster). In these cases, it can be given by i.v. infusion. Aciclovir may also be given orally despite its incomplete (15–30%) enteral absorption. In addition, it has topical uses. Because host DNA synthesis remains unaffected, adverse effects do not include bone marrow depression.

In **valaciclovir**, the hydroxyl group is esterified with the amino acid L-valine (p. 287**B**). This allows utilization of an enteral dipeptide transporter, leading to an enteral absorption rate almost double that of aciclovir. Subsequent cleavage of the valine residue yields aciclovir.

Famciclovir is an antiherpetic prodrug (active species *penciclovir*) with good oral bioavailability.

Ganciclovir (structure on p. 287**B**) is used in the treatment of severe infections with cytomegaly viruses (also belonging to the herpes group); these do not form thymidine kinase, phosphorylation being initiated by a different viral enzyme. Ganciclovir is less well tolerated and, not infrequently, produces leukopenia and thrombopenia. It is infused or administered orally as a valine ester (**valganciclovir**).

Foscarnet represents a diphosphate analogue. Incorporation of nucleotide into a DNA strand entails cleavage of a diphosphate residue. Foscarnet inhibits DNA polymerase by interacting with its binding site for the diphosphate group. *Indications:* systemic therapy in severe cytomegaly infections in AIDS patients; local therapy of herpes simplex infections.

Drugs against influenza viruses (C). *Amantadine* specifically affects the replication of influenza A (RNA) viruses, the causative agents of true influenza. These viruses are endocytosed into the cell. Release of viral RNA requires protons from the acidic content of endosomes to penetrate into the virus. Amantadine blocks a channel protein in the viral coat that permits influx of protons. Thus, "uncoating" is prevented. The drug is used for prophylaxis and, hence, must be taken before the outbreak of symptoms. It is also an antiparkinsonian drug (p. 188).

Neuraminidase inhibitors prevent the release of influenza A and B viruses. Normally, the viral neuraminidase splits off *N*-acetylneuraminic (sialic) acid residues on the cellular surface coat, thereby enabling newly formed viral particles to be detached from the host cell. *Zanamivir* is given by inhalation; *oseltamivir* is suitable for oral administration because it is an ester prodrug. Possible uses include treatment and prophylaxis of influenza virus infections.

A. Activation of acyclovir and inhibition of viral DNA synthesis

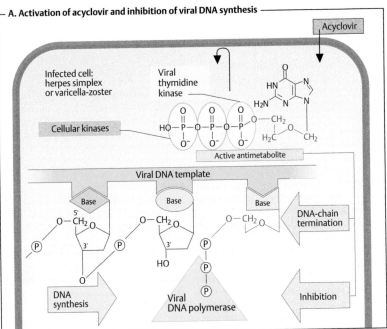

Acyclovir

Infected cell: herpes simplex or varicella-zoster

Viral thymidine kinase

Cellular kinases

Active antimetabolite

Viral DNA template

Base

Base

Base

DNA-chain termination

DNA synthesis

Viral DNA polymerase

Inhibition

B. Inhibitor of DNA-polymerase: Foscarnet

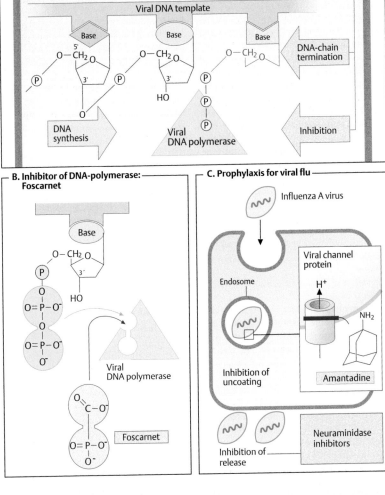

Base

Viral DNA polymerase

Foscarnet

C. Prophylaxis for viral flu

Influenza A virus

Viral channel protein

Endosome

H⁺

Amantadine

Inhibition of uncoating

Neuraminidase inhibitors

Inhibition of release

□ Drugs for the Treatment of AIDS

Replication of the human immunodeficiency virus (HIV), the causative agent of AIDS, is susceptible to targeted interventions because it entails several obligatory steps in virus-specific metabolism (**A**). First, the virus docks at the CD4 complex of T-helper lymphocytes by means of a glycoprotein in the viral coat (p. 304). A fusion protein is then extruded from the viral coat, by which fusion of the latter and the cell membrane is initiated. Next, viral RNA is transcribed into DNA, a step catalyzed by viral "reverse transcriptase." Double-stranded DNA is incorporated into the host genome with the help of viral integrase. Under control by viral DNA, viral replication can then be initiated, with synthesis of viral RNA and proteins (including enzymes such as reverse transcriptase and integrase, and structural proteins such as the matrix protein lining the inside of the viral envelope). These proteins are not assembled individually but in the form of *polyproteins*. An N-terminal fatty acid (myristoyl) residue promotes their attachment to the interior face of the plasmalemma. As the virus particle buds off the host cell, it carries with it the affected membrane area as its envelope. During this process, a protease contained within the polyprotein cleaves the latter into individual functionally active proteins.

I. Inhibitors of Reverse Transcriptase—Nucleoside Agents

Representatives of this group include **zidovudine**, **stavudine**, **zalcitabine**, **didanosine**, and **lamivudine**. They are nucleosides containing an abnormal sugar moiety and require bioactivation by phosphorylation (cf. zidovudine in **A**). As triphosphates, they inhibit reverse transcriptase and cause strand breakage following incorporation into viral DNA. The substances are administered orally. In part, they differ in their spectrum of adverse effects (e.g., leukopenia with zidovudine; peripheral neuropathy and pancreatitis with the others) and in the mechanisms

responsible for development of resistance. AIDS therapy mostly employs combinations of two members of this group plus either a nonnucleoside inhibitor (see below) or one to two protease inhibitors (see below).

Nonnucleoside Inhibitors

Nevirapine and **efavirenz** are active inhibitors of reverse transcriptase, that is, they do not require phosphorylation. Adverse reactions include rashes and interactions involving cytochrome P450 isozymes (CYP).

II. HIV protease Inhibitors

Inhibitors of viral protease prevent cleavage of inactive precursor proteins, and hence viral maturation. They are administered orally.

Saquinavir could be considered an abnormal peptide. Its bioavailability is low. **Ritonavir**, **indinavir**, **nelfinavir**, and **amprenavir** are other protease inhibitors that in part exhibit markedly higher bioavailability. Biotransformation of these drugs involves CYP enzymes and is therefore subject to interaction with various other drugs metabolized via this route. Prolonged administration may be associated with a peculiar redistribution of adipose tissue and metabolic disturbances (hyperlipidemia, insulin resistance, hyperglycemia).

III. Fusion Inhibitors

Enfuvirtide is a peptide that binds to the viral fusion protein in such a manner as to prevent the necessary change in conformation. It is a reserve drug.

A. AIDS drugs

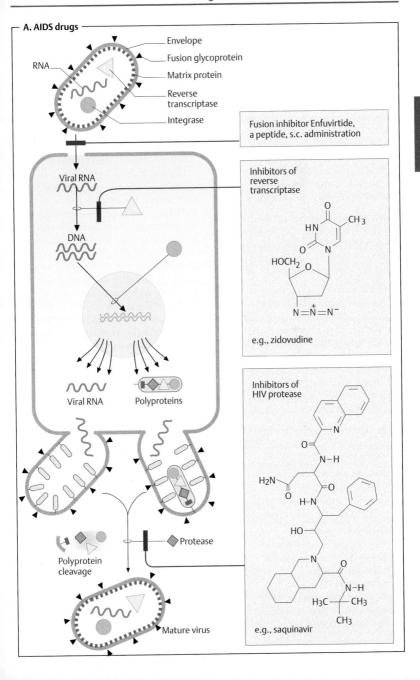

Envelope
Fusion glycoprotein
Matrix protein
RNA
Reverse transcriptase
Integrase

Fusion inhibitor Enfuvirtide, a peptide, s.c. administration

Viral RNA

DNA

Viral RNA   Polyproteins

Inhibitors of reverse transcriptase

e.g., zidovudine

Polyprotein cleavage   Protease

Mature virus

Inhibitors of HIV protease

e.g., saquinavir

□ Drugs for Treating Endoparasitic and Ectoparasitic Infestations

Adverse hygienic conditions favor human infestation with multicellular organisms (referred to here as parasites). Skin and hair are colonization sites for arthropod ectoparasites, such as insects (lice, fleas) and arachnids (mites). Against these, insecticidal and arachnicidal agents, respectively, can be used. Endoparasites invade the intestines or even internal organs and are mostly members of the phyla of flatworms and roundworms. They are combated with anthelmintics.

Antihelmintics. As shown in the table, the newer agents, *praziquantel* and *mebendazole*, are adequate for the treatment of diverse worm diseases. They are generally well tolerated, as are the other agents listed.

Insecticides. Whereas fleas can be effectively dealt with by disinfection of clothes and living quarters, lice and mites require the topical application of insecticides to the infested subject. The following agents act mainly by interfering with the activation or inactivation of neural voltage-gated insect sodium channels.

Chlorphenothane (DDT) kills insects after absorption of a very low amount, e. g., via foot contact with sprayed surfaces (contact insecticide). The cause of death is nervous system damage and seizures. In humans DDT causes acute neurotoxicity only after absorption of very large amounts. DDT is chemically stable and is degraded in the environment and the body at extremely slow rates. As a highly lipophilic substance, it accumulates in fat tissues. Widespread use of DDT in pest control has led to its accumulation in food chains to alarming levels. For this reason its use has now been banned in many countries.

Lindane is the active γ-isomer of hexachlorocyclohexane. It also exerts a neurotoxic action on insects (as well as humans). Irritation of skin or mucous membranes may occur after topical use. Lindane is active also against intradermal mites (*Sarcoptes scabiei*, causative agent of scabies), besides lice and fleas. Although it is more readily degraded than DDT, it should be used only as a second-line agent with appropriate precautions. In the United Kingdom its use for head lice has been banned; in the United States it is not recommended in young children and is contraindicated in premature infants.

Permethrin, a synthetic pyrethroid, exhibits similar antiectoparasitic activity and may be the drug of choice owing to its slower cutaneous absorption, fast hydrolytic inactivation, and rapid renal elimination.

Therapy of Worm Infestations	
Worms (helminths)	**Anthelminthic Drug of Choice**
Flatworms (platyhelminths)	
Tape worms (cestodes)	Praziquantel[a] or niclosamide
Flukes (trematodes),	Praziquantel
e. g., *Schistosoma* species (bilharziasis)	
Roundworms (nematodes)	
Pinworm (*Enterobius vermicularis*)	Mebendazole or pyrantel pamoate
Whipworm (*Trichuris trichiura*)	Mebendazole
Ascaris lumbricoides	Mebendazole or pyrantel pamoate
Trichinella spiralis[b]	Mebendazole and thiabendazole
Strongyloides stercoralis	Thiabendazole
Hookworms (*Necator americanus*, *Ancylostoma duodenale*)	Mebendazole or pyrantel pamoate

[a] Not for ocular or spinal cord cysticercosis.

[b] Thiabendazole in intestinal phase; mebendazole in tissue phase.

A. Endoparasites and ectoparasites: therapeutic agents

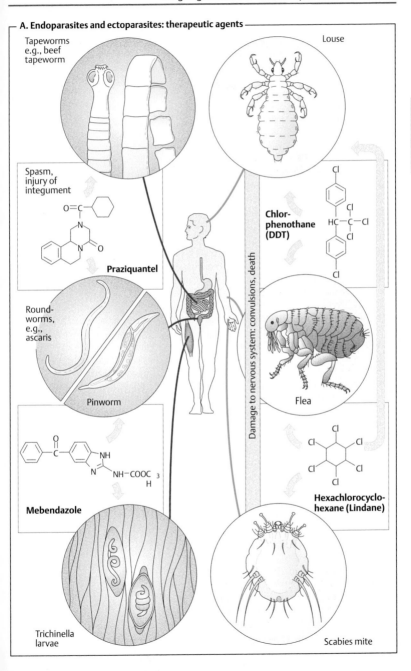

Tapeworms e.g., beef tapeworm

Louse

Spasm, injury of integument

O=C

Praziquantel

Chlor-phenothane (DDT)

Round-worms, e.g., ascaris

Pinworm

Flea

HC—C—Cl
Cl

Mebendazole

NH—COOC₃H

Hexachlorocyclo-hexane (Lindane)

Damage to nervous system: convulsions, death

Trichinella larvae

Scabies mite

□ Antimalarials

The causative agents of malaria are plasmodia, unicellular organisms (Order Hemosporidia, Class Protozoa). The infective form, the sporozoite, is inoculated into skin capillaries when infected female *Anopheles* mosquitoes (**A**) suck blood from humans. The sporozoites invade liver parenchymal cells, where they develop into primary tissue schizonts. These give rise to numerous merozoites that enter the blood. The preerythrocytic stage is asymptomatic. In blood, the parasite enters erythrocytes (erythrocytic stage), where it again multiplies by schizogony, resulting in the formation of more merozoites. Rupture of the infected erythrocytes releases the merozoites and pyrogens. A fever attack ensues and more erythrocytes are infected. The generation period for the next crop of merozoites determines the interval between fever attacks. With *Plasmodium vivax* and *P. ovale,* there can be a parallel multiplication in the liver (paraerythrocytic stage). Moreover, some sporozoites may become dormant in the liver as "hypnozoites" before entering schizogony.

Different **antimalarials** selectively kill the parasite's different developmental forms. The mechanism of action is known for some agents: *Chloroquine* and *quinine* accumulate within the acidic vacuoles of blood schizonts and inhibit polymerization of heme released from digested hemoglobin, free heme being toxic for the schizonts. *Pyrimethamine* inhibits protozoal dihydrofolate reductase (p. 274), as does *chlorguanide* (*proguanil*) via its active metabolite cycloguanil. The sulfonamide *sulfadoxine* inhibits synthesis of dihydrofolic acid (p. 274). Dihydrofolate reductase is also blocked by cycloguanil, the active form of *proguanil. Atoquavone* suppresses synthesis of pyrimidine bases, probably by interfering with mitochondrial electron transport. *Artemesinin derivatives* (artemether, artesunate) originate from the East Asian plant Qinghaosu (*Artemisia* sp.) Its antischizontal effect appears to involve a re-action between heme iron and the epoxide group of these compounds.

Antimalarial drug choice takes tolerability and plasmodial resistance into account.

Tolerability. The oldest antimalarial, quinine, has the smallest therapeutic margin. All newer agents are rather well tolerated.

Plasmodium falciparum, responsible for the most dangerous form of malaria, is particularly prone to develop **drug resistance**. The prevalence of resistant strains rises with increasing frequency of drug use. Resistance has been reported for chloroquine and also the combination pyrimethamine/sulfadoxine.

Drug choice for antimalarial chemoprophylaxis. In areas with a risk of malaria, continuous intake of antimalarials affords the best protection against the disease, though not against infection. Primaquine would be effective against primary tissue schizonts of all plasmodial species; however, it is not used for long-term prophylaxis because of unsatisfactory tolerability and the risk of plasmodial resistance. Instead, prophylactic regimens employ agents against blood schizonts. Depending on the presence of resistant strains, use can be made of chloroquine, and/or proguanil, mefloquine, the tetracycline doxycycline, as well as the combination of atoquavone and proguanil.

These drugs do not prevent the (symptom-free) hepatic infection but only the disease-causing infection of erythrocytes ("suppression therapy"). On a person's return from an endemic malaria region, a two-week course of primaquine is adequate for eradication of the late hepatic stages (*P. vivax* and *P. ovale*).

Protection from mosquito bites (with nets, skin-covering clothes, etc.) is a very important prophylactic measure.

Therapy. Antimalarial therapy employs the same agents, in addition to the combinations of artemether plus lumefantrine or pyrimethamine plus sulfadoxine.

A. Malaria: stages of the plasmodial life cycle in the human: therapeutic options

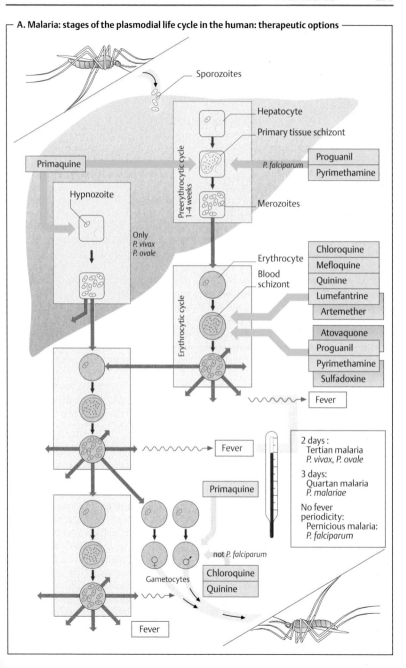

□ Other Tropical Diseases

In addition to malaria, other tropical diseases and their treatment will be considered for the following reasons. (1) Owing to the tremendous growth in global travel, inhabitants of temperate climatic zones have become exposed to the hazard of infection with tropical disease pathogens. (2) The spread of some tropical diseases is of unimaginable dimensions, with humans victims numbering in the millions. The pharmacotherapeutic possibilities known to date will be presented.

Amebiasis. The causative agent, *Entamoeba histolytica*, lives and multiplies in the colon (symptom: diarrhea), its cyst form residing also in the liver among other sites. In tropical regions, up to half the population can be infested, transmission occurring by the fecal–oral route. The most effective **treatment** against both intestinal infestation and systemic disease is administration of metronidazole. If monotherapy fails, combination therapy with chloroquine, emetine or tetracyclines may be indicated.

Leishmaniasis. The causative agents are flagellated protozoa that are transmitted by sand flies to humans. The parasites are taken up into phagocytes, where they remain in phagolysosomes and multiply until the cell dies and the parasites can infect new cells. **Symptoms:** A visceral form, known as *kala-azar*, and cutaneous or mucocutaneous forms exist (**A**). An estimated 12 million humans are affected. **Therapy** is difficult; pentavalent antimonial compounds, such as stibogluconate, must be given for extended periods. Adverse effects are pronounced.

Trypanosomiasis. The pathogens, *Trypanosoma brucei* (sleeping sickness) and *T. cruzi* (Chagas disease), are flagellated protozoa. *T. brucei* (**C**) is transmitted by the tsetse fly, distributed in West and East Africa. An initial stage (swelling of lymph nodes, malaise, hepatosplenomegaly, among others) is followed by invasion of the CNS with lethargy, extrapyramidal motor disturbances, Parkinson-like signs, coma, and death. **Therapy:** Long-term suramine i.v. or pentamidine (less effective); arsenicals (e.g., melarsoprol, highly toxic), when the CNS is involved. *T. cruzi* is confined to Central and South America and transmitted by blood-sucking reduviid bugs. These parasites preferentially infiltrate the cardiac musculature, where they cause damage to muscle fibers and the specialized conducting tissue. Death results from cardiac failure. **Therapy:** unsatisfactory.

Schistosomiasis (bilharziasis) (see also p. 292). The causative organisms are trematodes with a complex life cycle that need (aquatic) snails as intermediate hosts. Free-swimming larval cercariae penetrate the intact skin of humans. The adult worms (*Schistosoma mansoni*, **D**) live in the venous vasculature. **Occurrence:** tropical countries rich in aquatic habitats. About 200 million humans are afflicted. **Therapy:** praziquantel, 10–40 mg/kg, single dose, is highly effective with minimal adverse effects. Substances released from decaying worms may cause problems.

Filariasis. In its microform, *Wuchereria bancrofti* is transmitted by mosquitoes; the adult parasites live in the lymph system and cause inflammations and blockage of lymph drainage leading to elephantiasis in extreme cases (**B**). **Therapy:** diethylcarbamazepine for several weeks; adverse reactions are chiefly due to products from disintegrating worms.

Onchocerciasis ("River Blindness"). The causative organism is *Onchocerca volvulus*, a filaria transmitted by black flies (genus *Simulium*). The adult parasites (several centimeters long) form tangles and proliferating nodules (onchocercomas) in the skin and have a particular propensity for invading the eyeball, resulting in blindness. About 20 million people inhabiting banks of fast-flowing rivers are afflicted with river blindness. **Therapy:** ivermectin (0.15 mg/kg, single dose); adverse reactions are in part caused by disintegrating worms.

A. Cutaneous leishmaniasis
   Causative agent: *Leishmania major*

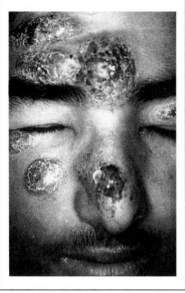

B. Elephantiasis
   Causative agent: *Wuchereria bancrofti*

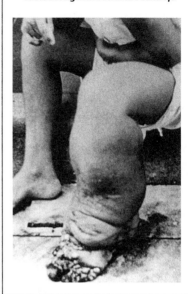

C. *Trypanosoma brucei*
   Causative agent of sleeping sickness

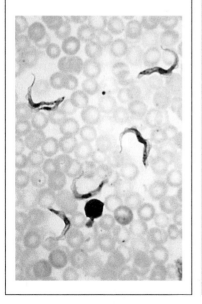

D. *Schistosoma mansoni*
   Causative agent of bilharziasis

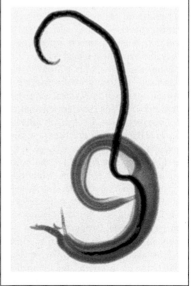

□ Chemotherapy of Malignant Tumors

A tumor (neoplasm) consists of cells that proliferate independently of the body's inherent "building plan." A malignant tumor (cancer) is present when the tumor tissue destructively invades healthy surrounding tissue or when dislodged tumor cells form secondary tumors (metastases) in other organs. A cure requires the elimination of all malignant cells (curative therapy). When this is not possible, attempts can be made to slow tumor growth and thereby prolong the patient's life or improve quality of life (palliative therapy). Chemotherapy is faced with the problem that the malignant cells are endogenous and almost lacking in specific metabolic properties.

Cytostatics (A) are cytotoxic substances that particularly affect proliferating or dividing (mitotic) cells. Rapidly dividing malignant cells are preferentially injured. Damage to mitotic processes not only retards tumor growth but also may initiate *apoptosis* (programmed cell death). Tissues with a low mitosis rate are largely unaffected; likewise, most healthy tissues. This, however, also applies to malignant tumors consisting of slowly dividing differentiated cells.

Tissues that have a physiologically high mitosis rate are bound to be affected by cytostatic therapy. Thus, **typical adverse effects** occur. *Loss of hair* results from injury to hair follicles; *gastrointestinal disturbances*, such as diarrhea, from inadequate replacement of enterocytes whose lifespan is limited to a few days; *nausea and vomiting* from stimulation of area postrema chemoreceptors (p. 342); and *lowered resistance to infection* from weakening of the immune system (p. 304). In addition, cytostatics cause *bone marrow depression*. Resupply of blood cells depends on the mitotic activity of bone marrow stem and daughter cells. When myeloid proliferation is arrested, the short-lived granulocytes are the first to be affected (neu-

tropenia), then blood platelets (thrombopenia) and, finally, the more long-lived erythrocytes (anemia). *Infertility* is caused by suppression of spermatogenesis or follicle maturation. Most cytostatics disrupt DNA metabolism. This entails the risk of a potential genomic alteration in healthy cells (*mutagenic* effect). Conceivably, the latter accounts for the occurrence of leukemias several years after cytostatic therapy (*carcinogenic* effect). Furthermore, congenital malformations are to be expected when cytostatics must be used during pregnancy (*teratogenic* effect).

Cytostatics possess different **mechanisms of action**.

Damage to the mitotic spindle (B). The contractile proteins of the spindle apparatus must draw apart the replicated chromosomes before the cell can divide. This process is prevented by the so-called *spindle poisons* (see also colchicine, p. 326) that arrest mitosis at metaphase by disrupting the assembly into spindle threads of microtubuli. These consist of the proteins α-and β-tubulin. Surplus tubuli are broken down, enabling the tubulin subunits to be recycled.

The vinca alkaloids, *vincristine* and *vinblastine* (from the periwinkle plant, *Vinca rosea*), inhibit the polymerization of tubulin subunits into microtubuli. Damage to the nervous system is a predicted adverse effect arising from injury to microtubule-operated axonal transport mechanisms.

Paclitaxel, from the bark of the pacific yew (*Taxus brevifolia*), inhibits disassembly of microtubules and induces formation of atypical ones, and thus impedes the reassemblage of tubulins into properly functioning microtubules. *Docetaxel* is a semisynthetic derivative.

A. Chemotherapy of tumors: principal and adverse effects

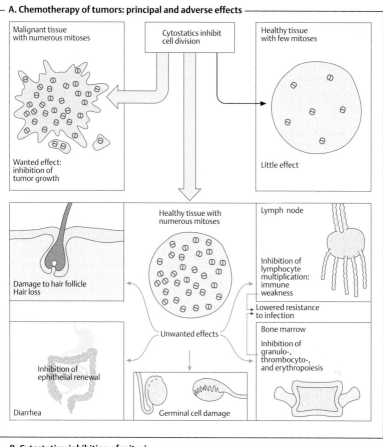

Malignant tissue with numerous mitoses

Cytostatics inhibit cell division

Healthy tissue with few mitoses

Wanted effect: inhibition of tumor growth

Little effect

Healthy tissue with numerous mitoses

Lymph node

Damage to hair follicle Hair loss

Inhibition of lymphocyte multiplication: immune weakness

Lowered resistance to infection

Bone marrow

Inhibition of granulo-, thrombocyto-, and erythropoiesis

Unwanted effects

Inhibition of ephithelial renewal

Diarrhea

Germinal cell damage

B. Cytostatics: inhibition of mitosis

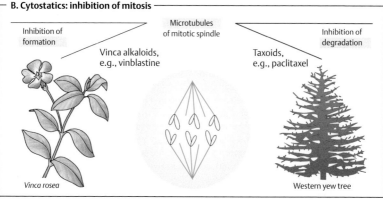

Inhibition of formation

Microtubules of mitotic spindle

Inhibition of degradation

Vinca alkaloids, e.g., vinblastine

Taxoids, e.g., paclitaxel

Vinca rosea

Western yew tree

Inhibition of DNA and RNA synthesis (A). Mitosis is preceded by replication of chromosomes (DNA synthesis) and increased protein synthesis (RNA synthesis). Existing DNA (gray) serves as a template for the synthesis of new (blue) DNA or RNA. De-novo synthesis may be inhibited by the following mechanisms.

Damage to the template (1). Alkylating cytostatics are reactive compounds that transfer alkyl residues into a covalent bond with DNA. For instance, *mechlorethamine* (*nitrogen mustard*) is able to cross-link double-stranded DNA on giving off its chlorine atoms. Correct reading of genetic information is thereby rendered impossible. Other alkylating agents are *chlorambucil, melphalan, thio-TEPA, cyclophosphamide, ifosfamide, lomustine,* and *busulfan.* Specific adverse reactions include irreversible pulmonary fibrosis due to busulfan and hemorrhagic cystitis caused by the cyclophosphamide metabolite acrolein (preventable by the uro-protectant mesna = sodium 2-mercaptoethanesulfonate). The **platinum-containing compounds** *cisplatin* and *carboplatin* release platinum, which binds to DNA.

Cystostatic antibiotics insert themselves into the DNA double strand; this may lead to strand breakage (e.g., with *bleomycin*). The *anthracycline antibiotics daunorubicin* and *adriamycin* (*doxorubicin*) may induce cardiomyopathy. Bleomycin can also cause pulmonary fibrosis.

Induction of strand breakage may result from inhibition of topoisomerase. **The epipodophyllotoxins** *etoposide* and *tenoposide* interact with topoisomerase II, which functions to split, transpose, and reseal DNA strands (p. 276); these agents cause strand breakage by inhibiting resealing. The "tecans" *topotecan* and *irinotecan* are derivatives of camptothecin from the fruits of a Chinese tree (*Camptotheca acuminata*). They inhibit topoisomerase I, which induces breaks in single-strand DNA.

Inhibition of nucleobase synthesis (2). Tetrahydrofolic acid (THF) is required for the synthesis of both purine bases and thymidine. Formation of THF from folic acid involves dihydrofolate reductase (p. 274). The *folate analogues aminopterin* and *methotrexate* (amethopterin) inhibit enzyme activity. Cellular stores of THF are depleted. The effect of these antimetabolites can be reversed by administration of folinic acid (5-formyl-THF, leucovorin, citrovorum factor). *Hydroxyurea* (*hydroxycarbamide*) inhibits ribonucleotide reductase that normally converts ribonucleotides into deoxyribonucleotides subsequently used as DNA building blocks.

Incorporation of false building blocks (3). Unnatural nucleobases (*6-mercaptopurine*; *5-fluorouracil*) or nucleosides with incorrect sugars (*cytarabine*) act as antimetabolites. They inhibit DNA/RNA synthesis or lead to synthesis of missense nucleic acids.

6-Mercaptopurine results from biotransformation of the inactive precursor *azathioprine* (p. 37). The uricostatic *allopurinol* (p. 327) inhibits the degradation of 6-mercaptopurine such that coadministration of the two drugs requires dose reduction of the latter.

Combination therapy. Cytostatics are frequently administered in complex therapeutic regimens designed to improve efficacy and tolerability of treatment.

Supportive therapy. Cancer chemotherapy can be supported by adjunctive medications. Thus, 5-HT$_3$ serotonin receptor antagonists (e.g., ondansetron, p. 342) afford effective protection against vomiting induced by highly emetogenic drugs such as cisplatin. Bone marrow depression can be counteracted by granulocyte and granulocyte/macrophage colony-stimulating factors (filgrastim and lenograstim and molgramostim, respectively).

A. Cytostatics: alkylating agents and cytostatic antibiotics (1), inhibitors of tetrahydrofolate synthesis (2), antimetabolites (3)

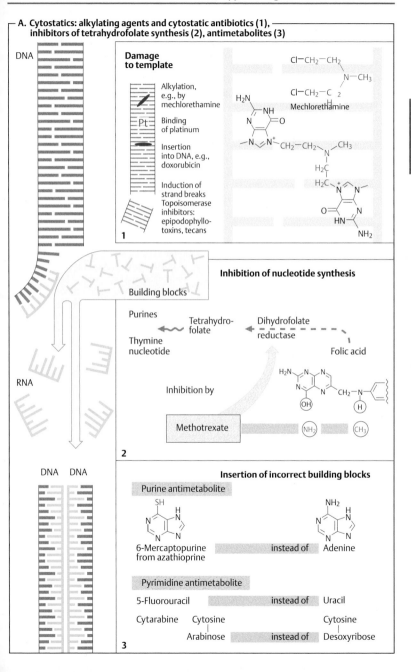

DNA

1

Damage to template

Alkylation, e.g., by mechlorethamine

Pt — Binding of platinum

Insertion into DNA, e.g., doxorubicin

Induction of strand breaks Topoisomerase inhibitors: epipodophyllo-toxins, tecans

Mechlorethamine

Inhibition of nucleotide synthesis

Building blocks

Purines

Thymine nucleotide

Tetrahydro-folate

Dihydrofolate reductase

Folic acid

RNA

Inhibition by

Methotrexate

2

DNA   DNA

Insertion of incorrect building blocks

Purine antimetabolite

6-Mercaptopurine from azathioprine   instead of   Adenine

Pyrimidine antimetabolite

5-Fluorouracil   instead of   Uracil

Cytarabine   Cytosine
Arabinose   instead of

Cytosine
Desoxyribose

3

☐ Targeting of Antineoplastic Drug Action (A)

When degenerating neoplastic cells display special metabolic properties *which are different from those of normal cells*, targeted pharmacotherapeutic intervention becomes possible.

Imatinib. Chronic myelogenous leukemia (CML) results from a genetic defect in the hematopoietic stem cells of the bone marrow. Nearly all CML patients possess the *Philadelphia chromosome.* It results from translocation between chromosomes 9 and 22 of the c-*abl* protooncogene, leading to the hybrid *bcr-abl* fusion gene on chromosome 22. The recombinant gene encodes a tyrosine kinase mutant with unregulated (constitutive), enhanced activity that promotes cell proliferation. Imatinib is a tyrosine kinase inhibitor that specifically affects this mutant but also interacts with some other kinases. It can be used orally in Philadelphia chromosome-positive CML.

Asparaginase cleaves the amino acid asparagine into aspartate and ammonia. Certain cells, in particular the tumor cells in acute lymphatic leukemia, require asparagine for protein synthesis and must take it up from the extracellular space, whereas many other cell types are themselves able to synthesize asparagine. Supply of the amino acid can be disrupted by administration of the asparagine-hydrolyzing enzyme. Consequently, protein synthesis and proliferation of neoplastic cells are inhibited. Asparaginase is obtained from *E. coli* bacteria or may be of plant origin (*Erwinia chrysanthemi*), when it is also named crisantaspase. Allergic reactions against the exogenous protein occur after parenteral administration.

Trastuzumab exemplifies a growing number of monoclonal antibodies that have become available for antineoplastic therapy. These are directed against cell surface proteins that are strongly expressed by cancer cells. Trastuzumab binds to HER2, the receptor for epidermal growth factor. The density of this receptor is greatly increased in some types of breast cancer. When the tumor cells have bound antibody, immune cells can recognize them as elements to be eliminated. Trastuzumab is indicated in advanced cases under certain conditions. The antibody is cardiotoxic; it is likely that cardiomyocytes also express HER2.

☐ Mechanisms of Resistance to Cytostatics (B)

Initial success can be followed by loss of effect because of the emergence of resistant tumor cells. Mechanisms of resistance are multifactorial.

- *Diminished cellular uptake* may result from reduced synthesis of a transport protein that may be needed for membrane penetration (e. g., methotrexate).
- *Augmented drug extrusion:* increased synthesis of the P-glycoprotein that extrudes drugs from the cell (e. g., anthracyclines, vinca alkaloids, epipodophyllotoxins, and paclitaxel) is responsible for multidrug resistance (*mdr1* gene amplification).
- *Diminished bioactivation of a prodrug*, e. g., cytarabine, which requires intracellular phosphorylation to become cytotoxic.
- *Change in site of action:* e. g., increased synthesis of dihydrofolate reductase may occur as a compensatory response to methotrexate.
- *Damage repair:* DNA repair enzymes may become more efficient in repairing defects caused by cisplatin. Inhibition of apoptosis due to activation of antiapoptotic cellular mechanisms.

A. Targeting of antineoplastic drug action

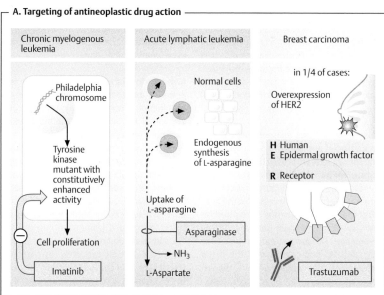

Chronic myelogenous leukemia

Philadelphia chromosome

Tyrosine kinase mutant with constitutively enhanced activity

Cell proliferation

⊖

Imatinib

Acute lymphatic leukemia

Normal cells

Endogenous synthesis of L-asparagine

Uptake of L-asparagine

Asparaginase

→ NH₃

L-Aspartate

Breast carcinoma

in 1/4 of cases:

Overexpression of HER2

H Human
E Epidermal growth factor
R Receptor

Trastuzumab

B. Mechanisms of cytostatic resistance

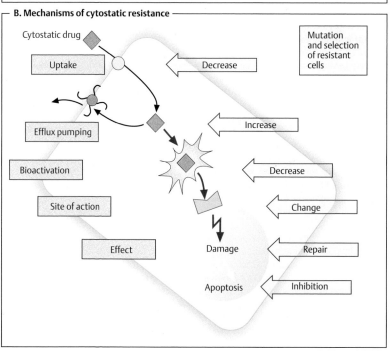

Cytostatic drug

Uptake

Mutation and selection of resistant cells

Decrease

Efflux pumping

Increase

Bioactivation

Decrease

Site of action

Change

Effect

Damage

Repair

Apoptosis

Inhibition

□ Inhibition of Immune Responses

Both the prevention of *transplant rejection* and the treatment of *autoimmune disorders* call for a suppression of immune responses. However, immune suppression also entails weakened defenses against infectious pathogens and a long-term increase in the risk of neoplasms.

A specific **immune response** begins with the binding of antigen by lymphocytes carrying specific receptors with the appropriate antigen-binding site. B-lymphocytes "recognize" antigen surface structures by means of membrane receptors that resemble the antibodies formed subsequently. T-lymphocytes (and naive B cells) require the antigen to be presented on the surface of macrophages or other cells in conjunction with the major histocompatibility complex (MHC); the latter permits recognition of antigenic structures by means of the T-cell receptor. T-helper (T_H) cells carry adjacent CD3 and CD4 complexes, cytotoxic T cells a CD8 complex. The CD proteins assist in docking to the MHC. Besides recognition of antigen, stimulation by cytokines plays an essential part in the activation of lymphocytes. Interleukin-1 is formed by macrophages, and various interleukins (IL), including IL-2, are made by T-helper cells. As antigen-specific lymphocytes proliferate, immune defenses are set into motion.

I. Interference with antigen recognition. **Muromonab CD3** is a monoclonal antibody directed against mouse CD3 that blocks antigen recognition by T-lymphocytes (use in graft rejection).

Glatirameracetate consists of peptides of varying lengths, polymerized in random sequence from the amino acids glutamine, lysine, alanine, and tyrosine. It can be used in the treatment of multiple sclerosis besides β-interferon. This disease is caused by a T-lymphocyte-mediated autoaggression directed against oligodendrocytes that form myelin sheaths of CNS axons. The culprit antigen appears to be myelin basic protein. Glatiramer resembles the latter; by blocking antigen receptors, it interferes with antigen recognition by lymphocytes.

II. Inhibition of cytokine production and action. Glucocorticoids modulate the expression of numerous genes; thus, the production of IL-1 and IL-2 is inhibited, which explains the suppression of T-cell-dependent immune responses. In addition, glucocorticoids interfere with inflammatory cytokines and signaling molecules at various other sites. Glucocorticoids are used in organ transplantations, autoimmune diseases, and allergic disorders. Systemic use carries the risk of iatrogenic Cushing syndrome (p. 244).

Ciclosporin and related substances inhibit the production of cytokines, in particular interleukin-2. In contrast to glucocorticoids, the plethora of accompanying metabolic effects is absent (see p. 306 for more details).

Daclizumab and **basiliximab** are monoclonal antibodies against the receptor for IL-2. They consist of murine Fab fragments and a human Fc-segment. They are used to suppress transplant rejection reactions.

Anakinra is a recombinant form of an endogenous antagonist at the interleukin-1 receptor; it is used in rheumatoid arthritis (p. 332).

III. Disruption of cell metabolism with inhibition of proliferation. At dosages below those needed to treat malignancies, some cytostatics are also employed for immunosuppression; e. g., azathioprine, methotrexate, and cyclophosphamide. The antiproliferative effect is not specific for lymphocytes and involves both T and B cells.

Mycophenolate mofetil has a more specific effect on lymphocytes than on other cells. It inhibits inosine monophosphate dehydrogenase, which catalyzes purine synthesis in lymphocytes. It is used in acute tissue rejection responses.

A. Immune reaction and immunosuppressives

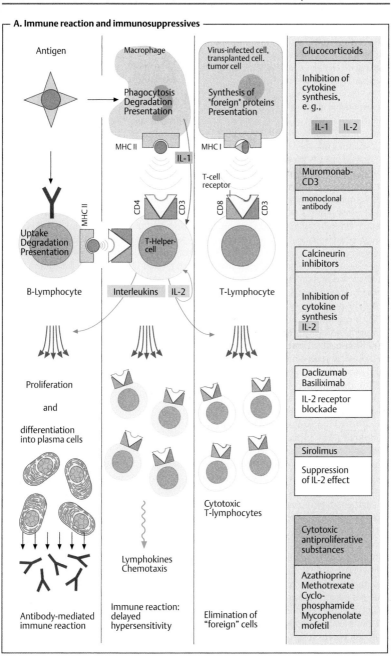

Antigen

Macrophage

Virus-infected cell, transplanted cell. tumor cell

Phagocytosis
Degradation
Presentation

Synthesis of "foreign" proteins
Presentation

MHC II

MHC I

IL-1

T-cell receptor

MHC II

Uptake
Degradation
Presentation

CD4   CD3

T-Helper-cell

CD8   CD3

B-Lymphocyte

Interleukins   IL-2

T-Lymphocyte

Proliferation

and

differentiation into plasma cells

Cytotoxic
T-lymphocytes

Lymphokines
Chemotaxis

Antibody-mediated immune reaction

Immune reaction: delayed hypersensitivity

Elimination of "foreign" cells

Glucocorticoids

Inhibition of cytokine synthesis, e. g.,

IL-1   IL-2

Muromonab-CD3

monoclonal antibody

Calcineurin inhibitors

Inhibition of cytokine synthesis IL-2

**Daclizumab
Basiliximab**

IL-2 receptor blockade

Sirolimus

Suppression of IL-2 effect

Cytotoxic antiproliferative substances

Azathioprine
Methotrexate
Cyclo-phosphamide
Mycophenolate mofetil

IV. Anti-T-cell immune serum is obtained from animals immunized with human T-lymphocytes. The antibodies bind to and damage T cells and can thus be used to attenuate tissue rejection.

Ciclosporin is of fungal origin; it is a cyclic peptide composed of 11, in part atypical, amino acids. Therefore, orally administered ciclosporin is not degraded by gastrointestinal proteases. In T-helper cells, it *inhibits the production of interleukin-2* by interfering at the level of transcriptional regulation. Normally, "nuclear factor of activated T cells," (NFAT) promotes the expression of interleukin-2. This requires dephosphorylation of the precursor, phosphorylated NFAT, by the *phosphatase calcineurin*, enabling NFAT to enter the cell nucleus from the cytosol. Ciclosporin binds to the protein *cyclophilin* in the cell interior; the complex inhibits calcineurin, hence the production of interleukin-2.

The breakthroughs in *modern transplantation medicine* are largely attributable to the introduction of ciclosporin. It is now also employed in certain autoimmune diseases, atopic dermatitis, and other disorders.

The predominant adverse effect of ciclosporin is *nephrotoxicity*. Its dosage must be titrated so that blood levels are neither too high (risk of renal injury) nor too low (rejection reaction). To complicate the problem, ciclosporin is a substance difficult to manage therapeutically. Oral bioavailability is incomplete. Back-transport of the drug into the gut lumen occurs via the P-glycoprotein efflux pump, in addition to metabolization by cytochrome oxidases of the 3A subfamily. Hepatic CYP3A4 enzymes contribute to presystemic elimination and are responsible for elimination of systemically available ciclosporin. Diverse drug interactions may occur by interference with CYP3A and P-glycoprotein. For optimal dosage adjustment, *monitoring of plasma levels* is mandatory.

Drug-mediated suppression of transplant rejection entails long-term treatment. Protracted immunosuppression carries an increased risk of malignomas. Risk factors for cardiovascular diseases may be adversely affected—a critical and important concern in long-term prognosis.

Tacrolimus is a macrolide antibiotic from *Streptomyces tsukubaensis*. In principle, it acts like ciclosporin. At the molecular level, however, its "receptor" is not cyclophilin but a so-called FK-binding protein. Tacrolimus is likewise used to prevent allograft rejection. Its epithelial penetrability is superior to that of ciclosporin, allowing topical application in atopic dermatitis.

Sirolimus (**rapamycin**) is another macrolide, produced by *Streptomyces hydroscopicus*. Its immunosuppressant action, evidently, does not appear to involve inhibition of calcineurin. It forms a complex with the FK protein, imparting a special conformation on it; and the complex then inhibits the mTOR (mammalian target of rapamycin) phosphatase. The latter operates in the signaling path leading from the interleukin-2 receptor to activation of mitosis in lymphocytes. Thus, sirolimus inhibits lymphocyte proliferation. It is approved for the prevention of transplant rejection.

A. Calcineurin inhibitors and sirolimus (rapamycin)

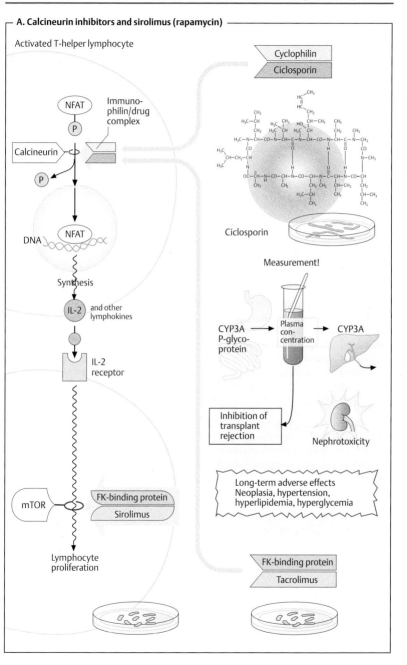

Activated T-helper lymphocyte

NFAT
P

Immuno-
philin/drug
complex

Calcineurin
P

DNA   NFAT

Synthesis

IL-2   and other
lymphokines

IL-2
receptor

mTOR   FK-binding protein
Sirolimus

Lymphocyte
proliferation

Cyclophilin
Ciclosporin

Ciclosporin

Measurement!

CYP3A
P-glyco-
protein   Plasma
con-
centration   CYP3A

Inhibition of
transplant
rejection   Nephrotoxicity

Long-term adverse effects
Neoplasia, hypertension,
hyperlipidemia, hyperglycemia

FK-binding protein
Tacrolimus

☐ Antidotes and Treatment of Poisonings

Drugs used to counteract drug overdosage are considered under the appropriate headings; e.g., physostigmine with atropine; naloxone with opioids; flumazenil with benzodiazepines; antibody (Fab fragments) with digitalis; and *N*-acetylcysteine with acetaminophen intoxication.

Chelating agents (**A**) serve as antidotes in poisoning with heavy metals. They act to complex and, thus, "inactivate" heavy metal ions. Chelates (from Greek: *chele* = pincer [of crayfish]) represent complexes between a metal ion and molecules that carry several binding sites for the metal ion. Because of their high affinity, chelating agents "attract" metal ions present in the organism. The chelates are nontoxic, are excreted predominantly via the kidney, and maintain a tight organometallic bond in the concentrated, usually acidic, milieu of tubular urine and thus promote the elimination of metal ions.

Na$_2$Ca-EDTA is used to treat lead poisoning. This antidote cannot penetrate through cell membranes and must be given parenterally. Because of its high binding affinity, the lead ion displaces Ca^{2+} from its bond. The lead-containing chelate is eliminated renally. Nephrotoxicity predominates among the unwanted effects. **Na$_3$Ca-pentetate** is a complex of diethylenetriaminopentaacetic acid (DPTA) and serves as antidote in lead and other metal intoxications.

Dimercaprol (BAL, British Anti-Lewisite) was developed in World War II as an antidote against vesicant organic arsenicals (**B**). It is able to chelate various metal ions. Dimercaprol forms a liquid, rapidly decomposing substance that is given intramuscularly in an oily vehicle. A related compound, both in terms of structure and activity, is **dimer-captopropanesulfonic acid**, whose sodium salt is suitable for oral administration. Shivering, fever, and skin reactions are potential adverse effects.

Deferoxamine derives from *Streptomyces pilosus*. The substance possesses a very high iron-binding capacity but does not withdraw iron from hemoglobin or cytochromes. It is poorly absorbed enterally and must be given parenterally to cause increased excretion of iron. Oral administration is indicated only if enteral absorption of iron is to be curtailed. Unwanted effects include allergic reactions.

It should be noted that bloodletting is the most effective means of removing iron from the body; however, this method is unsuitable for treating conditions of iron overload associated with anemia.

D-Penicillamine can promote the elimination of copper (e.g., in Wilson disease) and of lead ions. It can be given orally. Two additional indications are cystinuria and rheumatoid arthritis. In cystinuria, formation of cystine stones in the urinary tract is prevented because the drug can form a disulfide with cysteine that is readily soluble. In rheumatoid arthritis, penicillamine can be used as a basal regimen (p. 332). The therapeutic effect may result in part from a reaction with aldehydes, whereby polymerization of collagen molecules into fibrils is inhibited. Unwanted effects are cutaneous damage (diminished resistance to mechanical stress with a tendency to form blisters; p. 74), nephrotoxicity, bone marrow depression, and taste disturbances.

Apart from specific antidotes (if they exist), the treatment of poisonings also calls for **symptomatic measures** (control of blood pressure and blood electrolytes; monitoring of cardiac and respiratory function; prevention of toxin absorption by activated charcoal). An important step is early emptying of the stomach by gastric lavage and, if necessary, administration of an osmotic laxative. Use of emetics (saturated NaCl solution, ipecac syrup, apomorphine s.c.) is inadvisable.

A. Chelation of lead ions by EDTA

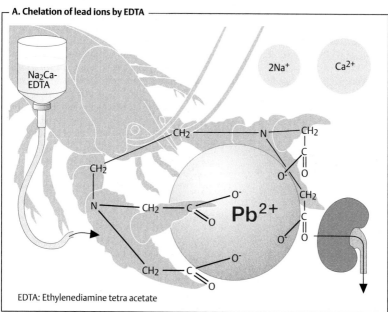

EDTA: Ethylenediamine tetra acetate

B. Chelators

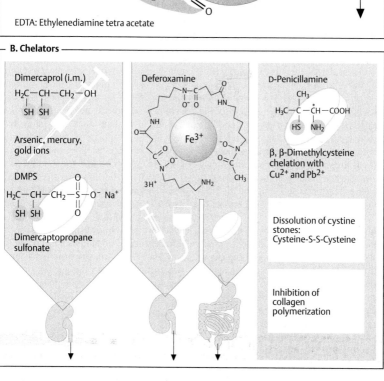

Dimercaprol (i.m.)

$$H_2C-CH-CH_2-OH$$
$$\quad|\quad\ |$$
$$\ SH\ \ SH$$

Arsenic, mercury, gold ions

DMPS

$$H_2C-CH-CH_2-\overset{\displaystyle O}{\underset{\displaystyle O}{\overset{\|}{\underset{\|}{S}}}}-O^-\ Na^+$$
$$\quad|\quad\ |$$
$$\ SH\ \ SH$$

Dimercaptopropane sulfonate

Deferoxamine

Fe^{3+}

$3H^+$ NH_2

D-Penicillamine

$$\begin{array}{c} CH_3 \\ | \\ H_3C-C-\overset{*}{C}H-COOH \\ |\quad\ \ | \\ HS\quad NH_2 \end{array}$$

β, β-Dimethylcysteine chelation with Cu^{2+} and Pb^{2+}

Dissolution of cystine stones:
Cysteine-S-S-Cysteine

Inhibition of collagen polymerization

Reactivators of phosphorylated acetylcholinesterase (AChE). Certain organic phosphoric acid compounds bind with high affinity to a serine OH group in the active center of AChE and thus block the hydrolysis of acetylcholine. As a result, the organism is poisoned with its own transmitter substance, acetylcholine. This mechanism operates not only in humans and warm-blooded animals but also in lower animals, ACh having been "invented" early in evolution. Thus, **organophosphates** enjoy widespread application as insecticides. Time and again, their use has led to human poisoning because these toxicants can enter the body through the intact skin or inhaled air. Depending on the severity, signs of poisoning include excessive parasympathetic tonus, ganglionic blockade, and inhibition of neuromuscular transmission leading to peripheral respiratory paralysis. Specific treatment of the intoxication consists in administration of extremely high doses of *atropine* and reactivation of acetylcholinesterase with *pralidoxime* or *obidoxime* (**A**).

Unfortunately, the organophosphates have been misused as biological weapons. In World War II, they were stockpiled on both sides but not deployed. The efficacy of the poisons was subsequently "demonstrated" in smaller local armed conflicts in developing countries. In the present global situation, the fear has arisen that organophosphates may be used by terrorist groups. Thus, understanding the signs of poisoning and the principles of treatment are highly important.

Tolonium chloride (toluidine blue). Brown-colored methemoglobin, containing trivalent instead of divalent iron, is incapable of carrying O_2. Under normal conditions, methemoglobin is produced continuously, but reduced again with the help of glucose-6-phosphate dehydrogenase. Substances that promote formation of methemoglobin (**B**) may cause a lethal deficiency of O_2. Tolonium chloride is a redox dye that can be given i.v. to reduce methemoglobin.

Antidotes for cyanide poisoning (B). Cyanide ions (CN^-) enter the organism in the form of hydrocyanic acid (HCN); the latter can be inhaled, released from cyanide salts in the acidic stomach juice, or enzymatically liberated from bitter almonds in the gastrointestinal tract. The lethal dose of HCN can be as low as 50 mg. CN^- binds with high affinity to trivalent iron and thereby arrests utilization of oxygen via mitochondrial cytochrome oxidases of the respiratory chain. Internal asphyxiation (*histotoxic hypoxia*) ensues while erythrocytes remain charged with O_2 (venous blood colored bright red).

In small amounts, cyanide can be converted to the relatively nontoxic thiocyanate (SCN^-) by hepatic "rhodanese" or sulfurtransferase. As a **therapeutic measure**, *sodium thiosulfate* can be given i.v. to promote formation of thiocyanate, which is eliminated in urine. However, this reaction is slow in onset. A more effective emergency treatment is the i.v. administration of the methemoglobin forming agent *4-dimethylaminophenol*, which rapidly generates trivalent iron from divalent iron in hemoglobin. Competition between methemoglobin and cytochrome oxidase for CN^- ions favors the formation of cyanmethemoglobin. Hydroxycobalamin (= vitamin B_{12a}) is an alternative, very effective antidote because its central cobalt atom binds CN^- with high affinity to generate cyanocobalamin (= vitamin B_{12}).

Ferric ferrocyanide ("Berlin blue" [B]) is used to treat poisoning with thallium salts (e.g., in rat poison), initial symptoms of which are gastrointestinal disturbances, followed by nerve and brain damage, as well as hair loss. Thallium ions present in the organism are secreted into the gut but undergo reabsorption. The insoluble, nonabsorbable colloidal Berlin blue binds thallium ions. It is given orally to prevent absorption of acutely ingested thallium or to promote clearance from the organism by intercepting thallium that is secreted into the intestines (**B**).

A. Reactivation of ACh-esterase by an oxime

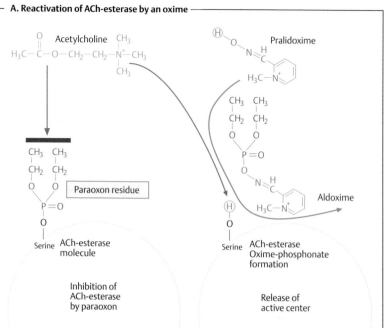

Acetylcholine

Pralidoxime

Paraoxon residue

Aldoxime

Serine ACh-esterase
molecule

Serine ACh-esterase
Oxime-phosphonate
formation

Inhibition of
ACh-esterase
by paraoxon

Release of
active center

B. Poisons and antidotes

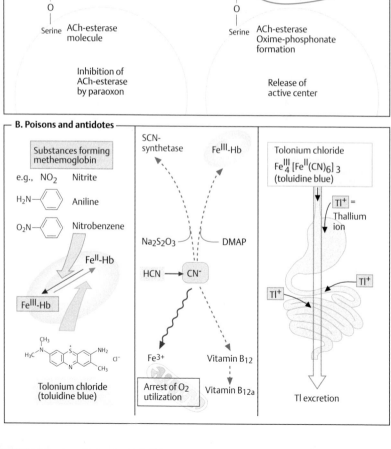

Substances forming
methemoglobin

e.g., NO_2 Nitrite

H_2N—⟨⟩   Aniline

O_2N—⟨⟩   Nitrobenzene

Fe^{II}-Hb

Fe^{III}-Hb

Tolonium chloride
(toluidine blue)

SCN-
synthetase

Fe^{III}-Hb

$Na_2S_2O_3$ DMAP

HCN → CN^-

Fe^{3+}

Arrest of O_2
utilization

Vitamin B_{12}

Vitamin B_{12a}

Tolonium chloride
$Fe^{III}_4 [Fe^{II}(CN)_6]_3$
(toluidine blue)

Tl^+ =
Thallium
ion

Tl^+

Tl^+

Tl excretion

Therapy of Selected Diseases

☐ Hypertension

Cardiovascular diseases are the leading cause of death in the Western world. Basically, atherosclerosis manifests itself in three major organs and thereby leads to severe secondary diseases. Coronary disease results from atherosclerosis of the coronary arteries and culminates in myocardial infarction when vessels are occluded by a thrombus. In the brain, atherosclerosis gives rise to arterial thrombi or ruptures that result in a stroke. Atherosclerosis in the kidney leads to renal failure. Since these diseases significantly lower life expectancy, early recognition and elimination of risk factors (hypertension, diabetes mellitus, hyperlipidemia, and smoking) that promote atherosclerosis are essential.

Hypertension is considered to be present when systolic blood pressure exceeds 140 mmHg and the diastolic value lies above 90 mmHg. Since cardiovascular risk increases over a wide range with increasing blood pressure, no "threshold value" exists that defines hypertension unequivocally. If other risk factors are present, blood pressure should be brought down to an even lower level (in diabetes mellitus below 130/80 mmHg). Therapeutic objectives comprise the prevention of organ damage and reduction of mortality. Because these target parameters cannot be measured in individual patients, the "surrogate parameter" of lowering of blood pressure is defined as the immediate goal. Before drug therapy is instituted, the patient has to be instructed to lower body weight (BMI <30), to reduce consumption of alcohol (in men <20–30 g ethanol/day; in women 10–20 g/day), to stop smoking, and to restrict the daily intake of NaCl (to 6 g/day).

The drugs of first choice in antihypertensive therapy are those that have been unambiguously shown in clinical studies to reduce mortality of hypertension—diuretics, ACE inhibitors and AT_1 antagonist, β-blockers, and calcium antagonists.

Among the diuretics, thiazides are particularly recommended for treatment of hypertension. To avoid undue loss of K^+, combination with triamterene or amiloride is often advantageous.

ACE inhibitors prevent the formation of angiotensin II by angiotensin-converting enzyme (ACE) and thereby reduce peripheral vascular resistance and blood pressure. In addition, ACE inhibitors prevent the effect of angiotensin II on protein synthesis in myocardial and vascular muscle cells, and thus diminish ventricular hypertrophy. As adverse effects, ACE inhibitors may provoke dry cough, impaired renal function, and hyperkalemia. When ACE inhibitors are poorly tolerated, an AT_1-receptor antagonist can be given.

From the group of antagonists at β-adrenoceptors, **$β_1$-selective blockers** are mainly used (e. g., metoprolol). Owing to blockade of $β_2$-receptors, β-blockers can impair pulmonary function, particularly in patients with chronic obstructive lung disease.

Among **calcium antagonists**, dihydropyridines with long half-lives are advantageous because short-acting drugs, which rapidly lower blood pressure, are prone to elicit reflex tachycardia.

Fewer that 50% of hypertensive patients are adequately managed by monotherapy. If the monotherapy fails, either the drug should be discontinued or two agents should be combined in reduced dosage (thiazide and β-blocker, or/and ACE inhibitor, or/and calcium-antagonist). Combinations that abolish the counterregulation against the primary antihypertensive drug are especially effective. For instance, diuretic-induced loss of Na^+ and water leads to a compensatory activation of the renin–angiotensin system that can be eliminated by ACE inhibitors or AT_1-antagonists.

A. Risk factors of atherosclerosis and secondary diseases

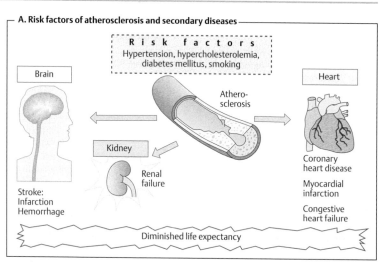

R i s k   f a c t o r s
Hypertension, hypercholesterolemia,
diabetes mellitus, smoking

Brain

Athero-
sclerosis

Heart

Kidney

Renal
failure

Coronary
heart disease

Myocardial
infarction

Congestive
heart failure

Stroke:
Infarction
Hemorrhage

Diminished life expectancy

B. Therapy of hypertension

H y p e r t e n s i o n > 1 4 0 / 9 0 m m H g

Healthy diet (low NaCl),
weight reduction, no smoking,
alcohol restriction, exercise

Thiazide diuretics

If antihypertensive effect insufficient, add:

β-Blocker or ACE inhibitor,
angiotensin receptor antagonist or calcium antagonist

If still not sufficient:

Combination therapy:
+ clonidine or α_1-antagonists or vasodilators

Therapeutic aim:
Lowering of blood pressure
(< 140/90, in diabetes < 130/80 mmHg);
and, hence, reduction in cardiovascular mortality

☐ Angina Pectoris

An anginal pain attack signals a transient hypoxia of the myocardium. As a rule, the *oxygen deficit* results from inadequate myocardial blood flow due to narrowing of larger coronary arteries. The underlying causes are most commonly an atherosclerotic change of the vascular wall (*coronary sclerosis* with exertional angina); very infrequently a spasmodic constriction of a morphologically healthy coronary artery (*coronary spasm* with angina at rest; variant angina); or more often a coronary spasm occurring in an atherosclerotic vascular segment.

The goal of treatment is to prevent myocardial hypoxia either by raising blood flow (*oxygen [O_2] supply*) or by lowering myocardial oxygen demand (O_2 *demand*) (**A**).

Factors determining oxygen supply. The force driving myocardial blood flow is the *pressure difference* between the coronary ostia (*aortic pressure*) and the opening of the coronary sinus (*right atrial pressure*). Blood flow is opposed by *coronary flow resistance*, which includes three components:

1. Owing to their large caliber, the *proximal coronary segments* do not normally contribute significantly to flow resistance. However, in coronary sclerosis or spasm, pathological obstruction of flow occurs here. Whereas the more common coronary sclerosis cannot be overcome pharmacologically, the less common coronary spasm can be relieved by appropriate vasodilators (nitrates, nifedipine).

2. The *caliber of arteriolar resistance vessels* controls blood flow through the coronary bed. Arteriolar caliber is determined by myocardial O_2 tension and local concentrations of metabolic products, and is "automatically" adjusted to the required blood flow (**B**, healthy subject). This *metabolic autoregulation* explains why anginal attacks in coronary sclerosis occur only during exercise (**B**, patient). At rest, the pathologically elevated flow resistance is

compensated by a corresponding decrease in arteriolar resistance, ensuring adequate myocardial perfusion. During exercise, further dilation of arterioles is impossible. As a result, there is ischemia associated with pain. Pharmacological agents that act to dilate arterioles would thus be inappropriate because at rest they may divert blood from underperfused into healthy vascular regions on account of redundant arteriolar dilation. The resulting "steal effect" could provoke an anginal attack.

3. The intramyocardial pressure, i. e., systolic squeeze, compresses the capillary bed. Myocardial blood flow is halted during systole and occurs almost entirely during diastole. *Diastolic wall tension* ("preload") depends on ventricular volume and filling pressure. The organic nitrates reduce preload by decreasing venous return to the heart.

Factors determining oxygen demand. The heart muscle cell consumes the most energy to generate contractile force. O_2 demand rises with an increase in (1) *heart rate*, (2) *contraction velocity*, (3) *systolic wall tension* ("afterload"). The last depends on ventricular volume and the systolic pressure needed to empty the ventricle. As peripheral resistance increases, aortic pressure rises and, hence, the resistance against which ventricular blood is ejected. O_2 demand is lowered by β-blockers and calcium-antagonists, as well as by nitrates (p. 318).

A. O$_2$ supply and demand of the myocardium

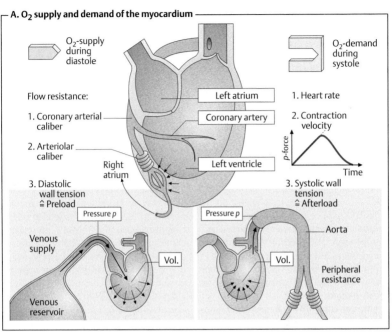

O$_2$-supply during diastole

Flow resistance:

1. Coronary arterial caliber
2. Arteriolar caliber
3. Diastolic wall tension $\hat{=}$ Preload

Venous supply

Venous reservoir

Pressure p

Vol.

Left atrium

Coronary artery

Right atrium

Left ventricle

Pressure p

Vol.

Aorta

Peripheral resistance

O$_2$-demand during systole

1. Heart rate
2. Contraction velocity

p-force · Time

3. Systolic wall tension $\hat{=}$ Afterload

B. Pathogenesis of exertion angina in coronary sclerosis

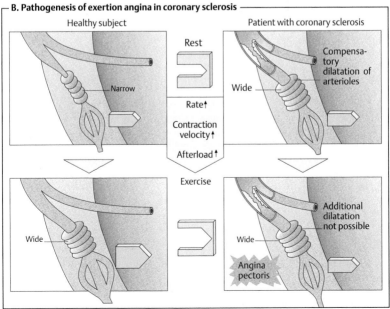

Healthy subject

Patient with coronary sclerosis

Rest

Narrow

Wide

Compensatory dilatation of arterioles

Rate↑

Contraction velocity↑

Afterload↑

Exercise

Wide

Wide

Additional dilatation not possible

Angina pectoris

☐ Antianginal Drugs

Antianginal agents derive from three drug groups, the pharmacological properties of which have already been presented in more detail: the organic nitrates (p.124), the calcium antagonists (p.126), and the β-blockers (p.96).

Organic nitrates (A) increase blood flow, hence O_2 supply, because diastolic wall tension (preload) declines as venous return to the heart is diminished. Thus, the nitrates enable myocardial flow resistance to be reduced even in the presence of coronary sclerosis with angina pectoris. In angina due to coronary spasm, arterial dilation overcomes the vasospasm and restores myocardial perfusion to normal. O_2 demand falls because of the ensuing decrease in the two variables that determine systolic wall tension (afterload): ventricular filling volume and aortic blood pressure.

Calcium antagonists (B) decrease O_2 demand by lowering aortic pressure, one of the components contributing to afterload. The dihydropyridine *nifedipine*, is devoid of a cardiodepressant effect, but may give rise to reflex tachycardia and an associated increase in O_2 demand. The catamphiphilic drugs *verapamil* and *diltiazem* are cardiodepressant. Reduced beat frequency and contractility contribute to a reduction in O_2 demand; however, AV-block and mechanical insufficiency can dangerously jeopardize heart function. In coronary spasm, calcium antagonists can induce spasmolysis and improve blood flow.

β-Blockers (C) protect the heart against the O_2-wasting effect of sympathetic drive by inhibiting β_1-receptor-mediated increases in cardiac rate and speed of contraction.

Uses of antianginal drugs (D). For relief of the **acute anginal attack**, rapidly absorbed drugs devoid of cardiodepressant activity are preferred. The drug of choice is *nitroglycerin* (NTG, 0.8–2.4 mg sublingually; onset of ac-

tion within 1–2 minutes; duration of effect ~30 minutes). Isosorbide dinitrate (ISDN) can also be used (5–10 mg sublingually); compared with NTG, its action is somewhat delayed in onset but of longer duration. Finally, nifedipine may be useful in chronic stable, or in variant angina (5–20 mg, capsule to be bitten and the content swallowed).

For sustained daytime **angina prophylaxis**, *nitrates* are of limited value because "nitrate pauses" of about 12 hours are appropriate if nitrate tolerance is to be avoided. If attacks occur during the day, ISDN, or its metabolite *isosorbide mononitrate*, may be given in the morning and at noon (e.g., ISDN 40 mg in extended-release capsules). Because of hepatic presystemic elimination, NTG is not suitable for oral administration. Continuous delivery via a transdermal patch would also not seem advisable because of the potential development of tolerance. With *molsidomine*, there is less risk of a nitrate tolerance; however, its clinical use is restricted owing to its potential carcinogenicity.

The choice between *calcium antagonists* must take into account the differential effect of nifedipine versus verapamil or diltiazem on cardiac performance (see above). When β-*blockers* are given, the potential consequences of reducing cardiac contractility (withdrawal of sympathetic drive) must be kept in mind. Since vasodilating β_2-receptors are blocked, an increased risk of vasospasm cannot be ruled out. Therefore, monotherapy with β-blockers is recommended only in angina due to coronary sclerosis, but not in variant angina.

A. Effects of nitrates

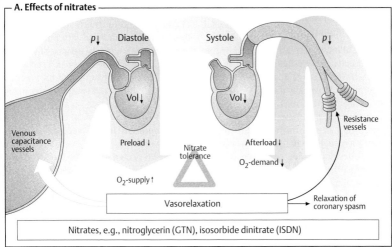

$p\downarrow$ Diastole   Systole $p\downarrow$

Vol↓   Vol↓

Resistance vessels

Venous capacitance vessels

Preload ↓   Afterload ↓

Nitrate tolerance

O_2-supply ↑ O_2-demand ↓

Vasorelaxation   Relaxation of coronary spasm

Nitrates, e.g., nitroglycerin (GTN), isosorbide dinitrate (ISDN)

B. Effects of Ca-antagonists

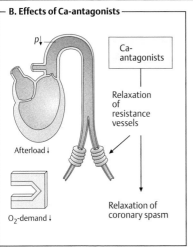

$p\downarrow$

Ca-antagonists

Relaxation of resistance vessels

Afterload ↓

O_2-demand ↓

Relaxation of coronary spasm

C. Effects of β-blockers

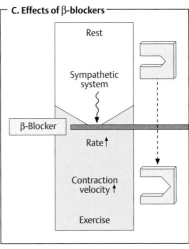

Rest

Sympathetic system

β-Blocker

Rate ↑

Contraction velocity ↑

Exercise

D. Clinical uses of antianginal drugs

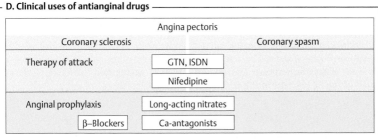

Angina pectoris	
Coronary sclerosis	Coronary spasm
Therapy of attack	
	GTN, ISDN
	Nifedipine
Anginal prophylaxis	Long-acting nitrates
β–Blockers	Ca-antagonists

☐ Acute Coronary Syndrome— Myocardial Infarction

Myocardial infarction (MI) is caused by the acute *thrombotic occlusion* of a coronary artery. The myocardial region that has been cut off from its blood supply dies within a short time owing to the lack of O_2 and glucose. The loss in functional muscle tissue results in reduced cardiac performance. In the infarct border zone, spontaneous pacemaker potentials may develop, leading to fatal ventricular fibrillation. The patient experiences severe pain, a feeling of annihilation, and fear of dying.

MI usually develops after rupture or erosion of an atherosclerotic plaque within a coronary blood vessel. At this site, the clotting cascade is activated and the resultant thrombus occludes the lumen. In all patients under suspicion of MI, **immediate therapy** has to be initiated by the emergency physician. To relieve the patient from severe pain and anxiety, morphine and a benzodiazepine need to be given. Antiplatelet drugs and heparin are necessary for preventing further formation of thrombi. Nitroglycerin can be used to reduce cardiac load. When blood pressure and heart rate have stabilized, a β-blocker can be administered to lower cardiac O_2 consumption and the risk of arrhythmias. Infusion of lidocaine is required to counter the threat of arrhythmias. The chance of survival of the MI patient depends on the interval between the onset of infarction and the start of therapy.

In the hospital, ECG and laboratory tests are performed promptly to determine the subsequent treatment strategy. When cardiomyocytes die, contractile proteins (troponin) or myocardial enzymes (creatine kinase, CK-MB) are liberated and can be detected in blood for diagnostic purposes. Marked elevation of the ST segment in the ECG raises the strong suspicion of a complete occlusion of a coronary artery (ST elevation MI, STEMI). In these MI patients, reperfusion of the affected area as early and as completely as possible may be life-saving. In this situation, removal of the coronary stenosis with a **balloon catheter** combined with implantation of a stent offers the best chance of survival but can be performed only in specialized cardiac centers. As dilatation of the vascular stenosis by the heart catheter liberates many thrombogenic mediators, platelet aggregation must be prevented by administration of **glycoprotein IIb/IIIa receptor antagonists** (p. 154).

If the MI patient cannot be transported to a cardiac center in time, **fibrinolytic treatment** of the coronary thrombus is instituted. For this purpose, fibrinolytics (streptokinase or recombinant tissue plasminogen activators) are given intravenously. Fibrinolysis is associated with an increased risk of bleeding; cerebral hemorrhages are of particular concern. A coronary **bypass operation** is available as a third therapeutic option.

Patients with persistent angina pectoris who lack an elevated ST segment in the ECG but show an elevated blood level of troponin may have a non-STEMI ("NSTEMI"). The most frequent cause is thrombi that have moved from the larger coronary arteries into smaller branches to produce a blockage there. If neither ST segment elevation nor biochemical MI markers can be ascertained, **unstable angina pectoris** is present, which is initially treated with antiplatelet drugs.

Post-MI management calls for strict adherence to a program of secondary prevention. Cardiac risk factors have to be excluded or modified, for instance, by reduction of overweight, cessation of smoking, optimal control of diabetes mellitus, and physical exercise (a dog that loves to run is an ideal training partner). Supportive pharmacotherapeutic measures include administration of platelet aggregation inhibitors, β-blockers, and ACE inhibitors.

A. Myocardial infarction: pharmacotherapeutic approaches

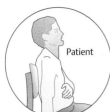

Patient

Acute symptoms:
severe pain
sense of impending
doom
fear of dying

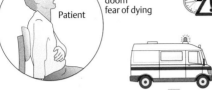

Acute care measures
– Nitroglycerin (reduction of
  pre- and afterload)
– Acetylsalicylic acid
  (if needed i.v.)
  (inhibition of platelet
  aggregation)
– Morphine (analgesia, sedation)
– Oxygen via nasal tube

Hospitalization
with minimal delay

Acute coronary syndrome
Angina pectoris > 20 min

Plaque rupture

Distal
thrombus

Thrombus

Hospital

ECG	ST-elevation	No ST-elevation	
Laboratory	CK-MB↑ Troponin-I, -T↑	Troponin-I, -T↑	–
Diagnosis	Myocardial infarction ("STEMI")	Myocardial infarction ("NSTEMI")	Unstable angina pectoris
Therapy	General: O₂, acetylsalicylic acid, heparin, nitrates, β-blocker, morphine		Acetylsalicylic acid, clopidrogel
	PTCA (Stent) GPIIb/IIIa-Antagonist or fibrinolysis or bypass surgery	PTCA (Stent) GPIIb/IIIa-Antagonist	Cardiac catheterization

Secondary prevention   Discharge

– Acetylsalicylic acid
– β-Blocker
– ACE inhibitor

possibly:
– Clopidrogel
– Phenprocoumon
– Statins

□ Congestive Heart Failure

In chronic congestive heart failure, cardiac pump performance falls below a level required by the body's organs for maintaining function and metabolism. The most common primary causes of heart failure are coronary disease, hypertension, volume overload, or cardiomyopathies. Diminished cardiac performance leads to a precardial congestion of venous blood. Congestion in front of the left ventricle causes dyspnea and pulmonary edema. Ankle edemas, enlarged liver, and ascites signal congestion in front of the right ventricle.

The degree of severity of myocardial failure is categorized according to the New York Heart Association (NYHA) Functional Classification System. Stages I–IV reflect an increasing level of disability.

The decrease in cardiac function activates several **compensatory mechanisms** that operate to maintain perfusion of organs. These include activation of the sympathetic nerve system and of the renin–angiotensin system. Increased release of norepinephrine raises cardiac rate and evokes peripheral vasoconstriction. Increased production of angiotensin II promotes both vasoconstriction and release of aldosterone from the adrenals. These compensations increase cardiac afterload and plasma volume is expanded because the kidney retains water and sodium. Although such "auxiliary" countermeasures afford transient help in maintaining cardiac output, (nor)epinephrine, aldosterone, and angiotensin II promote the progression of myocardial insufficiency: hypertrophy and fibrosis are the outcome. Successful therapy of chronic congestive failure is therefore contingent on **inhibition of compensation mechanisms**.

Although **β-blockers** were formerly held to be contraindicated, this drug class has been used successfully since the mid-1990s in the management of heart failure. A prerequisite is to begin therapy with very small daily doses. Every 2–3 weeks, the daily dose can be increased in small increments, as long as the patient does not develop bradycardia. Since bisoprolol, metoprolol, and carvedilol have proved effective in large clinical trials, these β-blockers would be the preferred choice for this indication.

ACE inhibitors are the appropriate agents for inhibiting the **renin–angiotensin II system**; they prevent the production of angiotensin II. The effect of angiotensin II receptor antagonists is equivalent to that of ACE inhibitors. Both interventions for attenuating compensatory mechanisms improve the clinical state of patients (less hospitalization) and increase life expectancy.

In edemas, dyspnea, and advanced myocardial insufficiency, **diuretics** are indispensable.

Digitalis glycosides augment contractile force and are likewise used in severe forms of insufficiency, specifically in the presence of concomitant atrial fibrillation. Because of the narrow margin of safety, the digoxin dose must be adjusted individually in each patient.

Drugs with an acute positive inotropic action (e.g., catecholamines or phosphodiesterase inhibitors) may be of transient help in sudden decompensation but must not be given in chronic congestive failure.

A. Congestive heart failure

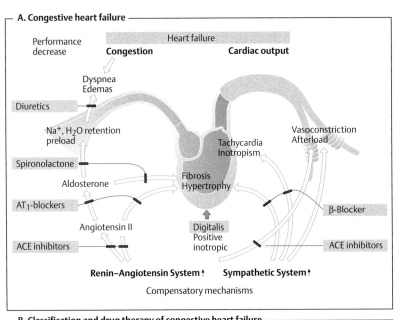

Heart failure

Performance decrease

Congestion   **Cardiac output**

Dyspnea
Edemas

Diuretics

Na$^+$, H$_2$O retention
preload

Spironolactone

Aldosterone

AT$_1$-blockers

Angiotensin II

ACE inhibitors

Tachycardia
Inotropism

Vasoconstriction
Afterload

Fibrosis
Hypertrophy

β-Blocker

Digitalis
Positive
inotropic

ACE inhibitors

Renin–Angiotensin System↑   **Sympathetic System↑**

Compensatory mechanisms

B. Classification and drug therapy of congestive heart failure

Impairment of cardiac function

NYHA Functional Class	I	II	III	IV
Clinical symptoms	—	slight	marked	at rest
ACE inhibitors	+	+	+	+
AT$_1$ blocker	when ACE inhibitors cause adverse effects, e.g., cough			
β-Blocker	Infarction Hypertension	+	+	+
Diuretics	Hypertension Edemas	+	+	+
Aldosterone antagonists	—	Hypokalemia	+	+
Digitalis	Atrial fibrillation	Atrial fibrillation	+	+

□ Hypotension

The venous side of the circulation accommodates ~85% of the total blood volume; because of the low venous pressure (mean ~15 mmHg), it is referred to as the *low-pressure system*. The arterial vascular beds, representing the *high-pressure system* (mean pressure ~100 mmHg), contain ~15%. The arterial pressure generates the driving force for perfusion of tissues and organs. Blood draining from these collects in the low-pressure system and is pumped back by the heart into the high-pressure system.

The arterial blood pressure (ABP) depends on: (1) the volume of blood per unit of time that is forced by the heart into the high-pressure system—cardiac output corresponding to the product of stroke volume and heart rate (beats/min), stroke volume being determined by, inter alia, venous filling pressure; (2) the counterforce opposing the flow of blood, i.e., peripheral resistance, which is a function of arteriolar caliber.

Chronic hypotension (recumbent systolic BP < 105 mmHg). *Primary idiopathic hypotension* generally has no clinical importance. If symptoms such as lassitude and dizziness occur, a program of physical exercise instead of drugs is advisable.

Secondary hypotension is a sign of an underlying disease that should be treated first. If stroke volume is too low, as in heart failure, a cardiac glycoside can be given to increase myocardial contractility and stroke volume. When stroke volume is decreased owing to insufficient blood volume, plasma substitutes will be helpful in treating blood loss, whereas aldosterone deficiency requires administration of a mineralocorticoid (e.g., fludrocortisone). The latter is the drug of choice for orthostatic hypotension due to autonomic failure. A parasympatholytic (or electrical pacemaker) can restore cardiac rate in bradycardia.

Acute hypotension. *Failure of orthostatic regulation.* A change from the recumbent to the erect position (orthostasis) will cause blood within the low-pressure system to sink toward the feet because the veins in body parts below the heart will be distended, despite a reflex venoconstriction, by the weight of the column of blood in the blood vessels. The fall in stroke volume is partly compensated by a rise in heart rate. The remaining reduction of cardiac output can be countered by elevating the peripheral resistance, enabling blood pressure and organ perfusion to be maintained. An orthostatic malfunction is present when counter-regulation fails and cerebral blood flow falls, with resultant symptoms, such as dizziness, "black-out," or even loss of consciousness. In the *sympathotonic form*, sympathetically-mediated circulatory reflexes are intensified (more pronounced tachycardia and rise in peripheral resistance, i.e., diastolic pressure); however, there is failure to compensate for the reduction in venous return. Prophylactic treatment with sympathomimetics would therefore hold little promise. Instead, cardiovascular fitness training would appear more important. An increase in venous return may be achieved in two ways. Increasing NaCl intake augments salt and fluid reserves and, hence, the blood volume (contraindications: hypertension, heart failure). Constriction of venous capacitance vessels might be produced by dihydroergotamine. Whether this effect could also be achieved by an α-sympathomimetic, remains debatable. In the very rare *asympathotonic form*, use of sympathomimetics would certainly be reasonable.

A. Treatment of hypotension

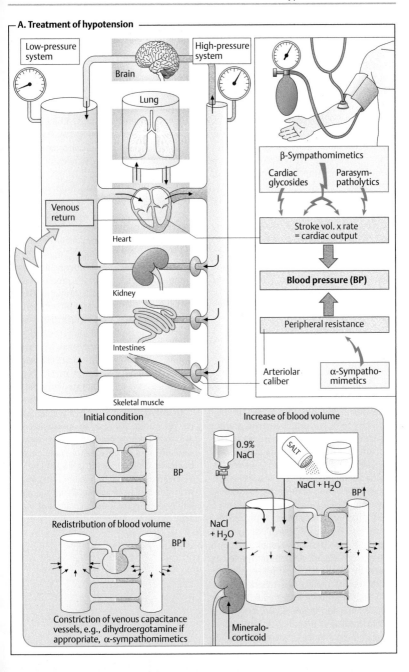

Low-pressure system

High-pressure system

Brain

Lung

Venous return

Heart

Kidney

Intestines

Skeletal muscle

β-Sympathomimetics

Cardiac glycosides

Parasympatholytics

Stroke vol. × rate = cardiac output

Blood pressure (BP)

Peripheral resistance

Arteriolar caliber

α-Sympathomimetics

Initial condition

BP

Increase of blood volume

0.9% NaCl

SALT

NaCl + H₂O

BP↑

Redistribution of blood volume

BP↑

NaCl + H₂O

Constriction of venous capacitance vessels, e.g., dihydroergotamine if appropriate, α-sympathomimetics

Mineralocorticoid

☐ **Gout**

Gout is an inherited metabolic disease that results from **hyperuricemia**, an elevation in the blood of uric acid, the end-product of purine degradation. Uric acid is not readily water-soluble; it therefore tends to crystallize at unphysiologically elevated concentrations, predominantly in bradytrophic tissues (such as the metatarsophalangeal joint). Like other crystals, urate crystals provide a strong stimulus for neutrophilic granulocytes and macrophages. Neutrophils are attracted (**1**) and phagocytose (**2**) this indigestible material. In the process, neutrophils release (**3**) proinflammatory cytokines. Macrophages also phagocytose the crystals, injure themselves, and liberate lysosomal enzymes that likewise promote inflammation and attack tissues. As a result, an acute and very painful gout attack may develop (**4**).

The **therapy** of gout is twofold: (1) treatment of the acute attack; and (2) chronic lowering of hyperuricemia.

1. The **acute attack** demands prompt action to relieve the patient from his painful state. The classical remedy (already used by Hippocrates) is **colchicine**, an alkaloid from the autumn crocus (*Colchicum autumnale*). This substance binds with high affinity to microtubular proteins and impairs their function, causing inter alia arrest of mitosis at metaphase ("spindle poison"). Its acute antigout activity is due to inhibition of neutrophil and macrophage reactions. The details of these mechanisms are not completely clear; at any rate, release of proinflammatory cytokines is prevented.

Colchicine is usually given orally (e.g., 0.5 mg hourly up to a maximum daily dose of 8 mg). Colchicine therapy is limited by injury to the gastrointestinal epithelium, which divides rapidly and therefore reacts with high sensitivity to the spindle poison. Nonsteroidal anti-inflammatory drugs, such as diclofenac and indometacin, are also effective; on occasion, glucocorticoids may be of additional help.

2. **Chronic lowering** of urate levels below 6 mg/l blood requires (a) an appropriate **diet** that avoids purine (cell nuclei)-rich foods (e.g., organ offal); and (b) **uricostatics for decreasing uric acid production.**

Allopurinol, as well as its accumulating metabolite, oxypurinol ("alloxanthine"), inhibits xanthine oxidase, which catalyzes urate formation from hypoxanthine via xanthine. These precursors are readily eliminated via the urine. Allopurinol is given orally (300–800 mg/day). Apart from infrequent allergic reactions, it is well tolerated and is the drug of choice for gout prophylaxis. Gout attacks may occur at the start of therapy but they can be prevented by concurrent administration of colchicine (0.5–1.5 mg/day).

Uricosurics, such as **probenecid** or **benzbromarone** (100 mg/day), promote renal excretion of uric acid. They saturate the organic acid transport system in the proximal renal tubules, making it unavailable for urate reabsorption. When underdosed, they inhibit only the acid secretory system, which has a smaller transport capacity. Urate elimination is then inhibited and a gout attack is possible. In patients with urate stones in the urinary tract, uricosurics are contraindicated.

Uricolytics. Nonprimates are able, via the enzyme urate oxidase, to metabolize uric acid to allantoin, a product with better water solubility and faster renal elimination. **Rasburicase**, a recombinant urate oxidase, can be given by infusion in patients with malignant neoplasias, in whom chemotherapy is liable to generate a massive amount of uric acid.

A. Gout and its therapy

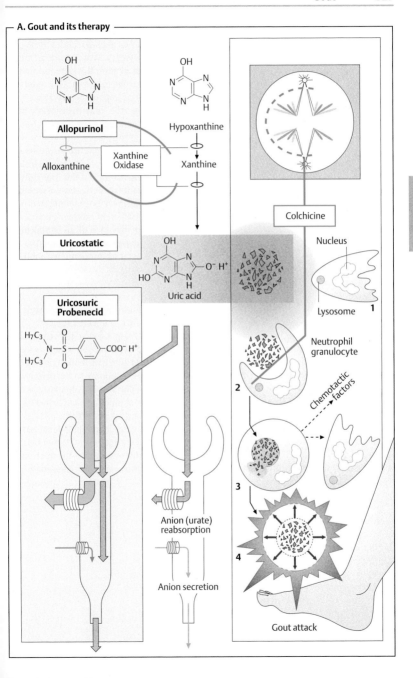

Allopurinol

Hypoxanthine

Xanthine Oxidase

Alloxanthine

Xanthine

Uricostatic

Colchicine

Uric acid

OH

$O^- H^+$

Nucleus

Lysosome **1**

Uricosuric Probenecid

H_7C_3

H_7C_3

$COO^- H^+$

Neutrophil granulocyte

2

Chemotactic factors

3

Anion (urate) reabsorption

Anion secretion

4

Gout attack

☐ Obesity—Sequelae and Therapeutic Approaches

In industrialized nations, a significant portion of the population is overweight. The **Body-Mass-Index** (BMI) provides a reliable and simple quantitative criterion for assessing this condition; it is calculated as follows:

$$BMI = \frac{\text{body weight in kg}}{\text{square of body height in m}}$$

Normal values range from 22 to 28. Values > 30 are indicative of an overweight condition. Obesity is always the consequence of a disturbed energy balance: caloric intake exceeds consumption. Almost unavoidably, excess body weight and obesity lead to diseases and a shortened lifespan.

The most important **secondary disorders** include development of type II diabetes mellitus, which alone shortens life, and hypertension, which together with disturbed lipid metabolism gives rise to atherosclerosis (angina pectoris, inadequate cerebral blood flow, etc.). Owing to the constant mechanical stress, weight-bearing joints suffer, resulting in arthrotic complaints. Finally, obesity gives rise to psychological problems that may overwhelm the coping ability of both adults and children.

The **treatment** of obesity—and it should be treated to safeguard normal life expectancy—is extraordinarily difficult. Although the principle "eat much less, move much more" is so simple, no more than a depressingly low percentage of patients can be relieved of their condition. Not until the obese individual, after sufficient counseling, realizes that he or she needs to make a change in lifestyle and can then muster sufficient self-discipline to stick to the "new life," will a return to normal body weight and protection from secondary diseases be achieved. Requisite changes include a diet low in fat with reduced caloric content (~ 1000 kcal/day), no snacks (sweets, potato chips, lemonades, beer, etc.), and plenty of physical exercise (sports, hiking, swimming, tennis, etc. instead of the TV easy-chair). Under these conditions, body weight will drop slowly; dramatic changes of several kilograms in a few days are not to be expected. This reduction therapy must be kept up for months.

Regrettably, the pharmacologist must confess that no drugs exist that can be recommended for the purpose of weight reduction. The so-called **appetite suppressants** (anorexiants) act only, if at all, for a limited period and are fraught with side effects. Most anorexiants are derivatives of methamphetamine that have been withdrawn from the market. A different mechanism of action is involved in the case of an **inhibitor of pancreatic lipase**, which is required in the intestines for fat absorption. This inhibitor (*orlistat*) diminishes fat absorption so that fats reach the lower bowel, where they can cause disturbances: flatulence, steatorrhea, and frequent need to relieve the bowels occur in about 30% of affected subjects. These symptoms correspond exactly to those seen in pancreatic hypofunction which are then usually treated with pancreatic lipase. Before an obese person submits to treatment with orlistat, he or she should voluntarily reduce the food fat content by one half to live free of such unpleasant adverse effects.

In summary, the obese individual has no choice but to normalize the energy balance under sympathetic guidance and by strength of will, and thus evade any secondary diseases.

A. Obesity: Sequelae and therapeutic approaches

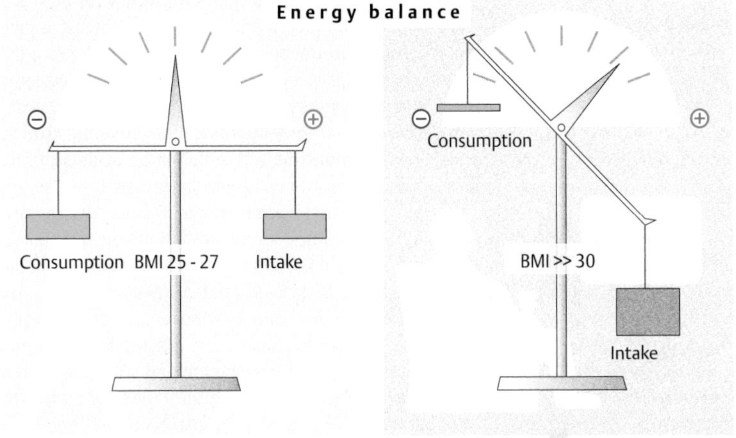

Energy balance

$\ominus$ Consumption BMI 25 - 27 Intake $\oplus$

$\ominus$ Consumption BMI >> 30 Intake $\oplus$

Consequences: life expectancy↓

Diabetes mellitus

Hyperlipoproteinemia

Hypertension

Joint mechanical stress

Psychosocial problems

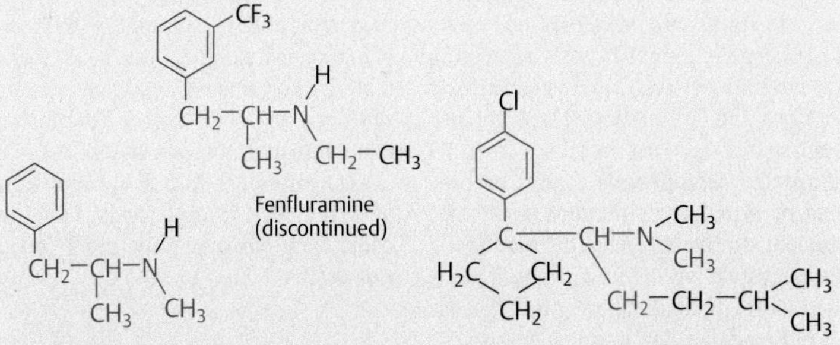

Therapy

Caloric restriction
Intensive psychological counseling,
much exercise

Drugs

Anorexiants
Methamphetamine
derivatives
Sibutramine

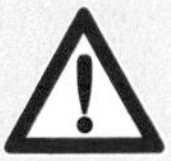

Lipase inhibitor orlistat

CF$_3$

CH$_2$-CH-N-CH$_2$-CH$_3$
   | |
   CH$_3$ H

Fenfluramine
(discontinued)

CH$_2$-CH-N-CH$_3$
   | |
   CH$_3$ H

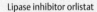

Methamphetamine (controlled substance)

Cl

C-CH-N-CH$_3$
        | |
        CH$_3$
H$_2$C CH$_2$
   CH$_2$ CH$_2$-CH$_2$-CH-CH$_3$
                        |
                        CH$_3$

Sibutramine

□ Osteoporosis

Osteoporosis is defined as a generalized decrease in bone mass (osteopenia) that equally affects bone matrix and mineral content and is associated with a change in spongiosal architecture. This condition predisposes to collapse of vertebral bodies and bone fractures with trivial trauma (e. g., hip fractures).

Bone substance is subject to continual remodeling. The equilibrium between bone formation and bone resorption is regulated in a complex manner: a remodeling cycle is initiated by osteoblasts when these stimulate uninucleated osteoclast precursor cells to fuse into large multinucleated cells. Stimulation occurs by direct cell-to-cell contact between osteoblasts and osteoclast precursor cells and is mediated by the RANK ligand on the surface of osteoblasts and its receptor on the osteoclasts (or their precursors), as well as cytokines secreted by osteoblasts. These processes are inhibited by estrogens and a protein secreted by osteoblasts (osteoprotegerin). The osteoclast creates an acidic milieu, enabling minerals to be solubilized, and then phagocytoses the organic matrix. Hormones regulate these events.

In hypocalcemia, the parathyroid increases its secretion of **parathormone**, resulting in enhanced liberation of Ca^{2+}. **Calcitonin** transfers active osteoclasts into a resting state. Calcitonin given therapeutically relieves pain associated with neoplastic bone metastases and vertebral body collapse. Estrogens diminish bone resorption by (a) inhibiting activation of osteoclasts by osteoblasts and (b) promoting apoptosis of osteoclasts.

Idiopathic osteoporosis cannot be prevented by prophylactic therapy, but its development can be delayed. This requires: a healthy lifestyle with plenty of physical exercise (sports, hiking), daily intake of calcium (1000 mg/day Ca^{2+}) and of vitamin D (1000 IU/day). The same principle holds for **postmenopausal osteoporosis**. Hormone replacement therapy in postmenopausal women has not been successful because of an increased incidence of breast cancers, thromboembolism, and other adverse effects (p. 250). Long-term hormone replacement therapy should no longer be carried out.

If osteoporosis has become clinically manifest, attempts can be made at improving the condition by means of drugs, or at least slowing down further deterioration. Besides administration of calcium and vitamin D, the following options are available.

Bisphosphonates (N-containing) structurally mimic endogenous pyrophosphate (see formulae), and like the latter are incorporated into the mineral substance of bone. During phagocytosis of the bone matrix, they are taken up by osteoclasts. There, the N-containing bisphosphonates inhibit prenylation of G-proteins and thus damage the cells. Accordingly, osteoclast activity levels are lowered by **alendronate** and **risedronate**, while osteoclast apoptosis is promoted. The result is a reduction in bone resorption and a decreased risk of bone fractures.

Raloxifene exerts an estrogen-like effect on bone, while acting as an estrogen antagonist in the uterus and breast tissue (p. 254). In terms of fracture prophylaxis, its effectiveness appears inferior to that of bisphosphonates. Thromboembolism and edema are reported as adverse effects.

It should also be mentioned that intermittent slight elevation in the plasma concentration of parathormone leads to increased formation of bone substance. The likely explanation is that, under this condition, stimulation of osteoblasts is sufficient to induce synthesis of bone matrix but not strong enough to activate osteoclasts. This strategy is applied therapeutically by administration of a fragment (amino acids 1–34) of recombinant human parathormone (**teriparatide**, s.c.).

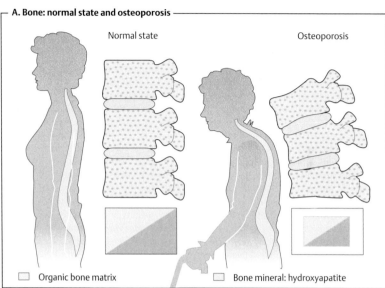

A. Bone: normal state and osteoporosis

Normal state

Osteoporosis

☐ Organic bone matrix

☐ Bone mineral: hydroxyapatite

B. Regulation of bone remodeling

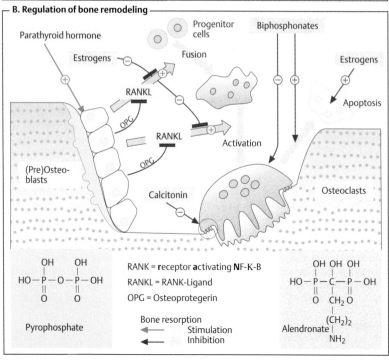

Parathyroid hormone

Estrogens ⊖

Progenitor cells

Biphosphonates

Fusion

Estrogens ⊕

RANKL

⊕

Apoptosis

OPG

⊖

RANKL

⊕

Activation

OPG

(Pre)Osteo-blasts

Calcitonin ⊖

Osteoclasts

$$HO-\overset{\overset{\displaystyle OH}{|}}{\underset{\underset{\displaystyle O}{||}}{P}}-O-\overset{\overset{\displaystyle OH}{|}}{\underset{\underset{\displaystyle O}{||}}{P}}-OH$$

Pyrophosphate

RANK = **r**eceptor **a**ctivating **N**F-K-B
RANKL = RANK-Ligand
OPG = Osteoprotegerin

Bone resorption
⟵ Stimulation
⟵ Inhibition

$$HO-\overset{\overset{\displaystyle OH}{|}}{\underset{\underset{\displaystyle O}{||}}{P}}-\overset{\overset{\displaystyle OH}{|}}{\underset{\underset{\displaystyle CH_2}{|}}{C}}-\overset{\overset{\displaystyle OH}{|}}{\underset{\underset{\displaystyle O}{||}}{P}}-OH$$

$(CH_2)_2$

Alendronate |
NH_2

□ Rheumatoid Arthritis

Rheumatoid arthritis or **chronic polyarthritis** (**A**) is a progressive inflammatory joint disease that intermittently attacks more and more joints, predominantly those of the fingers and toes. The probable cause of rheumatoid arthritis is a pathological reaction of the immune system. This malfunction can be promoted or triggered by various conditions, including genetic disposition, age-related wear and tear, hypothermia, and infection. An initial noxious stimulus elicits an **inflammation of synovial membranes** that, in turn, leads to release of antigens through which the inflammatory process is maintained.

The antigen is taken up by synovial antigen-presenting cells; lymphocytes, including T-helper cells (p. 304), are activated and start to proliferate. In the process of interaction between lymphocytes and macrophages, the intensity of inflammation increases. Macrophages release proinflammatory messengers; among these, interleukin-1 and tumor necrosis factor α (TNFα) are important. TNFα is able to elicit a multiplicity of proinflammatory actions (**B**) that benefit defense against infectious pathogens but are detrimental in rheumatoid arthritis. The cytokines stimulate gene expression for COX-2; inflammation-promoting prostanoids are produced. The inflammatory reaction increases activity of lymphocytes and macrophages, initiating a vicious circle. Synovial fibroblasts proliferate and release destructive enzymes; the inflamed characteristic pannus tissue develops and destructively invades joint cartilage and subjacent bone. Ultimately, ankylosis (loss of joint motion or bone fusion) with connective tissue scar formation occurs. Concomitant extra-articular disease may be superimposed. The disease process is associated with strong pain and restriction of mobility.

Pharmacotherapy. Acute relief of inflammatory symptoms can be achieved by **prostaglandin synthase inhibitors** (p. 200; nonselective COX inhibitors or COX-2 inhibitors) and by **glucocorticoids** (p. 244). The inevitably chronic use of both groups of substances is likely to cause significant *adverse effects*. Neither can halt the progressive destruction of joints.

Substances that are able to reduce the requirement for nonsteroidal anti-inflammatory drugs and to slow disease progression are labeled **disease-modifying agents**. Early use of these drugs is recommended. Their effect develops only after treatment for several weeks. Proliferation of lymphocytes can be slowed by **methotrexate** (p. 304) and **leflunomide**, which reduces the availability of pyrimidine nucleotides in lymphocytes (via inhibition of dihydroorotate dehydrogenase). For ciclosporin, see p. 306. In addition, use is made of immune suppressants such as **azathioprine** and **cyclophosphamide**. Intralysosomal accumulation and impaired phagocytic function may be involved in the action of chloroquine or **hydroxychloroquine**, as well as **gold compounds** (i.m.: aurothioglucose or aurothiomalate; oral: auranofin, less effective). The antibodies, **infliximab** and **adalimumab**, as well as the fusion protein **etanercept** intercept TNF-α molecules, preventing them from interacting with membrane receptors of target cells. **Anakinra** is a recombinant analogue of the endogenous interleukin-1 antagonist. The mechanisms of action of D-penicillamine and sulfasalazine are unknown. Same of the drugs mentioned possess considerable potential for adverse effects. **Sulfasalazine** and **methotrexate** exhibit a relatively favorable risk–benefit ratio. Combination of disease-modifying drugs is possible.

Surgical removal of the inflamed synovial membrane (synovectomy) frequently provides long-term relief. If feasible, this approach is preferred because all pharmacotherapeutic measures entail significant adverse effects.

A. Rheumatoid Arthritis

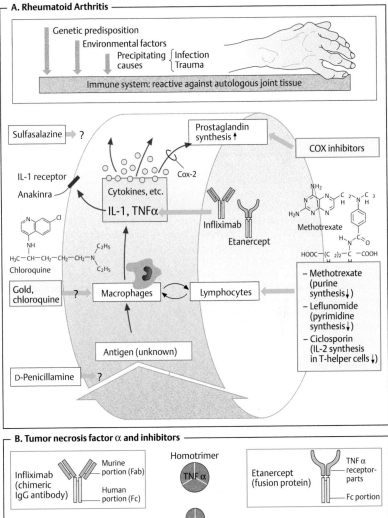

Genetic predisposition

Environmental factors

Precipitating causes { Infection / Trauma

Immune system: reactive against autologous joint tissue

Sulfasalazine → ?

Prostaglandin synthesis ↑

COX inhibitors

IL-1 receptor

Anakinra

Cytokines, etc.

Cox-2

IL-1, TNFα

Infliximab

Etanercept

Chloroquine

Methotrexate

Gold, chloroquine → ?

Macrophages ⇄ Lymphocytes

– Methotrexate (purine synthesis↓)
– Leflunomide (pyrimidine synthesis↓)
– Ciclosporin (IL-2 synthesis in T-helper cells ↓)

Antigen (unknown)

D-Penicillamine → ?

B. Tumor necrosis factor α and inhibitors

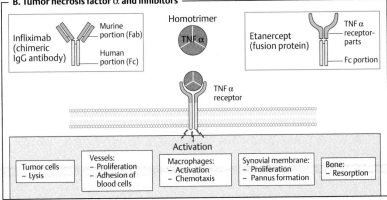

Infliximab (chimeric IgG antibody)

Murine portion (Fab)

Human portion (Fc)

Homotrimer

TNF α

Etanercept (fusion protein)

TNF α receptor-parts

Fc portion

TNF α receptor

Activation

| Tumor cells – Lysis | Vessels: – Proliferation – Adhesion of blood cells | Macrophages: – Activation – Chemotaxis | Synovial membrane: – Proliferation – Pannus formation | Bone: – Resorption |

☐ Migraine

Migraine is a syndrome characterized by recurrent attacks of intense headache and nausea that occur at irregular intervals and last for several hours. In classical migraine, the attack is typically heralded by an "aura" accompanied by spreading homonymous visual field defects with colored sharp edges ("fortification" spectra). In addition, the patient cannot focus on certain objects, has a ravenous appetite for particular foods, and is hypersensitive to odors (hyperosmia) or light (photophobia). The exact cause of these complaints is unknown; conceivably, the underlying pathogenetic mechanisms involve local release of proinflammatory mediators from nociceptive primary afferents (neurogenic inflammation) or a disturbance in cranial blood flow. In addition to an often inherited predisposition, precipitating factors are required to provoke an attack, e.g., psychic stress, lack of sleep, certain foods. Pharmacotherapy of migraine has two aims: stopping the acute attack and preventing subsequent ones.

Treatment of the attack. For symptomatic relief, headaches are treated with analgesics (acetaminophen, acetylsalicylic acid), and nausea is treated with metoclopramide (pp. 116, 342) or domperidone. Since there is delayed gastric emptying during the attack, drug absorption can be markedly retarded and hence effective plasma levels are not obtained. Because metoclopramide stimulates gastric emptying, it promotes absorption of ingested analgesic drugs and thus facilitates pain relief.

If acetylsalicylic acid is administered i.v. as the lysine salt, its bioavailability is complete. Therefore, i.v. injection may be advisable in acute attacks.

Should analgesics prove insufficiently effective, **sumatriptan** (prototype of the triptans) or **ergotamine** may help prevent an imminent attack in many cases. Both substances are effective in migraine and cluster headaches but not in other forms of headache. The probable common mechanism of action is a stimulation of serotonin receptors of the 5-HT$_{1D}$ subtype. Moreover, ergotamine has affinity for dopamine receptors (→nausea, emesis), as well as α-adrenoceptors and 5-HT$_2$ receptors (↑ vascular tone, ↑ platelet aggregation). With frequent use, the vascular side effects may give rise to severe peripheral ischemia (ergotism). Paradoxically, overuse of ergotamine (> once per week) may provoke "rebound" headaches, thought to result from persistent vasodilation. Though different in character (tension-type headache), these prompt further consumption of ergotamine. Thus, a vicious circle develops with chronic abuse of ergotamine or other analgesics that may end with irreversible disturbances of peripheral blood flow and impairment of renal function.

Administered orally, ergotamine and sumatriptan have only limited bioavailability. Dihydroergotamine may be given by i.m. or slow i.v. injection, sumatriptan subcutaneously, by nasal spray, or as a suppository. When given orally, other triptans such as **zolmitriptan**, **naratriptan**, and **rizatriptan** have higher bioavailability than sumatriptan.

Prophylaxis. Taken regularly over a longer period, a heterogeneous group of drugs comprising propranolol, nadolol, atenolol, and metoprolol (β-blockers), flunarizine (H$_1$-histamine, dopamine, and calcium antagonist), pizotifen (pizotyline, 5-HT antagonist with structural resemblance to tricyclic antidepressants), and methysergide (partial 5-HT antagonist) may decrease the frequency, intensity, and duration of migraine attacks. The drug of first choice is one of the β-blockers mentioned.

A: Migraine and its treatment

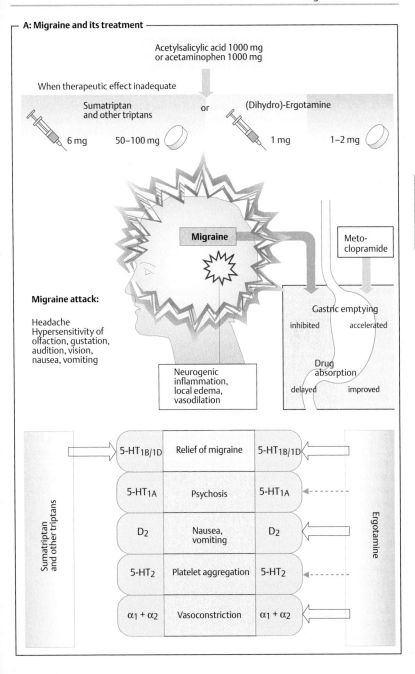

☐ Common Cold

The **common cold**—colloquially the flu, catarrh, or grippe (strictly speaking the rarer infection with influenza viruses)—is an acute infectious inflammation of the upper respiratory tract. Its symptoms—sneezing, running nose (due to rhinitis), hoarseness (laryngitis), difficulty in swallowing and sore throat (pharyngitis and tonsillitis), cough associated with first serous then mucous sputum (tracheitis, bronchitis), sore muscles, and general malaise—can be present individually or concurrently in varying combination or sequence. The term stems from an old popular belief that these complaints are caused by exposure to chilling or dampness. The causative pathogens are different viruses (rhino-, adeno-, and parainfluenza viruses) that may be transmitted by aerosol droplets produced by coughing and sneezing.

Therapeutic measures. Causal treatment with a *virustatic* is not possible at present. Since cold symptoms abate spontaneously, there is no compelling need to use drugs. However, conventional remedies are intended for *symptomatic relief.*

Rhinitis. Nasal discharge could be prevented by *parasympatholytics*; however, other atropine-like effects (p. 108) would have to be accepted. Parasympatholytics are threfore hardly ever used, although a corresponding action is probably exploited in the case of H_1-*antihistaminics*, an ingredient of many cold remedies. Locally applied (nasal drops), vasoconstricting α-sympathomimetics decongest the nasal mucosa and dry up secretions, clearing the nasal passage. Long-term use may cause damage to nasal mucous membranes (p. 94).

Sore throat, swallowing problems. Demulcent lozenges containing *surface anesthetics* such as lidocaine (caveat: benzocaine and tetracaine contain an allergenic *p*-aminophenyl group; p. 207) may provide short-term relief; however, the risk of allergic reactions should be kept in mind.

Cough. Since coughing serves to expel excess tracheobronchial secretions, suppression of this physiological reflex is justified only when coughing is dangerous (after surgery) or unproductive because of absent secretions. *Codeine* and *noscapine* (p. 210) suppress cough by a central action. A different, though incompletely understood, mechanism of action is evident in antitussives such as clobutinol, which do not derive from opium. The available clinical studies concerning the benefits of antitussives in common colds do not present a convincing picture.

Mucous airway obstruction. Expectorants are meant to promote clearing of bronchial mucus by a liquefying action that involves either cleavage of mucous substances (mucolytics) or stimulation of production of watery mucus (e. g., hot beverages). Whether mucolytics are indicated in the common cold and whether expectorants such as bromohexine or ambroxole effectively lower viscosity of bronchial secretions may be questioned. In clinical studies of chronic obstructive bronchitis (but not common cold infections), *N*-acetylcysteine was shown to have clinical effectiveness, as evidenced by a lowered incidence of exacerbations during chronic intake.

Fever. *Antipyretic analgesics* (acetylsalicylic acid, acetaminophen, p. 198) are indicated only when there is high fever. Fever is a natural response and useful in monitoring the clinical course of an infection.

Muscle aches and pains, headache. *Antipyretic analgesics* are effective in relieving these symptoms.

A. Drugs used in common cold

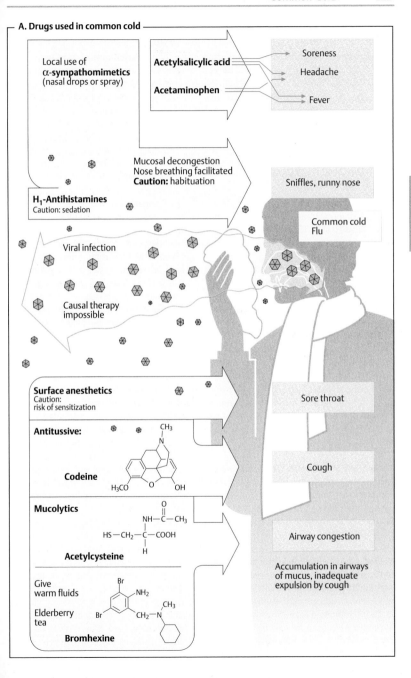

Local use of
α-sympathomimetics
(nasal drops or spray)

Acetylsalicylic acid → Soreness
→ Headache
Acetaminophen → Fever

Mucosal decongestion
Nose breathing facilitated
Caution: habituation

Sniffles, runny nose

H₁-Antihistamines
Caution: sedation

Common cold
Flu

Viral infection

Causal therapy
impossible

Surface anesthetics
Caution:
risk of sensitization

Sore throat

Antitussive:

CH₃

Codeine

H₃CO   O   OH

Cough

Mucolytics

O
‖
NH—C—CH₃
|
HS—CH₂—C—COOH
|
H

Acetylcysteine

Airway congestion

Give
warm fluids

Elderberry
tea

Br   NH₂

Br   CH₂—N   CH₃

Bromhexine

Accumulation in airways
of mucus, inadequate
expulsion by cough

□ Atopy and Antiallergic Therapy

Atopy denotes a hereditary predisposition for IgE-mediated allergic reactions. Clinical pictures include allergic rhinoconjunctivitis ("hay fever"), bronchial asthma, atopic dermatitis (neurodermatitis, atopic eczema) and urticaria. Evidently, differentiation of T-helper (TH) lymphocytes toward the TH$_2$ phenotype is the common denominator. Therapeutic interventions are aimed at different levels to influence pathophysiological events (**A**).

1. Specific immune therapy ("hyposensitization") with intracutaneous antigen injections is intended to shift TH cells in the direction of TH$_1$.

2. Inactivation of IgE can be achieved by means of the monoclonal antibody, omalizumab. This is directed against the Fc portion of IgE and prevents its binding to mast cells.

3. Stabilization of mast cells. *Cromolyn* prevents IgE-mediated release of mast cell mediators, although only after *chronic treatment*. It is applied *locally* to conjunctiva, nasal mucosa, the bronchial tree (inhalation), and intestinal mucosa (absorption is almost nil with oral intake). Indications: *prophylaxis of hay-fever, allergic asthma*, and *food allergies*. Nedocromil acts similarly.

4. Blockade of histamine receptors. Allergic reactions are predominantly mediated by H$_1$ receptors. *H$_1$-antihistaminics* (p.118) are mostly used orally. Their therapeutic effect is often disappointing. Indications: allergic rhinitis (*hay fever*).

5. Blockade of leukotriene receptors. Montelukast is an antagonist at receptors for (cysteinyl) leukotriene. Leukotrienes evoke intense bronchoconstriction and promote allergic inflammation of the bronchial mucosa. Montelukast is used for oral prophylaxis of bronchial asthma. It is effective in analgesia-induced asthma (pp. 200, 340) and exercise-induced bronchospasm.

6. Functional antagonists of mediators of allergy.

a **α-Sympathomimetics**, such as naphazoline, oxymetazoline, and tetrahydrozoline, are applied topically to the conjunctival and nasal mucosa to produce local vasoconstriction. Their use should be short-term at most.

b **Epinephrine**, given i.v., is the *most important drug in the management of anaphylactic shock*: it constricts blood vessels, reduces capillary permeability, and dilates bronchi.

c **β$_2$-Sympathomimetics**, such as terbutaline, fenoterol, and albuterol, are employed in *bronchial asthma*, mostly by inhalation, and parenterally in emergencies. Even after inhalation, effective amounts can reach the systemic circulation and cause side effects (e. g., palpitations, tremulousness, restlessness, hypokalemia). The duration of action of both salmeterol and formoterol, given by inhalation, is 12 hours. These long-acting β$_2$-mimetics are included in the treatment of severe asthma. Given at nighttime, they can prevent attacks that preferentially occur in the early morning hours.

d **Theophylline** belongs to the methylxanthines. Its effects are attributed to both inhibition of phosphodiesterase (cAMP increase, p.66) and antagonism at adenosine receptors. In *bronchial asthma*, theophylline can be given orally for prophylaxis or parenterally to control the attack. Manifestations of overdosage include tonic-clonic seizures and cardiac arrhythmias (blood level monitoring).

e **Glucocorticoids** (p.244) have significant antiallergic activity and probably interfere with different stages of the allergic response. Indications: *hay fever, bronchial asthma* (preferably local application of analogues with high presystemic elimination, e. g., beclomethasone dipropionate, budesonide, flunisolide, fluticasone propionate); and *anaphylactic shock* (i.v. in high dosage)—a probably nongenomic action of immediate onset.

A. Atopy and antiallergic therapy

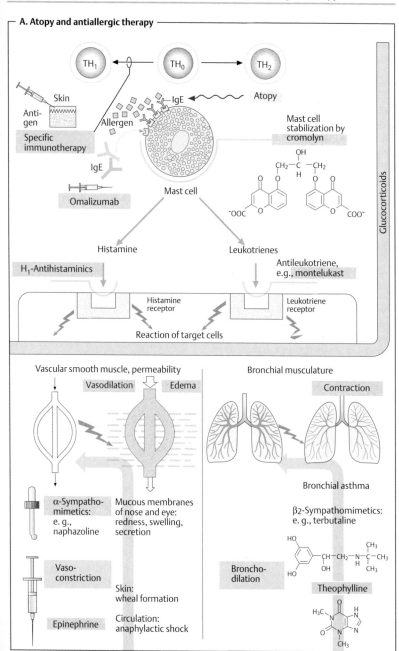

☐ Bronchial Asthma

Definition. A recurrent, episodic shortness of breath caused by bronchoconstriction arising from airway inflammation and hyperreactivity.

Pathophysiology. One of the main pathogenetic factors is an allergic inflammation of the bronchial mucosa. For instance, leukotrienes that are formed during an IgE-mediated immune response (p. 72) exert a chemotactic effect on inflammatory cells. As the inflammation develops, bronchi become globally hyperreactive to spasmogenic stimuli. Thus, stimuli other than the original antigen(s) can act as triggers (**A**); e. g., breathing of cold air is an important trigger in exercise-induced asthma. Cyclooxygenase inhibitors (p. 200) exemplify drugs acting as asthma triggers.

Management. Avoidance of asthma triggers is an important prophylactic measure, though not always feasible. Drugs that inhibit allergic inflammatory mechanisms or reduce bronchial hyperreactivity (*glucocorticoids,* "*mast-cell stabilizers,*" and *leukotriene antagonists*) attack crucial pathogenetic links. Bronchodilation is achieved by inhalation of β_2-sympathomimetics (with high presystemic elimination) or, in the case of chronic obstructive lung disease, the anticholinergic, tiotropium (long-acting; single daily dose).

The **step scheme** (**B**) illustrates successive levels of pharmacotherapeutic management at increasing degrees of disease severity.

Step 1. Medications of first choice for the acute attack are *short-acting, aerosolized β_2-sympathomimetics,* e. g., salbutamol or fenoterol. Their action occurs within minutes after inhalation and lasts for 4–6 hours.

Step 2. If β_2-mimetics have to be used more frequently than once a week, more severe disease is present. At this stage, management includes anti-inflammatory drugs, preferably an inhalable **glucocorticoid**

(p. 246). Inhalational treatment with glucocorticoids must be administered regularly, improvement being evident only after several weeks. With proper inhalational use of glucocorticoids undergoing high presystemic elimination, concern about systemic adverse effects ("cortisone fear") is unwarranted. Possible local adverse effects are oropharyngeal candidiasis and dysphonia. To minimize the risk of candidiasis, drug administration should occur before morning or evening meals. Alternatively, a "*mast-cell stabilizer*" (p. 118) given by inhalation may prove adequately successful. Oral administration of timed-release theophylline (p. 338) is considered a further alternative, particularly so since the effect of theophylline is thought to possess an additional inflammation-inhibiting component, apart from bronchodilation. The margin of safety is narrow (cardiac or CNS stimulation; plasma level controls!). A leukotriene antagonist (montelukast, p. 338) may also merit consideration.

Anti-inflammatory therapy is the more successful the less use is made of as-needed β_2-mimetic medication.

Step 3. Continuous bronchodilator treatment is added to the low-dose glucocorticoid regimen. Preference is given to local use of a *long-acting inhalable β_2-mimetic* (salmeterol or formoterol; p. 338). If this proves insufficient, the glucocorticoid dose is increased. Instead of a long-acting β_2-mimetic, oral administration of timed-release theophylline, of a controlled release β_2-agonist, or of a leukotriene antagonist would be possible.

Step 4. The dose of inhalable glucocorticoid is increased further. When this proves unsatisfactory, the active principles shown in (**B**) can be added on, including systemic administration of a glucocorticoid.

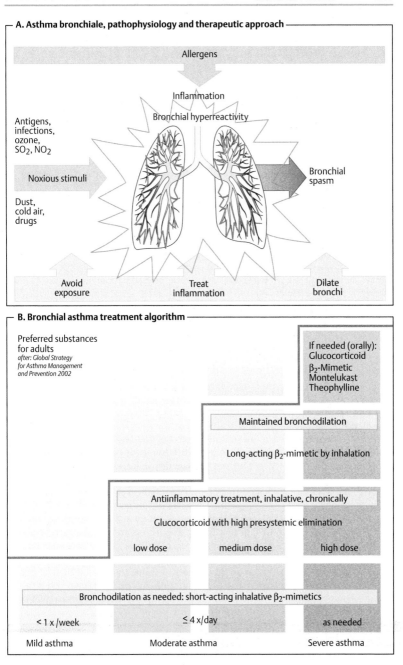

A. Asthma bronchiale, pathophysiology and therapeutic approach

Allergens

Inflammation
Bronchial hyperreactivity

Antigens,
infections,
ozone,
SO_2, NO_2

Noxious stimuli

Bronchial
spasm

Dust,
cold air,
drugs

Avoid
exposure

Treat
inflammation

Dilate
bronchi

B. Bronchial asthma treatment algorithm

Preferred substances
for adults
*after: Global Strategy
for Asthma Management
and Prevention 2002*

If needed (orally):
Glucocorticoid
β_2-Mimetic
Montelukast
Theophylline

Maintained bronchodilation

Long-acting β_2-mimetic by inhalation

Antiinflammatory treatment, inhalative, chronically

Glucocorticoid with high presystemic elimination

low dose   medium dose   high dose

Bronchodilation as needed: short-acting inhalative β_2-mimetics

< 1 x /week   ≤ 4 x/day   as needed

Mild asthma   Moderate asthma   Severe asthma

☐ Emesis

In emesis the stomach empties in a retrograde manner. The pyloric sphincter is closed while cardia and esophagus relax to allow gastric contents to be propelled orad by a forceful synchronous contraction of abdominal wall muscles and diaphragm. Closure of the glottis and elevation of the soft palate prevent entry of vomitus into the trachea and the nasopharynx. As a rule, there is prodromal salivation or yawning. Coordination between these different stages depends on the **medullary center for emesis**, which can be activated by diverse stimuli. These are conveyed via the **vestibular apparatus**, **visual**, **olfactory**, and **gustatory inputs**, as well as **viscerosensory afferents** from the upper alimentary tract. **Psychic stress** may also activate the emetic center. The mechanisms underlying **motion sickness** (kinetosis, sea sickness) and vomiting during pregnancy are still unclear.

Polar substances cannot reach the emetic center itself because it is protected by the blood–brain barrier. However, they can indirectly excite the center by activating chemoreceptors in the area postrema or receptors on peripheral vagal nerve endings.

Antiemetic therapy. Vomiting can be a useful reaction enabling the body to eliminate an orally ingested poison. Antiemetic drugs are used to prevent kinetosis, pregnancy vomiting, cytotoxic drug-induced or postoperative vomiting, as well as vomiting due to radiation therapy.

Motion sickness. Effective prophylaxis can be achieved with the parasympatholytic scopolamine (p. 110) and H_1-antihistaminics (p. 118) of the diphenylmethane type (e. g., diphenhydramine, meclizine). Antiemetic activity is not a property shared by all parasympatholytics or antihistaminics. The efficacy of the drugs mentioned depends on the actual situation of the individual (gastric filling, ethanol consumption), environmental conditions (e. g., the behavior of fellow travelers), and the type of motion experienced. The drugs should be taken 30 minutes before the start of travel and repeated every 4–6 hours. Scopolamine applied transdermally through an adhesive patch 6–8 hours before travel can provide effective protection for up to 3 days.

Pregnancy vomiting is prone to occur in the first trimester; thus, pharmacotherapy would coincide with the period of maximal fetal vulnerability to chemical injury. Accordingly, antiemetics (antihistaminics, or neuroleptics if required; p. 232) should be used only when continuous vomiting threatens to disturb electrolyte and water balance to a degree that places the fetus at risk.

Drug-induced vomiting. To prevent vomiting during anticancer chemotherapy (especially, with cisplatin), effective use can be made of $5-HT_3$ receptor antagonists (e. g., ondansetron, granisetron, and tropisetron), alone or in combination with glucocorticoids (methylprednisolone, dexamethasone). **Anticipatory nausea** and vomiting, resulting from inadequately controlled nausea and emesis in patients undergoing cytotoxic chemotherapy, can be attenuated by a benzodiazepine such as lorazepam. Dopamine agonist-induced nausea in parkinsonian patients (p. 188) can be counteracted with D_2-receptor antagonists that penetrate poorly into the CNS (e. g., domperidone, sulpiride). Metoclopramide is effective in nausea and vomiting of gastrointestinal origin ($5-HT_4$ receptor agonism) and at high dosage also in **chemotherapy-** and **radiation-induced sickness** (low potency antagonism at $5-HT_3$ and D_3-receptors). Phenothiazines (e. g., levomepromazine, trimeprazine, and perphenazine) or metoclopramide may suppress nausea/emesis that follows certain types of **surgery** or is due to opioid analgesics, gastrointestinal irritation, **uremia**, and diseases accompanied by **elevated intracranial pressure**.

The synthetic cannabinoids dronabinol and nabilone have antiemetic effects that may benefit AIDS and cancer patients.

A. Emetic stimuli and antiemetic drugs

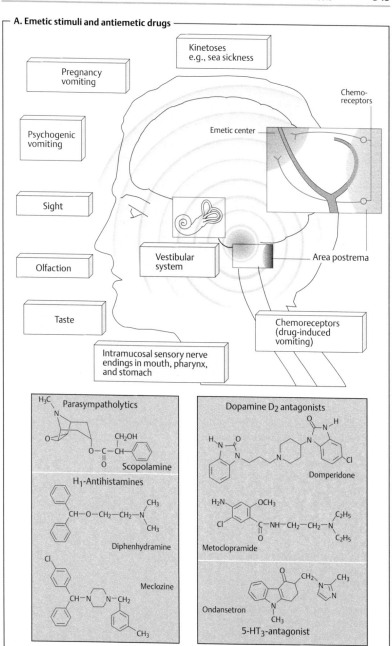

☐ Alcohol Abuse

Since prehistoric times, ethanol-containing beverages have enjoyed widespread use as a recreational luxury. What applies to any medicinal substance also holds for alcohol: the dose alone makes the poison (see p. 2). Excessive, long-term consumption of alcoholic drinks, or **alcohol abuse**, is harmful to the affected individual. Alcoholism must be considered a grave disorder that plays a major role in terms of numbers alone; for instance, in Germany 1 000 000 people are affected by this self-inflicted illness.

Ethanol is miscible with water and is well lipid-soluble, enabling it to penetrate easily through all barriers in the organism; the blood–brain barrier and the placental barrier are no obstacles. In liver cells, alcohol is broken down to acetic acid via acetaldehyde (**A**). Ethyl alcohol is never ingested as a chemically pure substance but in the form of an alcoholic beverage that contains flavoring agents and higher alcohols, depending on its origin. The effect desired by the consumer takes place in the brain: ethanol acts as a stimulant, it disinhibits, and it enhances sociability, as long as the beverage is enjoyed in moderate quantities. After higher doses, self-critical faculties are lost and motor function is impaired–the familiar picture of the drunk. Still higher doses induce a comatose state (caution: hypothermia and respiratory paralysis). The complex effects on the CNS cannot be ascribed to a simple mechanism of action. An inhibitory effect on the NMDA subtype of glutamate receptor appears to predominate.

In chronic alcohol abuse, mainly two organs are damaged:

1. In the **liver**, hepatocytes may initially undergo fatty degeneration, this process being reversible. With continued exposure, liver cells die and are replaced by connective tissue newly formed from myofibroblasts: liver cirrhosis. Hepatic blood flow is greatly reduced; the organ becomes unable to fulfill its detoxification function (danger of hepatic coma). Collateral circulation routes develop (bleeding from esophageal varicose veins) with production of ascites. Alcoholic liver cirrhosis is a severe, mostly progressive disease that permits only symptomatic therapy (**B**).

2. The functional capacity of the **brain** is impaired. Irreversible damage may manifest in a measurable fallout of neuronal cell bodies. Often delirium tremens develops (usually triggered by alcohol withdrawal), which can be managed with intensive therapy (clomethiazole, haloperidol, among others). In addition, alcoholic hallucinations and Wernicke–Korsakow syndrome occur. All of these are desolate states.

It must be pointed out specifically that alcohol abuse during pregnancy leads to (**embryo–fetal alcohol syndrome** (malformations, persistent intellectual deficits). This intrauterine intoxication is relatively common: one case per 1000 births (**C**).

Chronic alcohol abuse is an expression of true dependence. Thus, **therapy of this addiction** is difficult and frequently without success. There is no pharmacotherapeutic silver bullet (the NMDA receptor antagonist *acamprosate* may be worth trying). Above all, psychotherapeutic care, a change in milieu, and supportive treatment with benzodiazepines are important.

A. Alcoholism

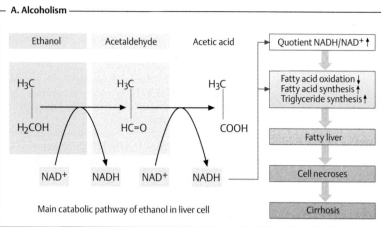

| Ethanol | Acetaldehyde | Acetic acid | Quotient NADH/NAD$^+$ ↑ |

H_3C — H_2COH → H_3C — $HC=O$ → H_3C — $COOH$

NAD$^+$ → NADH   NAD$^+$ → NADH

Fatty acid oxidation ↓
Fatty acid synthesis ↑
Triglyceride synthesis ↑

Fatty liver

Cell necroses

Cirrhosis

Main catabolic pathway of ethanol in liver cell

B. Liver cirrhosis

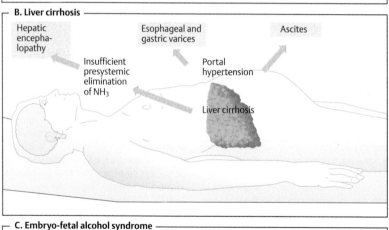

Hepatic encephalopathy

Esophageal and gastric varices

Ascites

Insufficient presystemic elimination of NH$_3$

Portal hypertension

Liver cirrhosis

C. Embryo-fetal alcohol syndrome

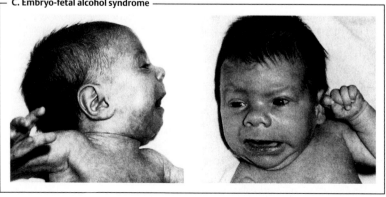

☐ Local Treatment of Glaucoma

Currently, glaucoma therapy remains focused on mechanisms designed to decrease intraocular pressure (IOP) and this approach is considered effective also in normal tension glaucoma.

Normal values of IOP lie between 15 and 20 mmHg, that is, above the venous pressure. IOP reflects the ratio of production and outflow of aqueous humor. Aqueous humor is secreted by the epithelial cells of the ciliary body and, following passage through the trabecular meshwork, is drained via the canal of Schlemm (blue arrows in **A**). This route is taken by 85–90% of aqueous humor; a smaller portion enters the uveoscleral vessels and, thus, the venous system. In the so-called **open-angle glaucoma**, passage of aqueous humor through the trabecular meshwork is impeded so that drainage through Schlemm's canal becomes inefficient. The much rarer primary **angle-closure glaucoma** features a narrowed iridocorneal angle or a tight contact between iris and lens ('pupillary block'). Secondarily, blockade by the iris of the trabecular meshwork may be due to various causes (e. g., synechiae). Topographical relationships in the chamber angle are shown enlarged in the red box.

For topical therapy of **open-angle glaucoma**, the following groups of drugs can be used: for reducing production of aqueous humor, β-blockers (e. g., timolol), α_2-agonists (clonidine, brimonidine), and inhibitors of carbonic anhydrase (dorzolamide, brinzolamide).

For promoting drainage through the trabecular meshwork, parasympathomimetics (e. g., pilocarpine) are effective, and through the uveoscleral route, prostaglandin derivatives. Pilocarpine excites the ciliary muscle and the pupillary sphincter. The contraction of both muscles widens the geometrical arrangement of trabeculae, resulting in improved drainage of aqueous humor. Uveoscleral drainage is augmented by the prostaglandin derivatives lanatoprost and bimatoprost. Both substances can be used for topical monotherapy or combined with other active principles. A peculiar side effect is notable: dark pigmentation of iris and eyelashes.

The therapy of **angle-closure glaucoma** involves chiefly reduction of aqueous humor production (osmotic agents, β-blockers) and surgical procedures.

The topical application of pharmaceuticals in the form of eye-drops is hampered by a pharmacokinetic problem. The drug must penetrate from the ocular surface (cornea and conjunctiva) to its target sites, namely, the smooth muscle of the ciliary body or the iris, the secretory epithelium of the ciliary body, or the uveoscleral vessels (**B**). The applied drug concentration is diluted by lacrimal fluid and drains via the tear duct to the nasal mucosa, where the drug may be absorbed. During permeation through the cornea, transport through blood vessels takes place. The drug concentration reaching the anterior chamber is diluted by aqueous humor and, finally, drug molecules are also transported away via Schlemm's canal. In order to reach the required concentrations at the target site (10^{-8} to 10^{-6} M, depending on the substance), the concentration needed in the eye drops is $\sim 10^{-2}$ M (equivalent to ~ 0.5 mg per droplet, depending on molecular weight). The amount of drug contained in a single drop is large enough to elicit a general reaction with systemic use. Even when applied properly, eye drops can therefore evoke side effects in the cardiovascular system or the bronchial space. This possibility leads to corresponding contraindications. Thus, in patients with severe congestive heart failure, bradycardia, or obstructive lung disease, eye drops containing β-blockers must be avoided at all times.

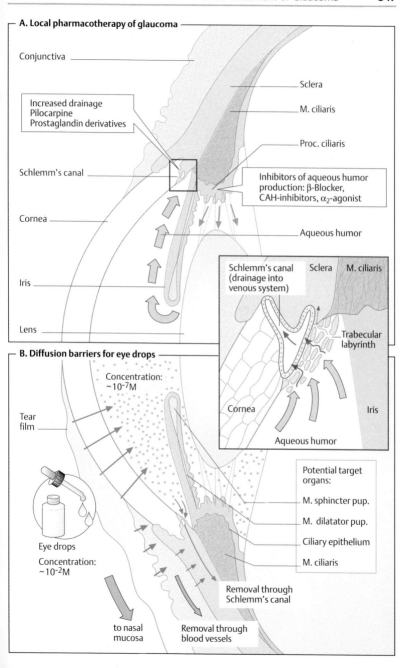

A. Local pharmacotherapy of glaucoma

Conjunctiva

Sclera

M. ciliaris

Increased drainage
Pilocarpine
Prostaglandin derivatives

Proc. ciliaris

Schlemm's canal

Inhibitors of aqueous humor production: β-Blocker, CAH-inhibitors, α_2-agonist

Cornea

Aqueous humor

Iris

Lens

Schlemm's canal (drainage into venous system)   Sclera   M. ciliaris

Trabecular labyrinth

Cornea

Iris

Aqueous humor

B. Diffusion barriers for eye drops

Concentration: ~10^{-7}M

Tear film

Eye drops
Concentration: ~10^{-2}M

Potential target organs:

M. sphincter pup.

M. dilatator pup.

Ciliary epithelium

M. ciliaris

Removal through Schlemm's canal

to nasal mucosa

Removal through blood vessels

Further Reading

□ Further Reading

Foundations and Basic Principles of Pharmacology

Foreman JC, Johansen T. Textbook of Receptor Pharmacology. 2nd ed. New York: McGraw-Hill; 2002.

Hardman JG, Limbird LE, Gilman A. Goodman & Gilman's The Pharmacological Basis of Therapeutics. 10th ed. New York: McGraw-Hill; 2001.

Katzung BG. Basic and Clinical Pharmacology. 9th ed. New York: Lange Medical Books/ McGraw-Hill; 2004.

Page CR, Curtis MJ, Sutter MC, Walker MJA, Hoffman BB. Integrated Pharmacology. 2nd ed. London: Mosby; 2002.

Pratt WB, Taylor P. Principles of Drug Action—The Basis of Pharmacology. 3rd ed. New York: Churchill Livingstone; 1990.

Rang HP, Dale MM, Ritter JM, Moore PK. Pharmacology. 5th ed. New York: Churchill Livingstone; 2003.

Clinical Pharmacology

Bennett PN, Brown MJ. Clinical Pharmacology. 9th ed. Edinburgh: Churchill Livingstone; 2003.

Caruthers SG, Hoffman BB, Melmon KL, Nierenberg DW. Melmon and Morelli's Clinical Pharmacology—Basic Principles in Therapeutics. 4th ed. New York: McGraw-Hill; 2000.

Clinical Pharmacology—Electronic Drug Reference. Tampa, Florida: Gold Standard Multimedia Inc. [Updated every 4 months].

Dipiro JT, Talbert RL, Yee GC, Matzke GR, Wells BG, Posey LM. Pharmacotherapy—A Pathophysiological Approach. New York: McGraw-Hill/Appleton and Lange; 2002.

Grahame-Smith D, Aronson J. Oxford Textbook of Clinical Pharmacology and Drug Therapy. 3rd ed. Oxford: Oxford University Press; 2002.

Drug Interactions and Adverse Effects

Davies DM, Ferner RE, de Glanville H. Davies' Textbook of Adverse Drug Reactions. 5th ed. London: Chapman and Hall; 1998.

Hansten PD, Horn JR. Drug interactions, Analysis and Management. Vancouver, WA: Applied Therapeutics Inc. [Updated every 4 months].

Websites
USA. FDA:
www.fda.gov/medwatch/index.html
UK. NHS: http://www.nhsdirect.nhs.uk/

Drugs in Pregnancy and Lactation

Briggs GG, Freeman RK, Yaffe SJ. Drugs in Pregnancy and Lactation: a Reference Guide to Fetal and Neonatal Risk. 6th ed. Baltimore: Williams and Wilkins; 2002.

Pharmacokinetics

Bauer LA. Applied Clinical Pharmacokinetics. New York: McGraw-Hill Med. Publ. Div.; 2001.

Boroujerdi M. Pharmacokinetics—Principles and Applications. New York: McGraw-Hill Med. Publ. Div.; 2002.

Shargel L, Yu A. Applied Biopharmaceutics and Pharmacokinetics. 4th ed. New York: McGraw-Hill Med. Publ. Div.; 1999.

Toxicology

Klaassen CD, Watkins J. Casarett and Doull's Toxicology: The Basic Science of Poisons. 7th ed. New York: McGraw-Hill; 2003.

□ Picture Credits

p. 75 Permission to use the two photographs in the plate on p. 75 was kindly granted by Professor Enno Christophers, Head of the Department of Dermatology, Venereology and Allergology at the University of Kiel.

p. 297 A and **B** taken from: Lang W, Löschner T. Tropenmedizin in Klinik und Praxis. 3rd ed. Stuttgart: Thieme; 1999.

p. 297 C taken from: Hof H, Dörries R. Medizinische Mikrobiologie. 2nd ed. Stuttgart: Thieme: 2002.

p. 297 D taken from: Kayser F, Bienz KA, Eckert J, Zinkernagel RM. Medizinische Mikrobiologie. 10th ed. Stuttgart: Thieme; 2001.

p. 345 C taken from: Murken J, Clevett. Humangenetik. 6th ed. Stuttgart: Enke; 1996.

Drug Indexes

Trade Name – Drug Name
(* denotes investigational status in the
United States)

A

Abbokinase®	Urokinase
Acantex®	Ceftriaxone
Accolate®	Zafirlukast
Accupril®	Quinapril
Acediur®	Captopril
Acephen®	Acetaminophen (= paracetamol)
Acepril®	Captopril
Achromycin®	Tetracycline
AcipHex®	Rabeprazole
Acnex®	Salicylic acid
Acthar®	Corticotropin
Acti-B₁₂®	Hydroxocobalamin
Actilyse®	Alteplase
Actimmune®	Interferon gamma
Actiprophen®	Ibuprofen
Activase®	t-PA (= alteplase)
Actonel®	Risedronate
Actos®	Pioglitazone
Actulin®	Repaglinide
Acular®	Ketorolac
Adalat®	Nifedipine
Adcortyl®	Triamcinolone
ADH®	Vasopressin
Adicort®	Triamcinolone acetonide
Adrenalin®	Epinephrine
Adriamycin®	Doxorubicin
Adriblastin®	Doxorubicin
Adrucil®	Fluorouracil
Advil®	Ibuprofen
Aegrosan®	Dimeticone
Aerius®	Desloratadine
Aerobid®	Flunisolide
Aerolate®	Theophylline
Afibrin®	ε-Aminocaproic acid
Afrin®	Oxymetazoline
Agenerase®	Amprenavir
Aggrastat®	Tirofiban
Agopton®	Lansoprazole
Airbron®	Acetylcysteine
Ak Pred®	Prednisolone
Akarpine®	Pilocarpine
Akineton®	Biperiden
Akinophyl®	Biperiden
Alazine®	Hydralazine
Albalon®	Naphazoline
Albego®	Camazepam
Albiotic®	Lincomycin
Albuterol®	Salbutamol
Alcoban®	Flucytosine
Aldactone®	Spironolactone
Aldecin®	Beclometasone
Aldinamide®	Pyrazinamide
Aldocorten®	Aldosterone

Aldomet®	Methyldopa
Aldrox®	Aluminum hydroxide
Aleve®	Naproxen
Alexan®	Cytarabine
Alfenta®	Alfentanil
Alflorone®	Fludrocortisone
Alfoten®	Alfuzosin
Algocalmin®	Dipyrone
Algocor®	Gallopamil
Alkeran®	Melphalan
Allegra®	Fexofenadine
Allerdryl®	Diphenhydramine
Allerest®	Oxymetazoline
Alloferin®	Alcuronium
Alloprin®	Allopurinol
Allvoran®	Diclofenac
Almocarpine®	Pilocarpine
Almodan®	Amoxicillin
Alocort®	Hydrocortisone (cortisol)
Alophen®	Phenolphthalein
Alopresin®	Captopril
Alphagan®	Brimonidine
Alpha-redisol®	Hydroxocobalamin
Altace®	Ramipril
Altracin®	Bacitracin
Alu-Cap®	Aluminum hydroxide
Aludrin®	Isoprenaline (= isoproterenol)
Alupent®	Metaproterenol (orciprenaline)
Alu-Tab®	Aluminum hydroxide
Alzapam®	Lorazepam
Ambaxine®	Amantadine
Ambien®	Zolpidem
Ambril®	Ambroxol
Amcill®	Ampicillin
Amen®	Medroxyprogesterone-acetate
Americaine®	Benzocaine
Amfebutamon(e)®	Bupropion
Amicar®	ε-Aminocaproic acid
Amidate®	Etomidate
Amidonal®	Aprindine
Amikin®	Amikacin
Aminomux®	Pamidronate
Aminopan®	Somatostatin
Amitril®	Amitriptyline
Ammuno®	Indometacin
Amoban®	Zopiclone
Amodopa®	Methyldopa
Amovane®	Zopiclone
Amoxil®	Amoxicillin
Amphipen®	Ampicillin
Amphojel®	Aluminum hydroxide
Amphozone®	Amphotericin B
Amycor®	Bifonazole

Anabactyl (A)®	Carbenicillin
Anabolin®	Nandrolone
Anacaine®	Benzocaine
Anacin-3®	Acetaminophen (= paracetamol)
Anacobin®	Cyanocobalamin
Anaesthesin®	Benzocaine
Anamid®	Kanamycin
Anaprox®	Naproxen
Ancotil®	Flucytosine
Andriol®	Testosterone undecanoate
Andro®	Testosterone enantate
Androcur®	Cyproterone-acetate
Androcyp®	Testosterone cypionate
Android®	Methyltestosterone
Androlone®	Nandrolone
Andronate®	Testosterone cypionate
Androviron®	Mesterolone
Anectine®	Succinylcholine
Anergan®	Promethazine
Anethaine®	Tetracaine
Anexate®	Flumazenil
Angettes®	Acetylsalicylic acid
Angionorm®	Dihydroergotamine
Ang-O-Span®	Nitroglycerin (glyceryl trinitrate)
Antagon®	Ganirelix
Antepsin®	Sucralfate
Antilirium®	Physostigmine
Antiminth®	Pyrantel pamoate
Antipressan®	Atenolol
Antivert®	Meclizine (meclozine)
Antocin®	Atosiban
Antrizine®	Meclizine (meclozine)
Apaurin®	Diazepam
Apocretin®	Etilefrine
Apresoline®	Hydralazine
Aprobal®	Alprenolol
Aprozide®	Hydrochlorothiazide
Apsin VK®	Pencillin V
Apsolox®	Oxprenolol
Aptine®	Alprenolol
Aralen®	Chloroquine
Aranesp®	Darbepoetin
Arava®	Leflunomide
Arduan®	Pipecuronium
Aredia®	Pamidronate
Arelix®	Piretanide
Arfonad®	Trimetaphan
Arhythmol®	Propafenone
Aricept®	Donepezil
Arimidex®	Anastrozole
Aristocort®	Triamcinolone
Arixtra®	Fondaparinux
Armazid®	Isoniazid
Arsumax®	Artesunate
Arteoptic®	Carteolol
Arterenol®	Norepinephrine (noradrenaline)
Arthrisin®	Acetylsalicylic acid
Articulose®	Prednisolone
Arumil®	Amiloride
Asacol®	Mesalamine (mesalazine)
Asadrine®	Acetylsalicylic acid
Ascotop®	Zolmitriptan
Aspenon®	Aprindine
Aspirin®	Acetylsalicylic acid
Astramorph®	Morphine sulfate
Atabrine®	Quinacrine
Atacand®	Candesartan
Atempol®	Nitrazepam
Atensine®	Diazepam
Ativan®	Lorazepam
Atridox®	Doxycycline
Atromid-S®	Clofibrate
Atropisol®	Atropine
Atrovent®	Ipratropium
Augmentan®	Amoxicillin + clavulanic acid
Augmentin®	Clavulanic acid + amoxicillin
Aureotan®	Aurothioglucose
Auromyose®	Aurothioglucose
Aurorix®	Moclobemide
Avandia®	Rosiglitazone
Avapro®	Irbesartan
Avicel®	Cellulose
Avinza®	Morphine sulfate
Avloclor®	Chloroquine
Avlosulfone®	Dapsone
Avodart®	Dutasteride
Avomine®	Promethazine
Azaline®	Salazosulfapyridine (sulfasalazine)
Azanin®	Azathioprine
Azlin®	Azlocillin
Azmacort®	Triamcinolone acetonide
Azopt®	Brinzolamide
Azulfidine®	Salazosulfapyridine (sulfasalazine)

B

Baciguent®	Bacitracin
Bactidan®	Enoxacin
Bactocill®	Oxacillin
Bactrim®	Co-trimoxazole
BAL in oil®	Dimercaprol
Barbita®	Phenobarbital
Bay-Bee®	Vitamin B_{12}
Baycol®	Cerivastatin
Bayer 205®	Suramine
Bayotensin®	Nitrendipine
Baypress®	Nitrendipine
Becloforte®	Beclometasone
Becodisks®	Beclometasone
Beconase®	Beclometasone
Becotide®	Beclometasone
Bedoz®	Cyanocobalamin
Bee Six®	Vitamin B_6
Bee-six®	Pyridoxine
Befizal®	Bezafibrate

Benadryl®	Diphenhydramine
Benemid®	Probenecid
Bentos®	Befunolol
Berkaprine®	Azathioprine
Berkatens®	Verapamil
Berkolol®	Propranolol
Berofor alpha 2®	Interferon alfa2
Berotec®	Fenoterol
Berubigen®	Vitamin B$_{12}$
Bestcall®	Cefmenoxime
Betaclar®	Befunolol
Betadran®	Bupranolol
Betadrenol®	Bupranolol
Betagon®	Mepindolol
Betalin 12®	Vitamin B$_{12}$
Betaloc®	Metoprolol
Betapen-VK®	Pencillin V
Betimol®	Timolol
Betoptic®	Betaxolol
Betriol®	Bunitrolol
Bextra®	Bucindolol
Bextra®	Valdecoxib
Bezalip®	Bezafibrate
Bezatol®	Bezafibrate
Biaxin®	Clarithromycin
Bicalm®	Zolpidem
Bicillin®	Penicillin G
Bicol®	Bisacodyl
Biltricide®	Praziquantel
Black Draught®	Senna
Blenoxane®	Bleomycin
Blocadren®	Timolol
Bofedrol®	Ephedrine
Bonamine®	Meclizine (meclozine)
Bonpyrin®	Dipyrone
Bopen-VK®	Pencillin V
Borotropin®	Atropine
Botox®	Botulinum toxin type A
Brethine®	Terbutaline
Brevibloc®	Esmolol
Brevital®	Methohexital
Bricanyl®	Terbutaline
Briclin®	Amikacin
Bromo-Seltzer®	Acetaminophen (= paracetamol)
Bronalide®	Flunisolide
Bronchaid®	Epinephrine
Bronchopront®	Ambroxol
Bronkodyl®	Theophylline
Broxalax®	Bisacodyl
Brufen®	Ibuprofen
Bumex®	Bumetanide
Buprene®	Buprenorphine
Burinex®	Bumetanide
Buscopan®	Butylscopolamine
Buscopan®	Hyoscine butyl bromide
Buspar®	Buspirone
Butylone®	Pentobarbital

C

Cabadon®	Vitamin B$_{12}$
Cabaseril®	Cabergoline
Cacit®	Calcium carbonate
Calabren®	Glibenclamide (= glyburide)
Calan®	Verapamil
Calchichew®	Calcium carbonate
Calcidrink®	Calcium carbonate
Calciferol®	Vitamin D
Calcimer®	Calcitonin
Calcimux®	Etidronate
Calciparin®	Heparin
Calcitare®	Calcitonin
Calderol®	Calcifediol
Calpol®	Acetaminophen (= paracetamol)
Calsan®	Calcium carbonate
Calsynar®	Calcitonin
Caltidren®	Carteolol
Caltrate®	Calcium carbonate
Calvepen®	Pencillin V
Camcolit®	Lithium carbonate
Camoquin®	Amodiaquine
Campral®	Acamprosate
Campto®	Irinotecan
Canasa®	Mesalamine (mesalazine)
Cancidas®	Caspofungin
Canesten®	Clotrimazole
Capastat®	Capreomycin
Caplenal®	Allopurinol
Capoten®	Captopril
Capramol®	ε-Aminocaproic acid
Caprolin®	Capreomycin
Carace®	Lisinopril
Carafate®	Sucralfate
Carbex®	Selegeline
Carbocaine®	Mepivacaine
Carbolite®	Lithium carbonate
Cardene®	Nicardipine
Cardinol®	Propranolol
Cardioqin®	Quinidine
Cardiorhythmino®	Ajmaline
Cardizem®	Diltiazem
Cardura®	Doxazosin
Carduran®	Doxazosin
Caridian®	Mepindolol
Carindapen®	Carbenicillin
Carteol®	Carteolol
Cartrol®	Carteolol
Casodex®	Bicalutamide
Catapres®	Clonidine
CCNU®	Lomustine
Cedocard®	Isosorbide dinitrate
Cedur®	Bezafibrate
CeeNu®	Lomustine
Cefmax®	Cefmenoxime
Celance®	Pergolide
Celebrex®	Celecoxib = Colecoxib
Celevac®	Methylcellulose

Celexa®	Citalopram
Celiomycin®	Viomycin
CellCept®	Mycophenolate mofetil
Cemix®	Cefmenoxime
Centrax®	Prazepam
Cephulac®	Lactulose
Cerebid®	Papaverine
Cerespan®	Papaverine
Cerubidine®	Daunorubicin
Cesamet®	Nabilone
Cesplon®	Captopril
Chloraminophene®	Chlorambucil
Chlorohist®	Xylometazoline
Chloromycetin®	Chloramphenicol
Chloroptic®	Chloramphenicol
Cholestabyl®	Colestipol
Cholestid®	Colestipol
Choloxin®	Thyroxine
Chronulac®	Lactulose
Cialis®	Tadalafil
Cibacalcin®	Calcitonin
Cidomycin®	Gentamicin
Cillimycin®	Lincomycin
Ciloxan®	Ciprofloxacin
Cimetrin®	Erythromycin-propionate
Cin-Quin®	Quinidine
Cipro®	Ciprofloxacin
Ciprobay®	Ciprofloxacin
Ciprox®	Ciprofloxacin
Ciproxin®	Ciprofloxacin
Circupon®	Etilefrine
Citanest®	Prilocaine
Citaprim®	Citalopram
Citrucell®	Methylcellulose
Claforan®	Cefotaxime
Clamoxyl®	Amoxicillin
Claripex®	Clofibrate
Claritin®	Loratadine
Clasteon®	Clodronate
Cleocin®	Clindamycin
Clexane®	Enoxaparin
Clomid®	Clomifene
Clonopin®	Clonazepam
Clont®	Metronidazole
Clopra®	Metoclopramide
Clotrimaderm®	Clotrimazole
Clovapen®	Cloxacillin
Clozan®	Clotiazepam
Clozaril®	Clozapine
Cobalin-H®	Hydroxocobalamin
Cobex®	Vitamin B_{12}
Cocillin-VK®	Pencillin V
Codelsol®	Prednisolone
Codicept®	Codeine
Cogentin®	Benztropine
Cognex®	Tacrine
Colchicine®	Colchicine
Coleb®	Isosorbide mononitrate
Colectril®	Amiloride
Collyrium®	Tetryzoline (= tetrahydrozoline)
Cologel®	Methylcellulose
Combactam®	Sulbactam
Combantrin®	Pyrantel pamoate
Complamin®	Xanthinol nicotinate
Complement	
Continus®	Pyridoxine
Comprecin®	Enoxacin
Comtan®	Entacapone
Comtess®	Entacapone
Concor®	Bisoprolol
Conducton®	Carazolol
Constant-T®	Theophylline
Contergan®	Thalidomide
Copaxone®	Glatimer acetate
Coracten®	Nifedipine
Coradus®	Isosorbide dinitrate
Cordanum®	Talinolol
Cordarex®	Amiloride
Cordarex®	Amiodarone
Cordarone®	Amiodarone
Cordilox®	Verapamil
Coreg®	Carvedilol
Corgal®	Gallopamil
Corgard®	Nadolol
Coricidin®	Oxymetazoline
Corindolan®	Mepindolol
Coronex®	Isosorbide dinitrate
Correctol®	Phenolphthalein
Cortalone®	Prednisolone
Cortate®	Hydrocortisone (cortisol)
Cortef®	Hydrocortisone (cortisol)
Cortelan®	Cortisone
Cortenema®	Hydrocortisone (cortisol)
Cortigel®	Corticotropin
Cortistab®	Cortisone
Cortogen®	Cortisone
Cortone®	Cortisone
Cortrophin®	Corticotropin
Corvaton®	Molsidomine
Coscopin®	Narcotine (= noscapine)
Coscopin®	Noscapine (= narcotine)
Coscotab®	Narcotine (= noscapine)
Coscotab®	Noscapine (= narcotine)
Cosmegen®	Dactinomycin
Coumadin®	Warfarin
Coversum®	Perindopril
Coversyl®	Perindopril
Cozaar®	Losartan
C-Pak®	Doxycycline
Crixivan®	Indinavir
Cryspen®	Penicillin G
Crystapen®	Penicillin G
Crystodigin®	Digitoxin
Cuemid®	Cholestyramine
Cuprimine®	D-Penicillamine
Cutivate®	Fluticasone
Cuvalit®	Lisuride
Cyanoject®	Vitamin B_{12}
Cyclogest®	Progesterone
Cyklokapron®	Tranexamic acid
Cymevene®	Ganciclovir
Cyomin®	Vitamin B_{12}

Cyprostat®	Cyproterone-acetate
Cytacon®	Cyanocobalamin
Cytamen®	Cyanocobalamin
Cytomel®	Triiodthyronine (= liothyronine)
Cytomel®	Liothyronine
Cytosar®	Cytarabine
Cytotec®	Misoprostol
Cytovene®	Ganciclovir
Cytoxan®	Cyclophosphamide

D

D.E.H.45®	Dihydroergotamine
Dagenan®	Sulfapyridine
Daktarin®	Miconazole
Dalacin®	Clindamycin
Dalcaine®	Lidocaine
Dalmane®	Flurazepam
Daneral®	Pheniramine
Dantrium®	Dantrolene
Daonil®	Glibenclamide (= glyburide)
Daraprim®	Pyrimethamine
Datril®	Acetaminophen (= paracetamol)
Daunoblastin®	Daunorubicin
DDAVP®	Desmopressin
Decadron®	Dexamethasone
Deca-Durabolin®	Nandrolone
Decapeptyl®	Triptorelin
Decapryn®	Doxylamine
Dedrogyl®	Calcifediol
Degest-2®	Naphazoline
Delapav®	Papaverine
Delatestryl®	Testosterone enantate
Delestrogen®	Estradiol-valerate
Delta-Cortef®	Prednisolone
Deltapen®	Penicillin G
Deltastab®	Prednisolone
Demerol®	Meperidine (pethidine)
Dendrid®	Idoxuridine
Depakene®	Valproic acid
Depen®	D-Penicillamine
Deponit®	Nitroglycerin (glyceryl trinitrate)
Depo-Provera®	Medroxyprogesterone-acetate
Deprenyl®	Selegeline
Dermonistat®	Miconazole
Deronil®	Dexamethasone
Deseril®	Methysergide
Desferal®	Deferoxamine
Desoxyn®	Methamphetamine
Desuric®	Benzbromarone
Desyrel®	Trazodone
Detensiel®	Bisoprolol
Detensol®	Propranolol
DiaBeta®	Glibenclamide (= glyburide)
Diabex®	Metformin

Diamox®	Acetazolamide
Diapid®	Lypressin
Diaqua®	Hydrochlorothiazide
Diarsed®	Diphenoxylate
Diastabol®	Miglitol
Diastat®	Diazepam
Dibenyline®	Phenoxybenzamine
Dibenzyline®	Phenoxybenzamine
Diclocil®	Dicloxacillin
Diclophlogont®	Diclofenac
Diflucan®	Fluconazole
Digacin®	Digoxin
Digibind®	Digoxin immune FAB
Digicor®	Digitoxin
Digimerck®	Digitoxin
Digitaline®	Digitoxin
Dihydergot®	Dihydroergotamine
Dihyzin®	Dihydralazine
Dilantin®	Phenytoin
Dilaudid®	Hydromorphone
Dimaval®	Dimercaptopropane-sulfonic acid
Dimetab®	Dimenhydrinate
Dinaplex®	Flunarizine
Diodronel®	Etidronate
Dioval®	Estradiol-valerate
Diovan®	Valsartan
Diphenasone®	Dapsone
Diphos®	Etidronate
Diprivan®	Propofol
Dirythmin®	Disopyramide
Distaquaine V-K®	Pencillin V
Distraneurin®	Clomethiazole
Diuchlor®	Hydrochlorothiazide
Diumax®	Piretanide
Divarine®	Dipyrone
Divegal®	Dihydroergotamine
Dixarit®	Clonidine
Dizac®	Diazepam
Dobutrex®	Dobutamine
Dolantine®	Meperidine (pethidine)
Dolophine®	Methadone
Domical®	Amitriptyline
Donnagel-MB®	Kaolin + pectin (= attapulgite)
Dopamet®	Methyldopa
Dopar®	Levodopa
Dopastat®	Dopamine
Dopergin®	Lisuride
Doral®	Quazepam
Doryl®	Carbachol
Doryx®	Doxycycline
Dostinex®	Cabergoline
Dowmycin®	Erythromycin-estolate
Doxicin®	Doxycycline
Dramamine®	Dimenhydrinate
Drisdol®	Vitamin D
Drisdol®	Ergocalciferol
Dristan®	Oxymetazoline
Drogenil®	Flutamide
Droleptan®	Droperidol
Droxia®	Hydroxyurea

Trade Name	Drug Name
Droxomin®	Hydroxocobalamin
Dryptal®	Furosemide
D-Tabs®	Colecalciferol (vitamin D₃)
Dulcolax®	Bisacodyl
Duoralith®	Lithium carbonate
Duphalac®	Lactulose
Duracoron®	Molsidomine
Duralutin®	Hydroxyprogesterone caproate
Duramorph®	Morphine sulfate
Duratest®	Testosterone cypionate
Durazanil®	Bromazepam
Durolax®	Bisacodyl
D-Vi-sol®	Vitamin D
Dymenate®	Dimenhydrinate
DynaCirc®	Isradipine
Dynapen®	Dicloxacillin
Dynaprin®	Imipramine
Dynastat®	Parecoxib
Dyneric®	Clomifene
Dyrenium®	Triamterene
Dyspamet®	Cimetidine
Dytac®	Triamterene

E

Trade Name	Drug Name
E605®	Nitrostigmine
Ebastel®	Ebastine
Econopred®	Prednisolone
Ecostatin®	Econazole
Ecotrin®	Acetylsalicylic acid
Edecrin®	Ethacrynic acid
Edronax®	Reboxetine
EES®	Erythromycin-ethyl-succinate
Efedron®	Ephedrine
Eferox®	Levothyroxine
Effectin®	Bitolterol
Effexor®	Venlafaxine
Effontil®	Etilefrine
Effortil®	Etilefrine
Effudex®	Fluorouracil
Effurix®	Fluorouracil
Elantan®	Isosorbide mononitrate
Elavil®	Amitriptyline
Eldepryl®	Selegeline
Eligard®	Leuprolide (leuprorelin)
Elimite®	Permethrin
Elixophyllin®	Theophylline
Eltroxin®	Thyroxine
Emcor®	Bisoprolol
Emex®	Metoclopramide
E-mycin®	Erythromycin
Enbrel®	Etanercept
Endak®	Carteolol
Endep®	Amitriptyline
Endophleban®	Dihydroergotamine
Endoxan®	Cyclophosphamide
Enoram®	Enoxacin
Enovil®	Amitriptyline

Trade Name	Drug Name
Enoxor®	Enoxacin
Entocort EC®	Budesonide
Entromone®	Chorionic gonadotropin (HCG)
Entrophen®	Acetylsalicylic acid
Epanutin®	Phenytoin
Epifin®	Epinephrine
Epimorph®	Morphine sulfate
Epinal®	Epinephrine
EpiPen®	Epinephrine
Epitol®	Carbamazepine
Epitrate®	Epinephrine
Epivir®	Lamivudine
Epogen®	Erythropoietin (= epoetin alfa)
Eporal®	Dapsone
Eprex®	Epoetin
Epsicapron®	ε-Aminocaproic acid
Ergocalm®	Lormetazepam
Ergomar®	Ergotamine
Ergotrate Maleate®	Ergometrine (= ergonovine)
Eridan®	Diazepam
Ermalate®	Ergometrine (= ergonovine)
Erwinase®	Asparaginase
Eryc®	Erythromcyin
Erymax®	Erythromcyin
Erymycin®	Erythromycin-stearate
Erythrocin®	Erythromycin-ethyl-succinate
Erythrocin®	Erythromycin-stearate
Erythromid®	Erythromycin
Erythroped®	Erythromcyin
Esidrix®	Hydrochlorothiazide
Eskalith®	Lithium carbonate
Espotabs®	Phenolphthalein
Estinyl®	Ethinylestradiol
Estrace®	Estradiol
Ethrane®	Enflurane
Ethyl Adrianol®	Etilefrine
Etibi®	Ethambutol
Etopophos®	Etoposide
Euciton®	Domperidone
Eudemine®	Diazoxide
Euglucon®	Glibenclamide (= glyburide)
Euhypnos®	Temazepam
Eulexin®	Flutamide
Eunal®	Lisuride
Euthyrox®	Levothyroxine
Evac-U-gen®	Phenolphthalein
Evac-U-Lax®	Phenolphthalein
Evastel®	Ebastine
Everone®	Testosterone enantate
Evipan®	Hexobarbital
Evista®	Raloxifene
Evoxin®	Domperidone
Exanta®	Ximelagatran
Exelon®	Rivastigmine
Ex-Lax®	Phenolphthalein

F

Fabrol®	Acetylcysteine
Factrel®	Gonadorelin
Falcigo®	Artesunate
Famvir®	Famciclovir
Fansidar®	Pyrimethamine + sulfadoxine
Fansidar®	Sulfadoxine + pyrimethamine
Farlutal®	Medroxyprogesterone-acetate
Fasigyn(CH)®	Tinidazol
Faslodex®	Fulvestrant
Fastject®	Epinephrine
Fasturtec®	Rasburicase
Faverin®	Fluvoxamine
F-Cortef®	Fludrocortisone
Felbatol®	Felbamate
Femara®	Letrozole
Femazole®	Metronidazole
Feminone®	Ethinylestradiol
Femogex®	Estradiol-valerate
Femotrone®	Progesterone
Femovan®	Gestoden + ethinyl-estradiol
Fenbid®	Ibuprofen
Fenestil®	Dimetindene
Fertodur®	Cyclofenil
Feverall®	Dipyrone
Fiblaferon 3®	Interferon beta
Fibocil®	Aprindine
Fiboran®	Aprindine
Flagyl®	Metronidazole
Flavoquine®	Amodiaquine
Fletcher's Castoria®	Senna
Flixonase®	Fluticasone
Flomax®	Tamsulosin
Flonase®	Fluticasone
Florinef®	Fludrocortisone
Flovent®	Fluticasone
Floxapen®	Flucloxacillin (floxacilline)
Floxifral®	Fluvoxamine
Fluagel®	Aluminum hydroxide
Fluctin®	Fluoxetine
Flugeral®	Flunarizine
Fluothane®	Halothane
Foldine®	Folic acid
Folex®	Methotrexate
Follutein®	Chorionic gonadotropin (HCG)
Folvite®	Folic acid
Fontego®	Bumetanide
Foradil®	Formoterol
Forane®	Isoflurane
Fordiuran®	Bumetanide
Fortaz®	Ceftazidime
Forteo®	Teriparatide
Fortovase®	Saquinavir
Fortral®	Pentazocine
Fortum®	Ceftazidime
Fosamax®	Alendronate
Foscavir®	Foscarnet
Fragmin®	Dalteparin
Fragmin®	Heparin, low molecular
Fraxiparin®	Heparin, low molecular
Frisium®	Clobazam
Fulcin®	Griseofulvin
Fulvicin®	Griseofulvin
Fungilin®	Amphotericin B
Fungizone®	Amphotericin B
Fusid®	Furosemide
Fuzeon®	Enfuvirtide

G

Gabitril®	Tiagabine
Gabren(e)®	Progabide
Gamazole®	Sulfamethoxazole
Ganal®	Fenfluramine
Ganphen®	Promethazine
Gantanol®	Sulfamethoxazole
Gantrisin®	Sulfisoxazole
Garamycin®	Gentamicin
Gardenal®	Phenobarbital
Gas.X®	Simethicone
Gastrozepin®	Pirenzepine
Gelafundin®	Gelatin-colloids
Gengraf®	Ciclosporin (= cyclosporine A)
Genna®	Senna
Genotropin®	Somatotropin
Genticin®	Gentamicin
Gentle Nature®	Senna
Geodon®	Ziprasidone
Geopen®	Carbenicillin
Germanin®	Suramine
Gestafortin®	Chlormadinone acetate
Gesterol L.A.®	Hydroxyprogesterone caproate
Gestone®	Progesterone
GHRH-Ferring®	Somatorelin
Gilurytmal®	Ajmaline
Gladem®	Sertraline
Glauconex®	Befunolol
Glaupax®	Acetazolamide
Glivec®	Imatinib
Glucophage®	Metformin
Granocyte®	Lenograstim (G-CSF)
Grisovin®	Griseofulvin
Gubernal®	Alprenolol
Gulfasin®	Sulfisoxazole
Gumbix®	Aminomethylbenzoic acid
Gyne-Lotrimin®	Clotrimazole
Gynergen®	Ergotamine
Gyno-Pevaryl®	Econazole
Gyno-Travogen®	Isoconazole

H

Trade Name	Drug Name
Haemaccel®	Gelatin-colloids
Halcion®	Triazolam
Haldol®	Haloperidol
Halfan®	Halofantrine
Hamarin®	Allopurinol
Hemineurin®	Clomethiazole
Hepalean®	Heparin
Hepsal®	Heparin
Herceptin®	Trastuzumab
Herpid®	Idoxuridine
Herplex®	Idoxuridine
Hespan®	Hetastarch (HES)
Hespan®	Hydroxyethyl starch
Hetrazan®	Diethylcarbamazepine
Hexa-Betalin®	Vitamin B₆
Hexa-Betalin®	Pyridoxine
Hexadrol®	Dexamethasone
Hexit®	Lindane
Hibanil®	Chlorpromazine
Hidroferol®	Calcifediol
Hismanal®	Astemizole
Hivid®	Zalcitabine
Homapin®	Homatropine
Honvol®	Diethylstilbestrol
Humalog®	Insulin
Humatin®	Paromomycin
Humira®	Adalimumab
Humulin®	Insulin
Hybalamine®	Hydroxocobalamin
Hybolin Decanoate®	Nandrolone
Hycamtin®	Topotecan
Hydeltrasol®	Prednisolone
Hyderm®	Hydrocortisone (cortisol)
Hydrea®	Hydroxyurea
Hydromal®	Hydrochlorothiazide
Hydromedin®	Ethacrynic acid
Hydrosaluric®	Hydrochlorothiazide
Hydrotricin®	Tyrothricin
Hygroton®	Chlorthalidone
Hylutin®	Hydroxyprogesterone caproate
Hymorphan®	Hydromorphone
Hyocort®	Hydrocortisone (cortisol)
Hyperstat®	Diazoxide
Hypertensin®	Angiotensinamide
Hypertil®	Captopril
Hypnomidate®	Etomidate
Hypnosedon®	Flunitrazepam
Hypnovel®	Midazolam
Hypovase®	Prazosin
Hyroxon®	Hydroxyprogesterone caproate
Hyskon®	Dextran
Hytrin®	Terazosin

I

Trade Name	Drug Name
Ifex®	Ifosfamide
Iktorivil®	Clonazepam
Iletin®	Insulin
Ilomedin®	Iloprost
Ilosone®	Erythromycin-estolate
Ilosone®	Erythromcyin
Imbrilon®	Indometacin
Imdur®	Isosorbide mononitrate
Imitrex®	Sumatriptan
Imodium®	Loperamide
Imovane®	Zopiclone
Importal®	Lactitol
Impril®	Imipramine
Imuran®	Azathioprine
Imurek®	Azathioprine
Inapsine®	Droperidol
Inderal®	Propranolol
Indocid®	Indometacin
Indocin®	Indometacin
Indomee®	Indometacin
Indomod®	Indometacin
Inflamase®	Prednisolone
Infumorph®	Morphine sulfate
Inhibace®	Cilazapril
Inhiston®	Pheniramine
Innovace®	Enalapril/enalaprilat
Innovar®	Fentanyl + droperidol
Inocor®	Amrinone
Insommal®	Diphenhydramine
Intal®	Cromoglycate (cromolyn)
Integriline®	Eptifibatide
Intron A®	Interferon alfa-2b
Intropin®	Dopamine
Invirase®	Saquinavir
I-Pilopine®	Pilocarpine
Ipral®	Trimethoprim
Isicom®	Carbidopa + levodopa
Ismelin®	Guanethidine
Ismo®	Isosorbide mononitrate
Isocaine®	Mepivacaine
Isocillin®	Phenoxybenzylpenicillin
Isoket®	Isosorbide dinitrate
Isoptin®	Verapamil
Isopto-Carpine®	Pilocarpine
Isordil®	Isosorbide dinitrate
Isotamine®	Isoniazid
Isoten®	Bisoprolol
Isotol®	Mannitol
Isotrate®	Isosorbide mononitrate
Isuprel®	Isoprenaline (= isoproterenol)
Itracol®	Itraconazole
Itrop®	Ipratropium

J

Trade Name	Drug Name
Janimine®	Imipramine
Jexin®	Tubocurarine

K

Kabikinase®	Streptokinase
Kabolin®	Nandrolone
Kadian®	Morphine sulfate
Kaletra®	Lopinavir
Kannasyn®	Kanamycin
Kanrenol®	Canrenone
Kantrex®	Kanamycin
Kaopectate®	Kaolin + pectin (= attapulgite)
Kaopectate II®	Loperamide
Karil®	Calcitonin
Keflex®	Cefalexin
Keftab®	Cefalexin
Kemicetine®	Chloramphenicol
Kenacort®	Triamcinolone
Kenalog®	Triamcinolone acetonide
Kenalone®	Triamcinolone acetonide
Kerecid®	Idoxuridine
Kerlone®	Betaxolol
Kertasin®	Etilefrine
Kestine®	Ebastine
Ketalar®	Ketamine
Key-Pred®	Prednisolone
Kiditard®	Quinidine
Kineret®	Anakinra
Kinidin®	Quinidine
Klebcil®	Kanamycin
Klot®	Tolonium chloride
Konakion®	Phytomenadione
Korostatin®	Nystatin
Kryptocur®	Gonadorelin
Kwell®	Lindane
Kwilldane®	Lindane
Kytril®	Granisetron

L

Lacril®	Methylcellulose
Ladropen®	Flucloxacillin (floxacilline)
Lamiazid®	Isoniazid
Lamictal®	Lamotrigine
Lampren®	Clofazimine
Lanacillin®	Penicillin G
Lanacillin-VK®	Penicillin V
Lanicor®	Digoxin
Lanoxin®	Digoxin
Lantus®	Insulin glargine
Lanzor®	Lansoprazole
Largactil®	Chlorpromazine
Lariam®	Mefloquine
Larodopa®	Levodopa
Lasix®	Furosemide
Lasma®	Theophylline
Laxabene®	Bisacodyl
Laxanin®	Bisacodyl
Lectopam®	Bromazepam
Ledercillin VK®	Penicillin V
Ledercort®	Triamcinolone

Lembrol®	Diazepam
Lendorm(A)®	Brotizolam
Lendormin®	Brotizolam
Lenoxin®	Digoxin
Lentin®	Carbachol
Lentizol®	Amitriptyline
Lescol®	Fluvastatin
Leucomax®	Molgramostim
Leucovorin®	Folic acid
Leukeran®	Chlorambucil
Leukomycin®	Chloramphenicol
Levate®	Amitriptyline
Levatol®	Penbutolol
Levitra®	Vardenafil
Levophed®	Norepinephrine (noradrenaline)
Levoprome®	Methotrimeprazine
Lexotan®	Bromazepam
Librium®	Chlordiazepoxide
Lidifen®	Ibuprofen
Lidopen®	Lidocaine
Likuden®	Griseofulvin
Lincocin®	Lincomycin
Lingraine Medihaler®	Ergotamine
Lioresal®	Baclofen
Lipitor®	Atorvastatin
Lipo-Merz®	Etofibrate
Lipostat®	Pravastatin
Liquamar®	Phenprocoumon
Liquemin®	Heparin
Lisino®	Loratadine
Liskonum®	Lithium carbonate
Litec®	Pizotifen = pizotyline
Lithane®	Lithium carbonate
Lithobid®	Lithium carbonate
Lithotabs®	Lithium carbonate
Lixil®	Bumetanide
Loceryl®	Amorolfin
Lomotil®	Diphenoxylate
Longum®	Sulfalen
Loniten®	Minoxidil
Looser®	Bupranolol
Lopid®	Gemfibrozil
Lopirin®	Captopril
Lopressor®	Metoprolol
Loramet®	Lormetazepam
Loraz®	Lorazepam
Lorinal®	Chloral hydrate
Losec®	Omeprazole
Lotensin®	Benazepril
Lovelco®	Probucol
Lovenox®	Enoxaparin
Ludiomil®	Maprotiline
Lumigan®	Bimatoprost
Lupron®	Leuprolide (leuprorelin)
Luvox®	Fluvoxamine
Lyclear®	Permethrin
Lynoral®	Ethinylestradiol
Lyophrin®	Epinephrine
Lysenyl®	Lisuride

M

Macrobin®	Clostebol
Madopar®	Levodopa + benserazide
Malarone®	Atoquavone + proguanil
Mallergan®	Promethazine
Marcumar®	Phenprocoumon
Marevan®	Warfarin
Marinol®	Dronabinol
Marmine®	Dimenhydrinate
Marvelon®	Desogestrel + ethinylestradiol
Mavik®	Trandolapril
Maxalt®	Rizatriptan
Maxeran®	Metoclopramide
Maxidex®	Dexamethasone
Maxolan®	Metoclopramide
Maxtrex®	Methotrexate
Mazepine®	Carbamazepine
Mectizam®	Ivermectin
Megacillin®	Penicillin G
Megacillin®	Phenoxybenzylpenicillin
Megaphen®	Chlorpromazine
Megestat®	Megestrol
Melarsen Oxide-BAL®	Melarsoprol
MelB®	Melarsoprol
Melipramin®	Imipramine
Menogon®	Menotropin
Menophase®	Mestranol
Mepron®	Atoquavone
Mercazol®	Methimazole (thiamazole)
Mercuval®	Dimercaptopropane-sulfonic acid
Mesacal®	Mesalamine (mesalazine)
Mesnex®	Mesna
Mestinon®	Pyridostigmine
Metacen®	Indometacin
Metahydrin®	Trichlormethiazide
Metalone®	Prednisolone
Metalyse®	Tenecteplase
Metandren®	Methyltestosterone
Metaprel®	Metaproterenol (orciprenaline)
Metenarin®	Methylergometrine (methylergonovine)
Meteosan®	Dimeticone
Methadose®	Methadone
Methampex®	Methamphetamine
Methanoxanol®	Sulfamethoxazole
Methergine®	Methylergometrine (methylergonovine)
Methofane®	Methoxyflurane
Methylergobrevin®	Methylergometrine (methylergonovine)
Meticorten®	Prednisone
Metilon®	Dipyrone
Metreton®	Prednisolone
Metronid®	Metronidazole
Mevacor®	Lovastatin
Meval®	Diazepam
Mevaril®	Amitriptyline
Mevinacor®	Lovastatin
Mexate®	Methotrexate
Mexitil®	Mexiletin
Mezlin®	Mezlocillin
Micardis®	Telmisartan
Micatin®	Miconazole
Micronase®	Glibenclamide (= glyburide)
Micronor®	Norethindrone (norethisterone)
Midamor®	Amiloride
Mielucin®	Busulfan
Mifegyne®	Mifepristone
Migril®	Ergotamine
Minipress®	Prazosin
Minirin®	Desmopressin
Minprog®	Alprostadil (= PGE_1)
Minprostin F2α®	Dinoprost
Mintezol®	Thiabendazole
Miocarpine®	Pilocarpine
Miostat®	Carbachol
Mistamine®	Mizolastine
Mitosan®	Busulfan
Mitoxana®	Ifosfamide
Mivacron®	Mivacurium
Mizollen®	Mizolastine
Mobenol®	Tolbutamide
Mobic®	Meloxicam
Modane®	Phenolphthalein
Moditen®	Fluphenazine
Moduret®	Amiloride + hydrochlorothiazide
Mogadon®	Nitrazepam
Molsidolat®	Molsidomine
Monistat®	Miconazole
Monitan®	Acebutolol
Monocor®	Bisoprolol
Monodox®	Doxycycline
Monomycin®	Erythromycin-succinate
Monopril®	Fosinopril
Monotrim®	Trimethoprim
Moronal®	Amphotericin B
Morphitec®	Morphine hydrochloride
Mosegor®	Pizotifen = pizotyline
Motilium®	Domperidone
Motrin®	Ibuprofen
Moxacin®	Amoxicillin
MSIR®	Morphine sulfate
MST Continus®	Morphine
Mucomyst®	Acetylcysteine
Mucosolvan®	Ambroxol
Murine®	Tetryzoline (= tetrahydrozoline)
Murocel®	Methylcellulose
Mustargen®	Mechlorethamine
Mutabase®	Diazoxide
Myambutol®	Ethambutol
Mycelex®	Clotrimazole
Mycifradin®	Neomycin
Myciguent®	Neomycin
Mycobutin®	Rifabutin

Mycospor® — Bifonazole
Mycosporan® — Bifonazole
Mycostatin® — Nystatin
Myidone® — Primidone
Mykinac® — Nystatin
Myleran® — Busulfan
Mylicon® — Simethicone
Myobid® — Papaverine
Myobloc® — Botulinum toxin type B
Mysoline® — Primidone
Nacom® — Carbidopa + levodopa

N

Nadopen-V® — Pencillin V
Naftin® — Naftifin
Nalador® — Sulprostone
Nalcrom® — Cromoglycate (Cromolyn)
Nalorex® — Naltrexone
Naprelan® — Naproxen
Napron® — Naproxen
Naprosyn® — Naproxen
Naqua® — Trichlormethiazide
Naramig® — Naratriptan
Narcan® — Naloxone
Narcaricin® — Benzbromarone
Narcozep® — Flunitrazepam
Narkotan® — Halothane
Nasalide® — Flunisolide
Nautamine® — Diphenhydramine
Nauzelin® — Domperidone
Navoban® — Tropisetron
Naxen® — Naproxen
Nebcin® — Tobramycin
Nefaclar® — Nefazodone
Negram® — Nalidixic acid
Nemasol Sodium® — 4-Aminosalicylic acid
Nembutal® — Pentobarbital
Neo-Codema® — Hydrochlorothiazide
Neo Epinin® — Isoprenaline (= isoproterenol)
Neo-Mercazole® — Carbimazole
Neoral® — Ciclosporin (= cyclosporine A)
Neo-Synephrine® — Oxymetazoline
Neosynephrine II® — Xylometazoline
Neo-Thyreostat® — Carbimazole
Nepresol® — Dihydralazine
Netillin® — Netilmicin
Netromycin® — Netilmicin
Neupogen® — Filgrastim
NeuroBloc® — Botulinum toxin type B
Neurontin® — Gabapentin
Nexium® — Esomeprazole
Niclocide® — Niclosamide
Nigalax® — Bisacodyl
Nilstat® — Nystatin
Nilurid® — Amiloride
Nimotop® — Nimodipine
Nipride® — Nitroprusside sodium

Nitrocap® — Nitroglycerin (glyceryl trinitrate)
Nitrogard® — Nitroglycerin (glyceryl trinitrate)
Nitronal® — Nitroglycerin (glyceryl trinitrate)
Nitropress® — Nitroprusside sodium
Nivaquine® — Chloroquine
Nivemycin® — Neomycin
Nix® — Permethrin
Nizoral® — Ketoconazol
Noan® — Diazepam
Nocinan® — Methotrimeprazine
Noctamid® — Lormetazepam
Noctec® — Chloral hydrate
Nogram® — Nalidixic acid
Nolvadex® — Tamoxifen
Norcuron® — Vecuronium
Nordox® — Doxycycline
Noriday® — Norethindrone (norethisterone)
Norlutin® — Norethindrone (norethisterone)
Normiflo® — Ardeparin
Normison® — Temazepam
Normodyne® — Labetalol
Normurat® — Benzbromarone
Noroxin® — Norfloxacin
Norpace® — Disopyramide
Norpramin® — Desipramine
Norprolac® — Quinagolide
Nor-Q D® — Norethindrone (norethisterone)
Norquen® — Mestranol
Norvasc® — Amlodipine
Norvir® — Ritonavir
Novalgin® — Dipyrone
Novamin® — Amikacin
Novamoxin® — Amoxicillin
Novarectal® — Pentobarbital
Novocaine® — Procaine
Novoclopate® — Clorazepate
Novodigoxin® — Digoxin
Novolin® — Insulin
Novolog® — Insulin aspart
Novomedopa® — Methyldopa
NovoNorm® — Repaglinide
Novopen-VK® — Pencillin V
Novopurol® — Allopurinol
Novorythro® — Erythromycin-estolate
Novotrimel® — Co-trimoxazole
Nubain® — Nalbuphine
Nu-Cal® — Calcium carbonate
Nuelin® — Theophylline
Nulicaine® — Lidocaine
Nuprin® — Ibuprofen
Nuromax® — Doxacurium
Nydrazid® — Isoniazid
Nystan® — Nystatin
Nystex® — Nystatin
Nytilax® — Senna

O

Octapressin®	Felypressin
Octostim®	Desmopressin
Oculinum®	Botulinum toxin type A
Ocupress®	Carteolol
Ocusert®	Pilocarpine
Olbemox®	Acipimox
Olbetam®	Acipimox
Omifin®	Clomifene
Omnipen®	Ampicillin
Oncovin®	Vincristine
Ondena®	Daunorubicin
Ondogyne®	Cyclofenil
Ondonid®	Cyclofenil
Opticrom®	Cromoglycate (cromolyn)
Optipranolol®	Metipranolol
Oragest®	Medroxyprogesterone-acetate
Oramide®	Tolbutamide
Oramorph®	Morphine
Orasone®	Prednisone
Oretic®	Hydrochlorothiazide
Orgalutran®	Ganirelix
Orgametril®	Lynestrenol
Orgaran®	Danaparoid
Orinase®	Tolbutamide
Orthoclone OKT3®	Muromonab-CD3
Osmitrol®	Mannitol
Ossiten®	Clodronate
Ostac®	Clodronate
Otrivin®	Xylometazoline
O-V Statin®	Nystatin
Ovastol®	Mestranol
Oxi®	Formoterol
Oxistat®	Oxiconazole
Oxpam®	Oxazepam

P

Paludrine®	Proguanil
Pamba®	Aminomethylbenzoic acid
Pamelor®	Nortriptyline
Panadol®	Acetaminophen (= paracetamol)
Panasol®	Prednisone
Panimit®	Bupranolol
Panwarfin®	Warfarin
Papacon®	Papaverine
Paralgin®	Dipyrone
Paraplatin®	Carboplatin
Parathion®	Nitrostigmine
Paraxin®	Chloramphenicol
Parcillin®	Penicillin G
Paregoric®	Opium tincture (laudanum)
Pariet®	Rabeprazole
Parlodel®	Bromocriptine
Parnate®	Tranylcypromine
Parsitan®	Ethopropazine

Parsitol®	Ethopropazine
Partergin®	Methylergometrine (methylergonovine)
Partusisten®	Fenoterol
Parvolex®	Acetylcysteine
Pathocil®	Dicloxacillin
Pavabid®	Papaverine
Pavadur®	Papaverine
Paveral®	Codeine
Pavulon®	Pancuronium
Paxil®	Paroxetine
Pectokay®	Kaolin + pectin (= attapulgite)
Pediapred®	Prednisolone
Pemavit®	Vitamin B_{12}
Penapar VK®	Penicillin V
Penapar-VK®	Penicillin V
Penbec-V®	Penicillin V
Penbritin®	Ampicillin
Pensorb®	Penicillin G
Pentacarinat®	Pentamidine
Pentanca®	Pentobarbital
Pentasa®	Mesalamine (mesalazine)
Pentazine®	Promethazine
Penthrane®	Methoxyflurane
Pentids®	Penicillin G
Pentostam®	Stibogluconate sodium
Pentothal®	Thiopental
Pen-VEE K®	Penicillin V
Pepcid®	Famotidine
Pepdul®	Famotidine
Pepto-Bismol®	Bismuth subsalicylate
Peptol®	Cimetidine
Pergotime®	Clomifene
Peridon®	Domperidone
Periostat®	Doxycycline
Permanone®	Permethrin
Permapen®	Penicillin G
Permax®	Pergolide
Pertofran®	Desipramine
Pethidine®	Meperidine
Petinimid®	Ethosuximide
Pevaryl®	Econazole
Pfizerpen VK®	Penicillin V
Pfizerpin®	Penicillin G
Phazyme®	Simethicone
Phenazine®	Promethazine
Phenergan®	Promethazine
Physeptone®	Methadone
Pilokair®	Pilocarpine
Pipracil®	Piperacillin
Pitocin®	Oxytocin
Pitressin®	Vasopressin
Plaquenil®	Hydroxychloroquine
Plasmotrim®	Artesunate
Platet®	Acetylsalicylic acid
Platinex®	Cisplatin
Platinol®	Cisplatin
Plavix®	Clopidogrel
Plendil®	Felodipine
Polamidon®	Levomethadone
Polycillin®	Ampicillin

Ponderal®	Fenfluramine
Ponderax®	Fenfluramine
Pondimin®	Fenfluramine
Pontocaine®	Tetracaine
POR 8®	Ornipressin
Pradin®	Repaglinide
Pravachol®	Pravastatin
Pravidel®	Bromocriptine
Precose®	Acarbose
Predate®	Prednisolone
Predcor®	Prednisolone
Predenema®	Prednisolone
Predfoam®	Prednisolone
Prednesol®	Prednisolone
Preferid®	Budesonide
Pregnesin®	Chorionic gonadotropin (HCG)
Pregnyl®	Chorionic gonadotropin (HCG)
Prelone®	Prednisolone
Prenalex®	Tertatolol
Prepidil®	Dinoprostone
Presinol®	Methyldopa
Pressunic®	Dihydralazine
Prevacid®	Lansoprazole
Prevalite®	Cholestyramine
Priadel®	Lithium carbonate
Primabolan®	Metenolone
Primaquine®	Primaquine
Primolut Depo®	Hydroxyprogesterone caproate
Primolut N®	Norethindrone (norethisterone)
Primperan®	Metoclopramide
Principen®	Ampicillin
Prinivil®	Lisinopril
Privine®	Naphazoline
Probalan®	Probenecid
Procan SR®	Procainamide
Procardia®	Nifedipine
Procorum®	Gallopamil
Procrit®	Erythropoietin (= epoetin alfa)
Procytox®	Cyclophosphamide
Pro-Depo®	Hydroxyprogesterone caproate
Progestasert®	Progesterone
Proglicem®	Diazoxide
Prograf®	Tacrolimus
Progynon®	Estradiol-benzoate
Progynova®	Estradiol-valerate
Prolixan®	Azapropazone
Prolixin®	Fluphenazine
Prolopa®	Levodopa + benserazide
Proloprim®	Trimethoprim
Prometh®	Promethazine
Promine®	Procainamide
Pronestyl®	Procainamide
Propaderm®	Beclometasone
Propasa®	Mesalamine (mesalazine)
Propecia®	Finasteride

Prophasi®	Chorionic gonadotropin (HCG)
Propulsid (discontinued)®	Cisapride
Propyl-Thyracil®	Propylthiouracil
Prorex®	Promethazine
Proscar®	Finasteride
Prostaphlin®	Oxacillin
Prostarmon®	Dinoprost
Prostigmin®	Neostigmine
Prostin E₂®	Dinoprostone
Prostin F₂ Alpha,®	Dinoprost
Prostin VR®	Alprostadil (= PGE₁)
Protonix®	Pantoprazole
Protopam Chloride®	Pralidoxime
Protostat®	Metronidazole
Protrin®	Co-trimoxazole
Provas®	Valsartan
Pro-Vent®	Theophylline
Provera®	Medroxyprogesterone-acetate
Provigan®	Promethazine
Proviron®	Mesterolone
Prozac®	Fluoxetine
Prulet®	Phenolphthalein
Pulmicort®	Budesonide
Pulsamin®	Etilefrine
Purinethol®	Mercaptopurine
Purodigin®	Digitoxin
Pyopen®	Carbenicillin
Pyrilax®	Bisacodyl
Pyronoval®	Acetylsalicylic acid
Pyroxine®	Vitamin B₆
Pyroxine®	Pyridoxine

Q

Quelicin®	Succinylcholine
Quellada®	Lindane
Questran®	Cholestyramine
Quibron-T®	Theophylline
Quinachlor®	Chloroquine
Quinalan®	Quinidine
Quinaminoph®	Quinine
Quinamm®	Quinine
Quine®	Quinine
Quinidex®	Quinidine
Quinite®	Quinine
Quinora®	Quinidine
Qvar®	Beclometasone

R

Rapamune®	Sirolimus
Rapilysin®	Reteplase
Rastinon®	Tolbutamide
Rebetol®	Ribavirin
Rebif®	Interferon beta-1a
Reclomide®	Metoclopramide

Trade Name	Drug Name
Recormon®	Epoetin
Rectocort®	Hydrocortisone (cortisol)
Redisol®	Vitamin B_{12}
Reductil®	Sibutramine
Redux®	Fenfluramine
Refludan®	Lepirudin
Refobacin®	Gentamicin
Regaine®	Minoxidil
Regitin®	Phentolamine
Reglan®	Metoclopramide
Regonol®	Pyridostigmine
Rehibin®	Cyclofenil
Relefact®	Gonadorelin
Relenza®	Zanamivir
Relpax®	Eletriptan
Remergil®	Mirtazepine
Remeron SolTab®	Mirtazepine
Remicade®	Infliximab
Reminyl®	Galantamine
Remsed®	Promethazine
Reomax®	Ethacrynic acid
ReoPro®	Abciximab
ReQuip®	Ropinirole
Rescriptor®	Delavirdine
Rescudose®	Morphine sulfate
Restandol®	Testosterone
Restoril®	Temazepam
Retardin®	Diphenoxylate
Retrovir®	Zidovudine
Revasc®	Desirudin
Reverin®	Rolitetracycline
Rezipas®	Mesalamine (mesalazine)
Rezulin®	Troglitazone
Rheumox®	Azapropazone
Rhinalar®	Flunisolide
Rhinocort®	Budesonide
Rhumalgan®	Diclofenac
Rhythmin®	Procainamide
Rhythmol®	Propafenone
Riamet®	Artemether + lumefantrine
Ridaura®	Auranofin
Rifadin®	Rifampin (rifampicin)
Rimactan®	Rifampin (rifampicin)
Rimifon®	Isoniazid
Rinatec®	Ipratropium
Riopan®	Magaldrate
Risperdal®	Risperidone
Rivotril®	Clonazepam
Rize®	Clotiazepam
Robicillin-VK®	Pencillin V
Rocaltrol®	Calcitriol
Rocephin®	Ceftriaxone
Roferon A3®	Interferon alpha-2a
Rogaine®	Minoxidil
Rogitin®	Phentolamine
Rohypnol®	Flunitrazepam
Romazicon®	Flumazenil
Roniacol®	Pyridylcarbinol
Ronicol®	Pyridylcarbinol
Rowasa®	Mesalamine (mesalazine)
Roxanol®	Morphine sulfate
RU 486®	Mifepristone
Rubesol®	Vitamin B_{12}
Rubion®	Cyanocobalamin
Rubramin®	Cyanocobalamin
Rulid®	Roxithromycin
Ryegonovin®	Methylergometrine (methylergonovine)
Rynacrom®	Cromoglycate (cromolyn)
Rythmodan®	Disopyramide

S

Trade Name	Drug Name
S.A.S.-500®	Salazosulfapyridine (sulfasalazine)
Sabril®	Vigabatrin
Saizen®	Somatotropin
Salazopyrin®	Salazosulfapyridine (sulfasalazine)
Saltucin®	Butizid
Sandimmune®	Ciclosporin (= cyclosporine A)
Sandomigran®	Pizotifen = pizotyline
Sandostatin®	Octreotide
Sandril®	Reserpine
Sang-35®	Ciclosporin (= cyclosporine A)
SangCya®	Ciclosporin (= cyclosporine A)
Sanocrisin®	Cyclofenil
Sansert®	Methysergide
Satric®	Metronidazole
Saventrine®	Isoprenaline (= isoproterenol)
Scabene®	Lindane
Scopoderm TTS®	Scopolamine
Sebcur®	Salicylic acid
Sectral®	Acebutolol
Securon®	Verapamil
Securopen®	Azlocillin
Seguril®	Furosemide
Seldane®	Terfenadine
Selectol®	Celiprolol
Sembrina®	Methyldopa
Sempera®	Itraconazole
Senokot®	Senna
Senolax®	Senna
Sepram®	Citalopram
Septra®	Co-trimoxazole
Serax®	Oxazepam
Serenace®	Haloperidol
Serevent®	Sameterol
Serlect®	Sertindole*
Sernyl®	Phencyclidine
Seromycin®	Cycloserine
Serono-Bagren®	Bromocriptine
Serophene®	Clomifene
Serpalan®	Reserpine
Serpasil®	Reserpine
Sertan®	Primidone
Serzone®	Nefazodone
Sevorane®	Sevoflurane

Sexovid®	Cyclofenil	Stresson®	Bunitrolol
Sibelium®	Flunarizine	Stromectol®	Ivermectin
Sifrol®	Pramipexole	Suacron®	Carazolol
Silain®	Simethicone	Sublimaze®	Fentanyl
Simplene®	Epinephrine	Succostrin®	Succinylcholine
Simplotan®	Tinidazol	Sufenta®	Sufentanil
Simulect®	Basiliximab	Sulcrate®	Sucralfate
Sinarest®	Oxymetazoline	Sulfabutin®	Busulfan
Sinemet®	Carbidopa + levodopa	Sulmycin®	Gentamicin
Singulair®	Montelukast	Sulpyrin®	Dipyrone
Sinthrome®	Acenocoumarin	Supasa®	Acetylsalicylic acid
	(= nicoumalone)	Supramycin®	Tetracycline
	Acenocoumarin	Suprane®	Desflurane
Sintrom®	(= nicoumalone)	Suprarenin®	Epinephrine
	Xylometazoline	Suprefact®	Buserelin
Sinutab®	Carbachol	Sustac®	Nitroglycerin
Sirtal®	Clofibrate		(glyceryl trinitrate)
Skleromexe®	Theophylline	Sustaine®	Xylometazoline
Slo-bid®	Theophylline	Sustaire®	Theophylline
Slo-Phyllin®	Chloramphenicol	Sustanon®	Testosterone
Sno Phenicol®	Clindamycin	Sustiva®	Efavirenz
Sobelin®	Warfarin	Suxamethonium®	Succinylcholine
Sofarin®	Canrenone	Suxinutin®	Ethosuximide
Soldactone®	Phenobarbital	Symmetrel®	Amantadine
Solfoton®	Aurothioglucose	Synflex®	Naproxen
Solganal®	Acetylsalicylic acid	Synkayvit®	Menadione
Solprin®	Amantadine	Synovir®	Thalidomide
Solu-Contenton®	Salicylic acid	Syntocinon®	Oxytocin
Soluver®	Reboxetine	Syntopressin®	Lypressin
Solvex®	Pegvisomant	Sytobex®	Cyanocobalamin
Somavert®	Nitrazepam	Sytobex®	Vitamin B_{12}
Somnite®	Chloral hydrate		
Somnos®	Theophylline		
Somophyllin-T®	Zaleplone	**T**	
Sonata®	Chloramphenicol		
Sopamycetin®	Bisoprolol		
Soprol®	Isosorbide dinitrate	Tacef®	Cefmenoxime
Sorbitrate®	Tinidazol	Tacicef®	Ceftazidime
Sorquetan®	Sotalol	Tactocile®	Atosiban
Sotacor®	Methylergometrine	Tagamet®	Cimetidine
Spametrin-M®	(methylergonovine)	Talwin®	Pentazocine
	Dexamethasone	Tambocor®	Flecainide
Spersadex®	Chloramphenicol	Tamiflu®	Oseltamivir
Spersanicol®	Tiotropium	Tamofen®	Tamoxifen
Spiriva®	Budesonide	Tapazole®	Methimazole
Spirocort®	Spironolactone		(thiamazole)
Spiroctan®	Itraconazole	Tardigal®	Digitoxin
Sporanox®	Buserelin	Tarivid®	Ofloxacin
Sprecur®	Pencillin V	Tasmar®	Tolcapone
Stabilin V-K®	Flucloxacillin	Tauredon®	Aurothiomalate sodium
Stafoxil®	(floxacilline)	Tavegil®	Clemastine
	Ambroxol	Tavist®	Clemastine
Stas Surfactal®	Morphine sulfate	Tavor®	Lorazepam
Statex®	Clostebol	Taxol®	Paclitaxel
Steranabol®	Diazepam	Taxotere®	Docetaxel
Stesolid®	Zolpidem	Tebrazid®	Pyrazinamide
Stilnox®	Diethylstilbestrol	Teebaconin®	Isoniazid
Stilphostrol®	Desmopressin	Tegison®	Etretinate
Stimate®	Idoxuridine	Tegopen®	Cloxacillin
Stoxil®	Streptomycin	Tegretol®	Carbamazepine
Strepolin®	Streptokinase	Telemin®	Bisacodyl
Streptase®	Streptomycin	Telfast®	Fexofenadine
Streptosol®		Temgesic®	Buprenorphine

Tempra®	Acetaminophen (= paracetamol)
Tenalin®	Carteolol
Tenormin®	Atenolol
Tensium®	Diazepam
Tensobon®	Captopril
Teoptic®	Carteolol
Testex®	Testosterone propionate
Testoject®	Testosterone cypionate
Testone®	Testosterone enantate
Testred®	Methyltestosterone
Teveten®	Eprosartan
Theelol®	Estratriol = estriol
Theolair®	Theophylline
Thesit®	Polidocanol
Thevier®	Levothyroxine
Thiotepa Lederle®	Thio-TEPA
Thorazine®	Chlorpromazine
Thrombinar®	Thrombin
Thrombostat®	Thrombin
Thyrogen®	Thyrotropin
Ticar®	Ticarcillin
Ticlid®	Ticlopidine
Tienor®	Clotiazepam
Tigason®	Etretinate
Tilade®	Nedocromil
Tildiem®	Diltiazem
Timentin®	Ticarcillin
Timonil®	Carbamazepine
Timoptic®	Timolol
Timoptol®	Timolol
Timox®	Oxcarbazepine
Toazul®	Tolonium chloride
Tobralex®	Tobramycin
Tobrex®	Tobramycin
Tofranil®	Imipramine
Tonocard®	Tocainide
Topamex®	Topiramate
Topitracin®	Bacitracin
Toposar®	Etoposide
Toradol®	Ketorolac
Tornalate®	Bitolterol
Totacillin®	Ampicillin
Totamol®	Atenolol
Toxogonin®	Obidoxime
Tracleer®	Bosentan
Tracrium®	Atracurium
Tramal®	Tramadol
Trandate®	Labetalol
Transcycline®	Rolitetracyclin
Transderm Scop®	Scopolamine
Trans-Ver-Sal®	Salicylic acid
Tranxene®	Clorazepate
Tranxilium N®	Nordazepam
Trapanal®	Thiopental
Trasicor®	Oxprenolol
Travogen®	Isoconazole
Travogyn®	Isoconazole
Trecalmo®	Clotiazepam
Trecator®	Ethionamide
Trelstar Depot®	Triptorelin
Tremblex®	Dexetimide

Trendar®	Ibuprofen
Trental®	Pentoxifylline
Trexan®	Naltrexone
Trialodine®	Trazodone
Triam-A®	Triamcinolone acetonide
Trichlorex®	Trichlormethiazide
Tricor®	Fenofibrate
Tridil®	Nitroglycerin (glyceryl trinitrate)
Trileptal®	Oxcarbazepine
Triludan®	Terfenadine
Trimpex®	Trimethoprim
Trimysten®	Clotrimazole
Triostat®	Liothyronine
Triptone®	Scopolamine
Trusopt®	Dorzolamide
Tryptizol®	Amitriptyline
Tubarine®	Tubocurarine
Tubasal®	4-Aminosalicylic acid
Tus®	Ambroxol
Tylenol®	Acetaminophen (= paracetamol)
Typramine®	Imipramine
Tyrozets®	Tyrothricin
Tyzine®	Tetryzoline (= tetrahydrozoline)

U

Udicil®	Cytarabine
Udolac®	Dapsone
Ukidan®	Urokinase
Ulcolax®	Bisacodyl
Ultair®	Pranlukast
Unacid®	Ampicillin + sulbactam
Unasyn®	Ampicillin + sulbactam
Unicort®	Hydrocortisone (cortisol)
Uniparin®	Heparin
Uniphyl®	Theophylline
Univer®	Verapamil
Uricovac®	Benzbromarone
Uritol®	Furosemide
Uromitexan®	Mesna
Urosin®	Allopurinol
UroXatral®	Alfuzosin
Uticillin-VK®	Pencillin V
Utinor®	Norfloxacin

V

Valadol®	Acetaminophen (= paracetamol)
Valcyte®	Valganciclovir
Valium®	Diazepam
Valorin®	Acetaminophen (= paracetamol)
Valtrex®	Valaciclovir
Vancocin®	Vancomycin
Vaponefrine®	Epinephrine
Vasal®	Papaverine

Vascardin®	Isosorbide dinitrate
Vasocon®	Naphazoline
Vasotec®	Enalapril/enalaprilat
Vatran®	Diazepam
Va-tro-nol®	Ephedrine
V-Cillin K®	Pencillin V
Vectavir®	Penciclovir
Veetids®	Pencillin V
Vegesan®	Nordazepam
Velacycline®	Rolitetracyclin
Velban®	Vinblastine
Velbe®	Vinblastine
Velosulin®	Insulin
Venactone®	Canrenone
VePesid®	Etoposide
Veratran®	Clotiazepam
Verelan®	Verapamil
Vermox®	Mebendazole
Versed®	Midazolam
Vestra®	Reboxetine
Viagra®	Sildenafil
Vibal®	Vitamin B_{12}
Vibal L.A.®	Hydroxocobalamin
Vibramycin®	Doxycycline
Videx®	Didanosine
Vidopen®	Ampicillin
Vigantol®	Colecalciferol (vitamin D_3)
Vigorsan®	Colecalciferol (vitamin D_3)
Vinactane®	Viomycin
Viocin®	Viomycin
Vionactane®	Viomycin
Vioxx®	Rofecoxib
Vira-A®	Vidarabine
Viracept®	Nelfinavir
Viramune®	Nevirapine
Virazole®	Ribavirin
Virilon®	Methyltestosterone
Virofral®	Amantadine
Visine®	Tetryzoline (= tetrahydrozoline)
Visken®	Pindolol
Vistacrom®	Cromoglycate (cromolyn)
Visutensil®	Guanethidine
Vitamine B_1®	Thiamin(e)
Vitrasert®	Ganciclovir
Vivol®	Diazepam
Volon®	Triamcinolone
Voltaren®	Diclofenac
Voltarol®	Diclofenac
VP-16®	Etoposide
Vumon®	Teniposide

W

Wandonorm®	Bopindolol
Welcovorin®	Leucovorin
Wellbatrin®	Bupropion
Wellbutrin®	Bupropion
Welldorm Elixir®	Chloral hydrate
Whevert®	Meclizine (meclozine)
Wincoram®	Amrinone
Wingom®	Gallopamil
Winpred®	Prednisone
Wyamycin®	Erythromycin-ethyl-succinate

X

Xalaten®	Lanatoprost
Xanax®	Alprazolam
Xanef®	Enalapril/Enalaprilat
Xenical®	Orlistat
Xolair®	Omalizumab
Xusal®	Levocetirizine
Xylocain®	Lidocaine
Xylocard®	Lidocaine
Xylonest®	Prilocaine

Y

Yal®	Sorbitol
Yomesan®	Niclosamide

Z

Zadstat®	Metronidazole
Zantac®	Ranitidine
Zapex®	Oxazepam
Zarontin®	Ethosuximide
Zebeta®	Bisoprolol
Zeldox®	Ziprasidone
Zemuron®	Rocuronium
Zenapax®	Daclizumab
Zepine®	Reserpine
Zerit®	Stavudine
Zestril®	Lisinopril
Zetria®	Ezetimibe
Ziagen®	Abacavir
Zimovane®	Zopiclone
Zinamide®	Pyrazinamide
Zithromax®	Azithromycin
Zocor®	Simvastatin
Zofran®	Ondansetron
Zoladex®	Goserelin
Zolim®	Mizolastine
Zoloft®	Sertraline
Zomig-ZMT®	Zolmitriptan
Zosyn®	Tazobactam + piperacillin
Zovirax®	Aciclovir
Zyban®	Bupropion
Zyloprim®	Allopurinol
Zyloric®	Allopurinol
Zyprexa®	Olanzapine
Zyvoxid®	Linezolide

Drug Name – Trade Name
(* denotes investigational status in the United States)

A

Abacavir	Ziagen®
Abciximab	ReoPro®
Acamprosate	Campral®
Acarbose	Precose®
Acebutolol	Monitan®, Sectral®
Acenocoumarin (= nicoumalone)	Sinthrome®, Sintrom®
Acetaminophen (= paracetamol)	Acephen®, Anacin-3®, Bromo-Seltzer®, Calpol®, Datril®, Panadol®, Tempra®, Tylenol®, Valadol®, Valorin®
Acetazolamide	Diamox®, Glaupax®
Acetylcysteine	Airbron®, Fabrol®, Mucomyst®, Parvolex®
Acetylsalicylic acid	Angettes®, Arthrisin®, Asadrine®, Aspirin®, Ecotrin®, Entrophen®, Platet®, Pyronoval®, Solprin®, Supasa®
Aciclovir (Acyclovir)	Zovirax®
Acipimox	Olbemox®, Olbetam®
ACTH	see Corticotropin®
Actinomycin D	see Dactinomycin®
ADH	see Vasopressin®
Adalimumab	Humira®
Adrenaline	see Epinephrine®
Adriamycin	see Doxorubicin®
Ajmaline	Cardiorhythmino®, Gilurytmal®
Albuterol	see Salbutamol®
Alcuronium	Alloferin®
Aldosterone	Aldocorten®
Alendronate	Fosamax®
Alfentanil	Alfenta®
Alfuzosin	Alfoten®, UroXatral®
Allopurinol	Alloprin®, Caplenal®, Hamarin®, Novopurol®, Urosin®, Zyloprim®, Zyloric ®
Alprazolam	Xanax®
Alprenolol	Aprobal®, Aptine®, Gubernal®
Alprostadil (= PGE₁)	Minprog®, Prostin VR®
Alteplase	Actilyse®
Aluminum hydroxide	Aldrox®, Alu-Cap®, Alu-Tab®, Amphojel®, Fluagel®
Amantadine	Ambaxine®, Solu-Contenton®, Symmetrel®, Virofral®

Ambroxol	Ambril®, Bronchopront®, Mucosolvan®, Stas Surfactal®, Tus®
Amfebutamon(e)	see Bupropion®
Amikacin	Amikin®, Briclin®, Novamin®
Amiloride	Arumil®, Colectril®, Cordarex®, Midamor®, Nilurid®
Amiloride + hydrochlorothiazide	Moduret®
ε-Aminocaproic acid	Afibrin®, Amicar®, Capramol®, Epsicapron®
Aminomethyl benzoic acid	Gumbix®, Pamba®
4-Aminosalicylic acid	Nemasol Sodium®, Tubasal®
5-Aminosalicylic acid	see Mesalamine (mesalazine)®
Amiodarone	Cordarex®, Cordarone®
Amitriptyline	Amitril®, Domical®, Elavil®, Endep®, Enovil®, Lentizol®, Levate®, Mevaril®, Tryptizol®
Amlodipine	Norvasc®
Amodiaquine	Camoquin®, Flavoquine®
Amorolfin	Loceryl®
Amoxicillin	Almodan®, Amoxil®, Clamoxyl®, Moxacin®, Novamoxin®
Amoxicillin + clavulanic acid	Augmentan®
Amphetamine	see Dextroamphetamine®
Amphotericin B	Amphozone®, Fungilin®, Fungizone®, Moronal®
Ampicillin	Amcill®, Amphipen®, Omnipen®, Penbritin®, Polycillin®, Principen®, Totacillin®, Vidopen®
Ampicillin + sulbactam	Unacid®, Unasyn®
Amprenavir	Agenerase®
Amrinone	Inocor®, Wincoram®
Anakinra	Kineret®
Anastrozole	Arimidex®
Angiotensinamide	Hypertensin®
Aprindine	Amidonal®, Aspenon®, Fibocil®, Fiboran®
Ardeparin	Normiflo®
Artemether + lumefantrine	Riamet®
Artesunate	Arsumax®, Falcigo®, Plasmotrim®
Asparaginase	Erwinase®
Astemizole	Hismanal®

Aspirin	*see* Acetylsalicylic acid®
Atenolol	Antipressan®, Tenormin®, Totamol®
Atoquavone	Mepron®
Atoquavone + proguanil	Malarone®
Atorvastatin	Lipitor®
Atosiban	Antocin®, Tactocile®
Atracurium	Tracrium®
Atropine	Atropisol®, Borotropin®
Auranofin	Ridaura®
Aurothioglucose	Aureotan®, Auromyose®, Solganal®
Aurothiomalate sodium	Tauredon®
Azapropazone	Prolixan®, Rheumox®
Azathioprine	Azanin®, Berkaprine®, Imuran®, Imurek®
Azidothymidine (AZT)	*see* Zidovudine®
Azithromycin	Zithromax®
Azlocillin	Azlin®, Securopen®

B

Bacitracin	Altracin®, Baciguent®, Topitracin®
Baclofen	Lioresal®
Basiliximab	Simulect®
Beclometasone	Aldecin®, Becloforte®, Becodisks®, Beconase®, Becotide®, Propaderm®, Qvar®
Befunolol	Bentos®, Betaclar®, Glauconex®
Benazepril	Lotensin®
Benserazide	Madopar (plus levodopa)®
Benzbromarone	Desuric®, Narcaricin®, Normurat®, Uricovac®
Benzocaine	Americaine®, Anacaine®, Anaesthesin®
Benztropine	Cogentin®
Betaxolol	Betoptic®, Kerlone®
Bezafibrate	Befizal®, Bezalip®, Bezatol®, Cedur®
Bicalutamide	Casodex®
Bifonazole	Amycor®, Mycospor®, Mycosporan®
Bimatoprost	Lumigan®
Biperiden	Akineton®, Akinophyl®
Bisacodyl	Bicol®, Broxalax®, Dulcolax®, Durolax®, Laxabene®, Laxanin®, Nigalax®, Pyrilax®, Telemin®, Ulcolax®
Bismuth subsalicylate	Pepto-Bismol®
Bisoprolol	Concor®, Detensiel®, Emcor®, Isoten®, Monocor®, Soprol®, Zebeta®
Bitolterol	Effectin®, Tornalate®

Bleomycin	Blenoxane®
Bopindolol	Wandonorm®
Bosentan	Tracleer®
Botulinum toxin type A	Botox®, Oculinum®
Botulinum toxin type B	Myobloc®, NeuroBloc®
Brimonidine	Alphagan®
Brinzolamide	Azopt®
Bromazepam	Durazanil®, Lectopam®, Lexotan®
Bromocriptine	Parlodel®, Pravidel®, Serono-Bagren®
Brotizolam	Lendorm(A)®, Lendormin®
Bucindolol	Bextra®
Budesonide	Entocort EC®, Preferid®, Pulmicort®, Rhinocort®, Spirocort®
Bumetanide	Bumex®, Burinex®, Fontego®, Fordiuran®, Lixil®
Bunitrolol	Betriol®, Stresson®
Bupranolol	Betadran®, Betadrenol®, Looser®, Panimit®
Buprenorphine	Buprene®, Temgesic®
Bupropion	Wellbatrin®, Wellbutrin®, Zyban®
Buserelin	Sprecur®, Suprefact®
Buspirone	Buspar®
Busulfan	Mielucin®, Mitosan®, Myleran®, Sulfabutin®
Butizid	Saltucin®
Butylscopolamine	Buscopan®

C

Cabergoline	Cabaseril®, Dostinex®
Calcifediol	Calderol®, Dedrogyl®, Hidroferol®
Calcitonin	Calcimer®, Calcitare®, Calsynar®, Cibacalcin®, Karil®
Calcitriol	Rocaltrol®
Calcium carbonate	Cacit®, Calchichew®, Calcidrink®, Calsan®, Caltrate®, Nu-Cal®
Camazepam	Albego®
Candesartan	Atacand®
Canrenone	Kanrenol®, Soldactone®, Venactone®
Capreomycin	Capastat®, Caprolin®
Captopril	Acediur®, Acepril®, Alopresin®, Capoten®, Cesplon®, Hypertil®, Lopirin®, Tensobon®
Carazolol	Conducton®, Suacron®
Carbachol	Doryl®, Lentin®, Miostat®, Sirtal®
Carbamazepine	Epitol®, Mazepine®, Tegretol®, Timonil®

Carbenicillin	Anabactyl (A)®, Carindapen®, Geopen®, Pyopen®
Carbidopa + levodopa	Isicom®, Nacom®, Sinemet®
Carbimazole	Neo-Mercazole®, Neo-Thyreostat®
Carboplatin	Paraplatin®
Carteolol	Arteoptic®, Caltidren®, Carteol®, Cartrol®, Endak®, Ocupress®, Tenalin®, Teoptic®
Carvedilol	Coreg®
Caspofungin	Cancidas®
Cefalexin	Keflex®, Keftab®
Cefmenoxime	Bestcall®, Cefmax®, Cemix®, Tacef®
Cefotaxime	Claforan®
Ceftazidime	Fortaz®, Fortum®, Tacicef®
Ceftriaxone	Acantex®, Rocephin®
Celecoxib = colecoxib	Celebrex®
Celiprolol	Selectol®
Cellulose	Avicel®
Cerivastatin	Baycol®
Chloral hydrate	Lorinal®, Noctec®, Somnos®, Welldorm Elixir®
Chlorambucil	Chloraminophene®, Leukeran®
Chloramphenicol	Chloromycetin®, Chloroptic®, Kemicetine Leukomycin®, Paraxin®, Sno Phenicol®, Sopamycetin®, Spersanicol®
Chlordiazepoxide	Librium®
Chlormadinone acetate	Gestafortin®
Chloroquine	Aralen®, Avloclor®, Nivaquine®, Quinachlor®
Chlorpromazine	Hibanil®, Largactil®, Megaphen®, Thorazine®
Chlorthalidone	Hygroton®
Cholestyramine	Cuemid®, Prevalite®, Questran®
Chorionic gonadotropin (HCG)	Entromone®, Follutein®, Pregnesin®, Pregnyl®, Prophasi®
Ciclosporin (= cyclosporine A)	Gengraf®, Neoral®, Sandimmune®, SangCya®, Sang-35®
Cilazapril	Inhibace®
Cimetidine	Dyspamet®, Peptol®, Tagamet®
Ciprofloxacin	Ciloxan®, Cipro®, Ciprobay®, Ciprox®, Ciproxin®
Cisapride	Propulsid (discontinued)®
Cisplatin	Platinex®, Platinol®
Citalopram	Celexa®, Citaprim®, Sepram®
Clarithromycin	Biaxin®
Clavulanic acid + amoxicillin	Augmentin®
Clemastine	Tavegil®, Tavist®
Clindamycin	Cleocin®, Dalacin®, Sobelin®
Clobazam	Frisium®
Clodronate	Clasteon®, Ossiten®, Ostac®
Clofazimine	Lampren®
Clofibrate	Atromid-S®, Claripex®, Skleromexe®
Clomethiazole	Distraneurin®, Hemineurin®
Clomifene	Clomid®, Dyneric®, Omifin®, Pergotime®, Serophene®
Clonazepam	Clonopin®, Iktorivil®, Rivotril®
Clonidine	Catapres®, Dixarit®
Clopidogrel	Plavix®
Clorazepate	Novoclopate®, Tranxene®
Clostebol	Macrobin®, Steranabol®
Clotiazepam	Clozan®, Rize®, Tienor®, Trecalmo®, Veratran®
Clotrimazole	Canesten®, Clotrimaderm®, Gyne-Lotrimin®, Mycelex® Trimysten®
Cloxacillin	Clovapen®, Tegopen®
Clozapine	Clozaril®
Codeine	Codicept®, Paveral®
Colchicine	Colchicine®
Colecalciferol (vitamin D₃)	D-Tabs®, Vigantol®, Vigorsan®
Colecoxib	*see* Celecoxib®
Colestipol	Cholestabyl®, Cholestid®
Corticotropin	Acthar®, Cortigel®, Cortrophin®
Cortisol	*see* Hydrocortisone®
Cortisone	Cortelan®, Cortistab®, Cortogen®, Cortone®
Co-trimoxazole	Bactrim®, Novotrimel®, Protrin®, Septra®
Cromoglycate (cromolyn)	Intal®, Nalcrom®, Opticrom®, Rynacrom®, Vistacrom®
Cyanocobalamin	Anacobin®, Bedoz®, Cytacon®, Cytamen®, Rubion®, Rubramin®, Sytobex®
Cyclofenil	Fertodur®, Ondogyne®, Ondonid®, Rehibin®, Sanocrisin®, Sexovid®
Cyclophosphamide	Cytoxan®, Endoxan®, Procytox®
Cycloserine	Seromycin®
Cyclosporine A	*see* Ciclosporin®
Cyproterone-acetate	Androcur®, Cyprostat®
Cytarabine	Alexan®, Cytosar®, Udicil®

D

Daclizumab	Zenapax®
Dactinomycin	Cosmegen®
Dalteparin	Fragmin®
Danaparoid	Orgaran®
Dantrolene	Dantrium®
Dapsone	Avlosulfone®, Eporal®, Diphenasone®, Udolac®
Darbepoetin	Aranesp®
Daunorubicin	Cerubidine®, Daunoblastin®, Ondena®
Deferoxamine	Desferal®
Delavirdine	Rescriptor®
Desflurane	Suprane®
Desipramine	Norpramin®, Pertofran®
Desirudin	Revasc®
Desloratadine	Aerius®
Desmopressin	DDAVP®, Minirin®, Octostim®, Stimate®
Desogestrel + ethinylestradiol	Marvelon®
Dexamethasone	Decadron®, Deronil®, Hexadrol®, Maxidex®, Spersadex®
Dexetimide	Tremblex®
Dextran	Hyskon®
Diazepam	Apaurin®, Atensine®, Diastat®, Dizac®, Eridan®, Lembrol®, Meval®, Noan®, Stesolid®, Tensium®, Valium®, Vatran®, Vivol®
Diazoxide	Eudemine®, Hyperstat®, Mutabase®, Proglicem®
Diclofenac	Allvoran®, Diclophlogont®, Rhumalgan®, Voltaren®, Voltarol®
Dicloxacillin	Diclocil®, Dynapen®, Pathocil®
Didanosine	Videx®
Diethylcarbamazepine	Hetrazan®
Diethylstilbestrol	Honvol®, Stilphostrol®
Digitoxin	Crystodigin®, Digicor®, Digimerck®, Digitaline®, Purodigin®, Tardigal®
Digoxin	Digacin®, Lanicor®, Lanoxin®, Lenoxin®, Novodigoxin®
Digoxin immune FAB	Digibind®
Dihydralazine	Dihyzin®, Nepresol®, Pressunic®
Dihydroergotamine	Angionorm®, D.E.H.45®, Dihydergot®, Divegal®, Endophleban®
Diltiazem	Cardizem®, Tildiem®
Dimenhydrinate	Dimetab®, Dramamine®, Dymenate®, Marmine®
Dimercaprol	BAL in oil®

Dimercaptopropane-sulfonic acid	Dimaval®, Mercuval®
Dimethylaminophenol	4-DMAP®
Dimeticone	Aegrosan®, Meteosan®
Dimetindene	Fenistil®
Dinoprost	Minprostin F2α®, Prostarmon®, Prostin F₂ Alpha®
Dinoprostone	Prepidil®, Prostin E₂®
Diphenhydramine	Allerdryl®, Benadryl®, Insommal®, Nautamine®
Diphenoxylate	Diarsed®, Lomotil®, Retardin®
Dipyrone	Algocalmin®, Bonpyrin®, Divarine®, Feverall®, Metilon®, Novalgin®, Paralgin®, Sulpyrin®
Disopyramide	Dirythmin®, Norpace®, Rythmodan®
Dobutamine	Dobutrex®
Docetaxel	Taxotere®
Domperidone	Euciton®, Evoxin®, Motilium®, Nauzelin®, Peridon®
Donepezil	Aricept®
Dopamine	Dopastat®, Intropin®
Dorzolamide	Trusopt®
Doxacurium	Nuromax®
Doxazosin	Cardura®, Carduran®
Doxorubicin	Adriamycin®, Adriblastin®
Doxycycline	Atridox®, C-Pak®, Doryx®, Doxicin®, Monodox®, Nordox®, Periostat®, Vibramycin®
Doxylamine	Decapryn®
Dronabinol	Marinol®
Droperidol	Droleptan®, Inapsine®
Dutasteride	Avodart®

E

Ebastine	Ebastel®, Evastel®, Kestine®
Econazole	Ecostatin®, Gyno-Pevaryl®, Pevaryl®
Efavirenz	Sustiva®
Eletriptan	Relpax®
Enalapril/enalaprilat	Innovace®, Vasotec®, Xanef®
Enflurane	Ethrane®
Enfuvirtide	Fuzeon®
Enoxacin	Bactidan®, Comprecin®, Enoram®, Enoxor®
Enoxaparin	Clexane®, Lovenox®
Entacapone	Comtan®, Comtess®
Ephedrine	Bofedrol®, Efedron®, Va-tro-nol®

Epinephrine	Adrenalin®, Bronchaid®, Epifin®, Epinal®, EpiPen®, Epitrate®, Fastject®, Lyophrin®, Simplene®, Suprarenin®, Vaponefrine®
Epoetin	Eprex®, Recormon®
Eprosartan	Teveten®
Eptifibatide	Integriline®
Ergocalciferol	Drisdol®
Ergometrine (= ergonovine)	Ergotrate Maleate®, Ermalate®
Ergotamine	Ergomar®, Gynergen®, Lingraine Medihaler®, Migril®
Erythromcyin	E-mycin®, Eryc®, Ery-max®, Erythromid®, Erythroped®, Ilosone®
Erythromycin-estolate	Dowmycin®, Ilosone®, Novorythro®
Erythromycin-ethylsuccinate	EES®, Erythrocin®, Wyamycin®
Erythromycin-propionate	Cimetrin®
Erythromycin-stearate	Erymycin®, Erythrocin®
Erythromycin-succinate	Monomycin®
Erythropoietin (=epoetin alfa)	Epogen®, Procrit®
Esmolol	Brevibloc®
Esomeprazole	Nexium®
Estradiol	Estrace®
Estradiol-benzoate	Progynon®
Estradiol-valerate	Delestrogen®, Dioval®, Femogex®, Progynova®
Estratriol (= estriol)	Theelol®
Etanercept	Enbrel®
Ethacrynic acid	Edecrin®, Hydromedin®, Reomax®
Ethambutol	Etibi®, Myambutol®
Ethinylestradiol	Estinyl®, Feminone®, Lynoral®
Ethionamide	Trecator®
Ethopropazine	Parsitan®, Parsitol®
Ethosuximide	Petinimid®, Suxinutin®, Zarontin®
Etidronate	Calcimux®, Diodronel®, Diphos®
Etilefrine	Apocretin®, Circupon®, Effontil®, Effortil®, Ethyl Adrianol®, Kertasin®, Pulsamin®
Etofibrate	Lipo-Merz®
Etomidate	Amidate®, Hypnomi-date®
Etoposide	Etopophos®, Toposar®, VePesid®, VP-16®
Etretinate	Tegison®, Tigason®
Ezetimibe	Zetria®

F

Famciclovir	Famvir®
Famotidine	Pepcid®, Pepdul®
Felbamate	Felbatol®
Felodipine	Plendil®
Felypressin	Octapressin®
Fenfluramine	Ganal®, Ponderal®, Ponderax®, Pondimin®, Redux®
Fenofibrate	Tricor®
Fenoterol	Berotec®, Partusisten®
Fentanyl	Sublimaze®
Fentanyl + droperidol	Innovar®
Fexofenadine	Allegra®, Telfast®
Filgrastim	Neupogen®
Finasteride	Propecia®, Proscar®
Flecainide	Tambocor®
Flucloxacillin (floxacilline)	Floxapen®, Ladropen®, Stafoxil®
Fluconazole	Diflucan®
Flucytosine	Alcoban®, Ancotil®
Fludrocortisone	Alflorone®, F-Cortef®, Florinef®
Flumazenil	Anexate®, Romazicon®
Flunarizine	Dinaplex®, Flugeral®, Sibelium®
Flunisolide	Aerobid®, Bronalide®, Nasalide®, Rhinalar®
Flunitrazepam	Hypnosedon®, Narco-zep®, Rohypnol®
Fluorouracil	Adrucil®, Effudex®, Effurix®
Fluoxetine	Fluctin®, Prozac®
Fluphenazine	Moditen®, Prolixin®
Flurazepam	Dalmane®
Flutamide	Drogenil®, Eulexin®
Fluticasone	Cutivate®, Flixonase®, Flonase®, Flovent®
Fluvastatin	Lescol®
Fluvoxamine	Faverin®, Floxifral®, Luvox®
Folic acid	Foldine®, Folvite®, Leucovorin®
Fondaparinux	Arixtra®
Formoterol	Foradil®, Oxi®
Foscarnet	Foscavir®
Fosinopril	Monopril®
Fulvestrant	Faslodex®
Furosemide	Dryptal®, Fusid®, Lasix®, Seguril®, Uritol®

G

Gabapentin	Neurontin®
Galantamine	Reminyl®
Gallopamil	Algocor®, Corgal®, Procorum®, Wingom®

Ganciclovir	Cymevene®, Cytovene®, Vitrasert®
Ganirelix	Antagon®, Orgalutran®
Gelatin-colloids	Gelafundin®, Haemaccel®
Gemfibrozil	Lopid®
Gentamicin	Cidomycin®, Garamycin®, Genticin®, Refobacin®, Sulmycin®
Gestoden + ethinyl estradiol	Femovan®
Glatimer acetate	Copaxone®
Glibenclamide (= glyburide)	Calabren®, Daonil®, DiaBeta®, Euglucon®, Micronase®
Glyceryl trinitrate	see Nitroglycerin®
Gonadorelin	Factrel®, Kryptocur®, Relefact®
Goserelin	Zoladex®
Granisetron	Kytril®
Griseofulvin	Fulcin®, Fulvicin®, Grisovin®, Likuden®
Guanethidine	Ismelin®, Visutensil®

H

Halofantrine	Halfan®
Haloperidol	Haldol®, Serenace®
Halothane	Fluothane®, Narkotan®
HCG	see Chorionic gonadotropin®
Heparin	Calciparin®, Hepalean®, Hepsal®, Liquemin®, Uniparin®
Heparin®, low molecular	Fragmin®, Fraxiparin®
Hetastarch (HES)	Hespan®
Hexachlorophane	see Lindane®
Hexobarbital	Evipan®
Homatropine	Homapin®
Hydralazine	Alazine®, Apresoline®
Hydrochlorothiazide	Aprozide®, Diaqua®, Diuchlor®, Esidrix®, Hydromal®, Hydrosaluric®, Neo-Codema®, Oretic®
Hydrocortisone (cortisol)	Alocort®, Cortate®, Cortef®, Cortenema®, Hyderm®, Hyocort®, Rectocort®, Unicort®
Hydromorphone	Dilaudid®, Hymorphan®
Hydroxocobalamin	Acti-B₁₂®, Alpha-redisol®, Cobalin-H®, Droxomin®, Hybalamine®, Vibal L.A.®
Hydroxychloroquine	Plaquenil®
Hydroxyethyl starch	Hespan®
Hydroxyprogesterone caproate	Duralutin®, Gesterol L.A.®, Hylutin®, Hyroxon®, Primolut Depo®, Pro-Depo®

Hydroxyurea	Droxia®, Hydrea®
Hyoscine butyl bromide	Buscopan®

I

Ibuprofen	Actiprophen®, Advil®, Brufen®, Fenbid®, Lidifen®, Motrin®, Nuprin®, Trendar®
Idoxuridine	Dendrid®, Herpid®, Herplex®, Kerecid®, Stoxil®
Ifosfamide	Ifex®, Mitoxana®
Iloprost	Ilomedin®
Imatinib	Glivec®
Imipramine	Dynaprin®, Impril®, Janimine®, Melipramin®, Tofranil®, Typramine®
Indinavir	Crixivan®
Indometacin	Ammuno®, Imbrilon®, Indocid®, Indocin®, Indomee®, Indomod®, Metacen®
Infliximab	Remicade®
Insulin	Humalog®, Humulin®, Iletin®, Novolin®, Velosulin®
Insulin aspart	Novolog®
Insulin glargine	Lantus®
Interferon alfa-2	Berofor alpha 2®
Interferon alfa-2a	Roferon A3®
Interferon alfa-2b	Intron A®
Interferon beta	Fiblaferon 3®
Interferon beta-1a	Rebif®
Interferon gamma	Actimmune®
Ipratropium	Atrovent®, Itrop®, Rinatec®
Irbesartan	Avapro®
Irinotecan	Campto®
Isoconazole	Gyno-Travogen®, Travogen®, Travogyn®
Isoflurane	Forane®
Isoniazid	Armazid®, Isotamine®, Lamiazid®, Nydrazid®, Rimifon®, Teebaconin®
Isoprenaline (= isoproterenol)	Aludrin®, Isuprel®, Neo Epinin®, Saventrine®
Isosorbide dinitrate	Cedocard®, Coradus®, Coronex®, Isoket®, Isordil®, Sorbitrate®, Vascardin®
Isosorbide mononitrate	Coleb®, Elantan®, Imdur®, Ismo®, Isotrate®
Isradipine	DynaCirc®
Itraconazole	Itracol®, Sempera®, Sporanox®
Ivermectin	Mectizam®, Stromectol®

K

Kanamycin	Anamid®, Kannasyn®, Kantrex®, Klebcil®
Kaolin + pectin (=attapulgite)	Donnagel-MB®, Kaopectate®, Pectokay®
Ketamine	Ketalar®
Ketoconazole	Nizoral®
Ketorolac	Acular®, Toradol®

L

Labetalol	Normodyne®, Trandate®
Lactitol	Importal®
Lactulose	Cephulac®, Chronulac®, Duphalac®
Lamivudine	Epivir®
Lamotrigine	Lamictal®
Lanatoprost	Xalaten®
Lansoprazole	Agopton®, Lanzor®, Prevacid®
Leflunomide	Arava®
Lenograstim	(G-CSF)®, Granocyte®
Lepirudin	Refludan®
Letrozole	Femara®
Leucovorin	Welcovorin®
Leuprolide (leuprorelin)	Eligard®, Lupron®
Levocetirizine	Xusal®
Levodopa	Dopar®, Larodopa®
Levodopa + benserazide	Madopar®, Prolopa®
Levodopa + carbidopa	Sinemet®
Levomethadone	Polamidon®
Levothyroxine	Eferox®, Euthyrox®, Thevier®
Lidocaine	Dalcaine®, Lidopen®, Nulicaine®, Xylocain®, Xylocard®
Lincomycin	Albiotic®, Cillimycin®, Lincocin®
Lindane	Hexit®, Kwell®, Kwilldane®, Quellada®, Scabene®
Linezolide	Zyvoxid®
Liothyronine	Cytomel®, Triostat®
Lisinopril	Carace®, Prinivil®, Zestril®
Lisuride	Cuvalit®, Dopergin®, Eunal®, Lysenyl®
Lithium carbonate	Camcolit®, Carbolite®, Duoralith®, Eskalith®, Liskonum®, Lithane®, Lithobid®, Lithotabs®, Priadel®
Lomustine	CCNU®, CeeNu®
Loperamide	Imodium®, Kaopectate II®
Lopinavir	Kaletra®
Loratadine	Claritin®, Lisino®
Lorazepam	Alzapam®, Ativan®, Loraz®, Tavor®
Lormetazepam	Ergocalm®, Loramet®, Noctamid®
Losartan	Cozaar®
Lovastatin	Mevacor®, Mevinacor®
Lumefantrine (= benflumetol)	see Artemether®
Lynestrenol	Orgametril®
Lypressin	Diapid®, Syntopressin®

M

Magaldrate	Riopan®
Mannitol	Isotol®, Osmitrol®
Maprotiline	Ludiomil®
Mebendazole	Vermox®
Mechlorethamine	Mustargen®
Meclizine (meclozine)	Antivert®, Antrizine®, Bonamine®, Whevert®
Medroxyprogesterone-acetate	Amen®, Depo-Provera®, Farlutal®, Oragest®, Provera®
Mefloquine	Lariam®
Megestrol	Megestat®
Melarsoprol	MelB®, Melarsen Oxide-BAL®
Meloxicam	Mobic®
Melphalan	Alkeran®
Menadione	Synkayvit®
Menotropin	Menogon®
Meperidine (pethidine)	Demerol®, Dolantine®
Mepindolol	Betagon®,Caridian®, Corindolan®
Mepivacaine	Carbocaine®, Isocaine®
Mercaptopurine	Purinethol®
Mesalamine (mesalazine)	Asacol®, Canasa®, Mesacal®, Pentasa®, Propasa®, Rezipas®, Rowasa®
Mesna	Mesnex®, Uromitexan®
Mesterolone	Androviron®, Proviron®
Mestranol	Menophase®, Norquen®, Ovastol®
Metamizol	see Dipyrone®
Metaproterenol (orciprenaline)	Alupent®, Metaprel®
Metenolone	Primabolan®
Metformin	Diabex®, Glucophage®
Methadone	Dolophine®, Methadose®, Physeptone®
Methamphetamine	Desoxyn®, Methampex®
Methimazole (thiamazole	Tapazole®, Mercazol®
Methohexital	Brevital®
Methotrexate	Folex®, Maxtrex®, Mexate®
Methotrimeprazine	Levoprome®, Nocinan®
Methoxyflurane	Methofane®, Penthrane®

Methylcellulose	Celevac®, Citrucell®, Cologel®, Lacril®, Murocel®
Methyldopa	Aldomet®, Amodopa®, Dopamet®, Novomedopa®, Presinol®, Sembrina®
Methylergometrine (methyl ergonovine)	Metenarin®, Methergine®, Methylergobrevin®, Partergin Ryegonovin®, Spametrin-M®
Methyltestosterone	Android®, Metandren®, Testred®, Virilon®
Methysergide	Deseril®, Sansert®
Metipranolol	Optipranolol®
Metoclopramide	Clopra®, Emex®, Maxeran®, Maxolan®, Primperan®, Reclomide®, Reglan®
Metoprolol	Betaloc®, Lopressor®
Metronidazole	Clont®, Femazole®, Flagyl®, Metronid®, Protostat®, Satric®, Zadstat®
Mexiletin	Mexitil®
Mezlocillin	Mezlin®
Miconazole	Daktarin®, Dermonistat®, Micatin®, Monistat®
Midazolam	Hypnovel®, Versed®
Mifepristone	RU 486®, Mifegyne®
Miglitol	Diastabol®
Minoxidil	Loniten®, Regaine®, Rogaine®
Mirtazepine	Remergil®, Remeron SolTab®
Misoprostol	Cytotec®
Mivacurium	Mivacron®
Mizolastine	Mistamine®, Mizollen®, Zolim®
Moclobemide	Aurorix®
Molgramostim	Leucomax®
Molsidomine	Corvaton®, Duracoron®, Molsidolat®
Montelukast	Singulair®
Morphine	MST Continus®, Oramorph®
Morphine hydro-chloride	Morphitec®
Morphine sulfate	Astramorph®, Avinza®, Duramorph®, Epimorph®, Infumorph®, Kadian®, MSIR®, Roxanol®, Rescudose®, Statex®
Muromonab-CD3	Orthoclone OKT3®
Mycophenolate mofetil	CellCept®

N

Nabilone	Cesamet®
Nadolol	Corgard®
Naftifin	Naftin®
Nalbuphine	Nubain®
Nalidixic acid	Negram®, Nogram®
Naloxone	Narcan®
Naltrexone	Nalorex®, Trexan®
Nandrolone	Anabolin®, Androlone®, Deca-Durabolin®, Hybolin Decanoate®, Kabolin®
Naphazoline	Albalon®, Degest-2®, Privine®, Vasocon®
Naproxen	Aleve®, Anaprox®, Naprelan®, Napron®, Naprosyn®, Naxen®, Synflex®
Naratriptan	Naramig®
Narcotine (= noscapine)	Coscopin®, Coscotab®
Nedocromil	Tilade®
Nefazodone	Nefaclar®, Serzone®
Nelfinavir	Viracept®
Neomycin	Mycifradin®, Myciguent®, Nivemycin®
Neostigmine	Prostigmin®
Netilmicin	Netillin®, Netromycin®
Nevirapine	Viramune®
Nicardipine	Cardene®
Niclosamide	Niclocide®, Yomesan®
Nifedipine	Adalat®, Coracten®, Procardia®
Nimodipine	Nimotop®
Nitrazepam	Atempol®, Mogadon®, Somnite®
Nitrendipine	Bayotensin®, Baypress®
Nitroglycerin	Ang-O-Span®, Deponit®, Nitrocap®, Nitrogard®, Nitronal®, Sustac®, Tridil®
Nitroprusside sodium	Nipride®, Nitropress®
Nitrostigmine	E605®, Parathion®
Nordazepam	Tranxilium N®, Vegesan®
Norepinephrine (noradrenaline)	Arterenol®, Levophed®®
Norethindrone (norethisterone)	Micronor®, Noriday®, Norlutin®, Nor-Q D®, Primolut N®
Norfloxacin	Noroxin®, Utinor®
Nortriptyline	Pamelor®
Noscapine (= narcotine)	Coscopin®, Coscotab®
Nystatin	Korostatin®, Mycostatin®, Mykinac®, Nilstat®, Nystan®, Nystex®, O-V Statin®

O

Obidoxime	Toxogonin®
Octreotide	Sandostatin®
Ofloxacin	Tarivid®
Olanzapine	Zyprexa®

Omalizumab	Xolair®
Omeprazole	Losec®
Ondansetron	Zofran®
Opium tincture (laudanum)	Paregoric®
Orciprenaline	see Metaproterenol®
Orlistat	Xenical®
Ornipressin	POR 8®
Oseltamivir	Tamiflu®
Oxacillin	Bactocill®, Prostaphlin®
Oxazepam	Oxpam®, Serax®, Zapex®
Oxcarbazepine	Timox®, Trileptal®
Oxiconazole	Oxistat®
Oxprenolol	Apsolox®, Trasicor®
Oxymetazoline	Afrin®, Allerest®, Coricidin®, Dristan®, Neo-Synephrine®, Sinarest®
Oxytocin	Pitocin®, Syntocinon®

P

Paclitaxel	Taxol®
Pamidronate	Aminomux®, Aredia®
Pancuronium	Pavulon®
Pantoprazole	Protonix®
Papaverine	Cerebid®, Cerespan®, Delapav®, Myobid®, Papacon®, Pavabid®, Pavadur®, Vasal®
Paracetamol	see Acetaminophen®
Parecoxib	Dynastat®
Paromomycin	Humatin®
Paroxetine	Paxil®
Pegvisomant	Somavert®
Penbutolol	Levatol®
Penciclovir	Vectavir®
D-Penicillamine	Cuprimine®, Depen®
Penicillin G	Bicillin®, Cryspen®, Crystapen®, Deltapen®, Lanacillin®, Megacillin®, Parcillin®, Pensorb®, Pentids®, Permapen®, Pfizerpin®
Penicillin V	Apsin VK®, Betapen-VK®, Bopen-VK®, Calvepen®, Cocillin-VK®, Distaquaine V-K®, Lanacillin-VK®, Ledercillin VK®, Nadopen-V®, Novopen-VK®, Pen-Vee K®, Pen-VEE K Penapar VK®, Penapar-VK®, Penbec-V®, Pfizerpen VK®, Robicillin-VK®, Stabillin V-K®, Uticillin-VK®, V-Cillin K®, Veetids®
Pentamidine	Pentacarinat®
Pentazocine	Fortral®, Talwin®
Pentobarbital	Butylone®, Nembutal®, Novarectal®, Pentanca®
Pentoxifylline	Trental®
Pergolide	Celance®, Permax®

Perindopril	Coversum®, Coversyl®
Permethrin	Elimite®, Lyclear®, Nix®, Permanone®
Pethidine	see Meperidine®
Phencyclidine	Sernyl®
Pheniramine	Daneral®, Inhiston®
Phenobarbital	Barbita®, Gardenal®, Solfoton®
Phenolphthalein	Alophen®, Correctol®, Espotabs®, Evac-U-gen®, Evac-U-Lax®, Ex-Lax®, Modane®, Prulet®
Phenoxybenzamine	Dibenyline®, Dibenzyline®
Phenoxybenzyl penicillin	Isocillin®, Megacillin®
Phenprocoumon	Liquamar®, Marcumar®
Phentolamine	Regitin®, Rogitin®
Phenytoin	Dilantin®, Epanutin®
Physostigmine	Antilirium®
Phytomenadione	Konakion®
Pilocarpine	Akarpine®, Almocarpine®, I-Pilopine®, Isopto-Carpine®, Miocarpine®, Ocusert®, Pilokair®
Pindolol	Visken®
Pioglitazone	Actos®
Pipecuronium	Arduan®
Piperacillin	Pipracil®
Pirenzepine	Gastrozepin®
Piretanide	Arelix®, Diumax®
Pizotifen = pizotyline	Litec®, Mosegor®, Sandomigran®
Polidocanol	Thesit®
Pralidoxime	Protopam Chloride®
Pramipexole	Sifrol®
Pranlukast	Ultair®
Pravastatin	Lipostat®, Pravachol®
Prazepam	Centrax®
Praziquantel	Biltricide®
Prazosin	Hypovase®, Minipress®
Prednisolone	Ak Pred®, Articulose®, Codelsol®, Cortalone®, Delta-Cortef®, Deltastab®, Econopred®, Hydeltrasol®, Inflamase®, Key-Pred®, Metalone®, Metreton®, Pediapred®, Predate®, Predcor®, Predenema®, Predfoam®, Prednesol®, Prelone®
Prednisone	Meticorten®, Orasone®, Panasol®, Winpred®
Prilocaine	Citanest®, Xylonest®
Primaquine	Primaquine®
Primidone	Myidone®, Mysoline®, Sertan®
Probenecid	Benemid®, Probalan®
Probucol	Lovelco®
Procainamide	Procan SR®, Promine®, Pronestyl®, Rhythmin®

Procaine	Novocaine®
Progabide	Gabren(e)®
Progesterone	Cyclogest®, Femotrone®, Gestone®, Progestasert®
Proguanil	Paludrine®
Promethazine	Anergan®, Avomine®, Ganphen®, Mallergan®, Pentazine®, Phenazine®, Phenergan®, Prometh®, Prorex®, Provigan®, Remsed®
Propafenone	Arhythmol®, Rhythmol®
Propofol	Diprivan®
Propranolol	Berkolol®, Cardinol®, Detensol®, Inderal®
Propylthiouracil	Propyl-Thyracil®
Pyrantel pamoate	Antiminth®, Comban-trin®
Pyrazinamide	Aldinamide®, Tebrazid®, Zinamide®
Pyridostigmine	Mestinon®, Regonol®
Pyridoxine	Bee-six®, Complement Continus®, Hexa-Beta-lin®, Pyroxine®
Pyridylcarbinol	Roniacol®, Ronicol®
Pyrimethamine	Daraprim®
Pyrimethamine + sulfadoxine	Fansidar®

Q

Quazepam	Doral®
Quinacrine	Atabrine®
Quinagolide	Norprolac®
Quinapril	Accupril®
Quinidine	Cardioqin®, Cin-Quin®, Kiditard®, Kinidin®, Quinalan®, Quinidex®, Quinora®
Quinine	Quinaminoph®, Quinamm®, Quine®, Quinite®

R

Rabeprazole	AcipHex®, Pariet®
Raloxifene	Evista®
Ramipril	Altace®
Ranitidine	Zantac®
Rapamycin	see Sirolimus®
Rasburicase	Fasturtec®
Reboxetine	Edronax®, Solvex®, Vestra®
Repaglinide	Actulin®, NovoNorm®, Pradin®
Reserpine	Sandril®, Serpalan®, Serpasil®, Zepine®
Reteplase	Rapilysin®
Ribavirin	Rebetol®, Virazole®
Rifabutin	Mycobutin®

Rifampin (rifampicin)	Rifadin®, Rimactan®
Risedronate	Actonel®
Risperidone	Risperdal®
Ritonavir	Norvir®
Rivastigmine	Exelon®
Rizatriptan	Maxalt®
Rocuronium	Zemuron®
Rofecoxib	Vioxx®
Rolitetracycline	Reverin®, Transcycline®, Velacycline®
Ropinirole	ReQuip®
Rosiglitazone	Avandia®
Roxithromycin	Rulid®

S

Salazosulfapyridine (sulfasalazine)	Azaline®, Azulfidine®, S. A.S.-500®, Salazopyrin®
Salbutamol	see Albuterol®
Salicylic acid	Acnex®, Sebcur®, Sol-uver®, Trans-Ver-Sal®
Sameterol	Serevent®
Saquinavir	Fortovase®, Invirase®
Scopolamine	Scopoderm TTS®, Trans-derm Scop®, Triptone®
Selegeline	Carbex®, Deprenyl®, Eldepryl®
Senna	Black Draught®, Fletch-er's Castoria®, Genna®, Gentle Nature®, Nytilax®, Senokot®, Senolax®
Sertindole*	Serlect®
Sertraline	Gladem®, Zoloft®
Sevoflurane	Sevorane®
Sibutramine	Reductil®
Sildenafil	Viagra®
Simethicone	Gas.X®, Mylicon®, Phazyme®, Silain®
Simvastatin	Zocor®
Sirolimus	Rapamune®
Somatorelin	GHRH-Ferring®
Somatostatin	Aminopan®
Somatotropin	Genotropin®, Saizen®
Sorbitol	Yal®
Sotalol	Sotacor®
Spironolactone	Aldactone®, Spiroctan®
Stavudine	Zerit®
Stibogluconate sodium	Pentostam®
Streptokinase	Kabikinase®, Streptase®
Streptomycin	Strepolin®, Streptosol®
Succinylcholine	Anectine®, Quelicin®, Succostrin®
Sucralfate	Antepsin®, Carafate®, Sulcrate®
Sufentanil	Sufenta®
Sulbactam	Combactam®
Sulfadoxine + pyri-methamine	Fansidar®
Sulfalen	Longum®

Sulfamethoxazole	Gamazole®, Gantanol®, Methanoxanol®
Sulfapyridine	Dagenan®
Sulfisoxazole	Gantrisin®, Gulfasin®
Sulfasalazine	see Salazosulfapyridine®
Sulprostone	Nalador®
Sumatriptan	Imitrex®
Suramine	Bayer 205®, Germanin®
Suxamethonium	see Succinylcholine®

T

t-PA (= alteplase)	Activase®
Tacrine	Cognex®
Tacrolimus	Prograf®
Tadalafil	Cialis®
Talinolol	Cordanum®
Tamoxifen	Nolvadex®, Tamofen®
Tamsulosin	Flomax®
Tazobactam + piperacillin	Zosyn®
Telmisartan	Micardis®
Temazepam	Euhypnos®, Normison®, Restoril®
Tenecteplase	Metalyse®
Teniposide	Vumon®
Terazosin	Hytrin®
Terbutaline	Brethine®, Bricanyl®
Terfenadine	Seldane®, Triludan®
Teriparatide	Forteo®
Tertatolol	Prenalex®
Testosterone	Restandol®, Sustanon®
Testosterone cypionate	Androcyp®, Andronate®, Duratest®, Testoject®
Testosterone enantate	Andro®, Delatestryl®, Everone®, Testone®
Testosterone propionate	Testex®
Testosterone undecanoate	Andriol®
Tetracaine	Anethaine®, Pontocaine®
Tetracycline	Achromycin®, Supramycin®
Tetryzoline (= tetrahydrozoline)	Collyrium®, Murine®, Tyzine®, Visine®
Thalidomide	Contergan®, Synovir®
Theophylline	Aerolate®, Bronkodyl®, Constant-T®, Elixophyllin®, Lasma®, Nuelin®, Pro-Vent®, Quibron-T®, Slo-bid®, Slo-Phylli®, Somophyllin-T®, Sustaire®, Theolair®, Uniphyl®
Thiabendazole	Mintezol®
Thiamazole	see Methimazole®
Thiamine	Vitamine B₁®
Thiopental	Pentothal®, Trapanal®
Thio-TEPA	Thiotepa Lederle®
Thrombin	Thrombinar®, Thrombostat®
Thyrotropin	Thyrogen®

Thyroxine	Choloxin®, Eltroxin®
Tiagabine	Gabitril®
Ticarcillin	Ticar®, Timentin®
Ticlopidine	Ticlid®
Timolol	Betimol®, Blocadren®, Timoptic®, Timoptol®
Tinidazol	Fasigyn(CH)®, Simplotan®, Sorquetan®
Tiotropium	Spiriva®
Tirofiban	Aggrastat®
Tobramycin	Nebcin®, Tobralex®, Tobrex®
Tocainide	Tonocard®
Tolbutamide	Mobenol®, Oramide®, Orinase®, Rastinon®
Tolcapone	Tasmar®
Tolonium chloride	Klot®, Toazul®
Topiramate	Topamex®
Topotecan	Hycamtin®
Tramadol	Tramal®
Trandolapril	Mavik®
Tranexamic acid	Cyklokapron®
Tranylcypromine	Parnate®
Trastuzumab	Herceptin®
Trazodone	Desyrel®, Trialodine®
Triamcinolone	Adcortyl®, Aristocort®, Kenacort®, Ledercort®, Volon®
Triamcinolone acetonide	Adicort®, Azmacort®, Kenalog®, Kenalone®, Triam-A®
Triamterene	Dyrenium®, Dytac®
Triazolam	Halcion®
Trichlormethiazide	Metahydrin®, Naqua®, Trichlorex®
Triiodthyronine (= liothyronine)	Cytomel®
Trimetaphan	Arfonad®
Trimethoprim	Ipral®, Monotrim®, Proloprim®, Trimpex®
Triptorelin	Decapeptyl®, Trelstar Depot®
Troglitazone	Rezulin®
Tropisetron	Navoban®
Tubocurarine	Jexin®, Tubarine®
Tyrothricin	Hydrotricin®, Tyrozets®

U

Urokinase	Abbokinase®, Ukidan®

V

Valaciclovir	Valtrex®
Valdecoxib	Bextra®
Valganciclovir	Valcyte®
Valproic acid	Depakene®
Valsartan	Diovan®, Provas®
Vancomycin	Vancocin®
Vardenafil	Levitra®

Vasopressin — Pitressin®
Vecuronium — Norcuron®
Venlafaxine — Effexor®
Verapamil — Berkatens®, Calan®, Cordilox®, Isoptin®, Securon®, Univer®, Verelan®
Vidarabine — Vira-A®
Vigabatrin — Sabril®
Vinblastine — Velban®, Velbe®
Vincristine — Oncovin®
Viomycin — Celiomycin®, Vinactane®, Viocin®, Vionactane®
Vitamin B₆ — Bee Six®, Hexa-Betalin®, Pyroxine®
Vitamin B₁₂ — Bay-Bee®, Berubigen®, Betalin 12®, Cabadon®, Cobex®, Cyanoject®, Cyomin®, Pemavit®, Redisol®, Rubesol®, Sytobex®, Vibal®
Vitamin D — Calciferol®, Drisdol®, D-Vi-sol®

W

Warfarin — Coumadin®, Marevan®, Panwarfin®, Sofarin®

X

Xanthinol nicotinate — Complamin®
Ximelagatran — Exanta®
Xylometazoline — Chlorohist®, Neosynephrine II®, Otrivin®, Sinutab®, Sustaine®

Z

Zafirlukast — Accolate®
Zalcitabine — Hivid®
Zaleplone — Sonata®
Zanamivir — Relenza®
Zidovudine — Retrovir®
Ziprasidone — Geodon®, Zeldox®
Zolmitriptan — Ascotop®, Zomig-ZMT®
Zolpidem — Ambien®, Bicalm®, Stilnox®
Zopiclone — Amoban®, Amovane®, Imovane®, Zimovane®

Subject Index

Subject Index